AYURVEDA in

Nepal

The Teachings of Vaidya Mana Bajra Bajracharya

Volume One

Principles, Diagnosis, and Treatment

Text and Illustrations by
Vaidya Mana Bajra Bajracharya

Edited by Vaidya Madhu Bajra Bajracharya,
Alan Tillotson, and Todd Caldecott

PhytoAlchemy Press

Vancouver, BC, Canada

Ayurveda in Nepal
The Teachings of Vaidya Mana Bajra Bajracharya
Volume One: Ayurveda Principles, Diagnosis, and Treatment
Edited by Vaidya Madhu Bajra Bajracharya,
Alan Tillotson, and Todd Caldecott

Second edition – June 2017
ISBN: 978-0-9868935-1-3

Printed in the U.S.A.

Table of Contents

CHAPTER 12: DISEASES OF THE DIGESTIVE SYSTEM (ANNAVAHASROTA ROGA) 157

CHAPTER 17: DISEASES OF THE KIDNEYS (MUTRAVAHASROTA ROGA) 201

CHAPTER 18: DISEASES OF MALE SEXUAL FUNCTION (PURUSHAJANENDRIYA ROGA) 211

CHAPTER 19: DISEASES OF FEMALE SEXUAL FUNCTION (STRI ROGA)
219

CHAPTER 20: DISEASES OF THE NERVES (SNAYUKANDARA ROGA)
227

CHAPTER 21: DISEASES OF THE SKIN (CHARMA ROGA) 235

CHAPTER 22: DISEASES OF TISSUE METABOLISM (SAPTADHATU ROGA) 253

CHAPTER 23: DISEASES OF PREGNANCY AND DELIVERY (GARBHA ROGA)   265

CHAPTER 24: DISEASES OF CHILDHOOD (BALA ROGA)   271

CHAPTER 25: DISEASES OF THE MOUTH, THROAT, NOSE, AND EARS

283

Important Notice

The information contained in this book is intended to authentically represent the medical knowledge held by the venerable Bajracharya tradition of Nepal, as taught and practiced by Vaidya Mana Bajra Bajracharya. It is not designed to diagnose or treat individual health problems or ailments, and nor should it be taken as medical advice or treatment. Simply by purchasing or reading this book does not give permission nor confer any right for health care providers to adopt the methods or use the medications described herein — it takes years of supervised study and practice to implement the principles and practices of Ayurveda correctly. Just as there are risks associated with the use of prescription medications, remedies in Ayurveda also need to be used with caution and with experienced supervision. In particular, the alchemical preparations referred to as 'bhasma' or 'rasa' that are prepared with heavy metals are potentially toxic and frequently illegal to import, prescribe, or use in many countries. Some traditional remedies too mentioned in this text, such as the herb Kushtha, deer musk, and elephant teeth, are illegal to import as they come from threatened or endangered species. Other remedies may contain substances such as animal urine, blood and other excretions, which if not prepared properly, may contain pathogenic bacteria, chemicals, and viruses. It is therefore important to read this text with this warning in mind, and always and only use this information in a responsible way, only after consulting with a fully trained and licensed health care practitioner.

The Editors

Autobiography of Dr. Mana Bajra Bajracharya

I was born February 3rd, 1930 in a family of Bajracharya (Buddhist priests). My father, Durga Bajra Bajracharya, and mother Tirthakumari Bajracharya have five sons. I am the fourth one. We are members of a Bihara called Kanaka Chaitya Mahabihar, one of the most famous Biharas in Kathmandu Valley. Our Bihar was established about seven hundred years ago in front of the ancient Chaitya of Kanakmuni Buddha.

By caste, we are Shakya related to the Shakya of Kapilavastu, the birthplace of Lord Gautama Buddha. During the medieval period, following the principles of Bajrayana – the third advanced stage of Buddhism (following Hinayana and Mahayana) – our ancestors received the consecration of Bajrayana. This consecration bestows the title

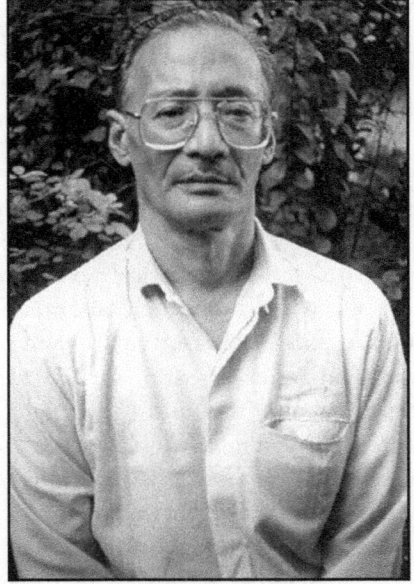

Vaidya Mana Bajra Bajracharya, 1994

of Bajracharya. To have this title, one must follow the principles of the Heruka Chaka Samvara Tantra. Those with the title of Bajracharya are the priests of the Newari Buddhists, one of the ancient inhabitants of Kathmandu Valley.

In 1937, I received my formal initiation as a Bajracharya, which I needed to be a member of the Bihara. In 1944, I received my consecration as Bajrayana, which I needed to be an authorized Bajracharya. In 1945, I married with Gyani Devi Bajracharya. Marriage is essential for Bajrayana practice. We have a son and four daughters.

In addition to being priests, my family has also carried forward the tradition of Ayurveda, running unbroken from generation to generation during these seven hundred years. Our family maintains our original vows to help mankind, and especially to maintain the health of the Newari Buddhists who live around the Bihara. During all this time, we have never charged for a medical consultation. We have a very good traditional education system in our home to study Buddhism and Ayurveda side by side. We have an extensive Sanskrit family library of Ayurveda that contains many unpublished texts.

My grandfather, Nila Bajra Bajracharya, was a specialist in Spiritual Healing (Bhuta Vidya). In his time, he was the royal physician of Nepal. In his field, religious approaches are used to cure diseases such as paralysis, meningitis, children's diseases and mental illness. My father was a specialist in Internal Medicine (Kaya Chikitsa Tantra). However, he died at an early age in an accident. This tragedy actually made our family very strong. My eldest brother, Divya Bajra Bajracharya, who had already completed his studies in Internal Medicine, continued his work and study, and with the help of my grandfather, achieved a high level in Internal Medicine. He passed his knowledge to his brothers, and I am one of those who chose to specialize in the Internal Medicine field.

For six years, I studied Sanskrit from my brother and his friends. Almost all of the Buddhist and Ayurveda texts are written in Sanskrit, so it is necessary to achieve complete fluency. During this period of study, I also had to help my grandfather and my brothers run our medical clinic, and learned the practical basics of diagnosis, botany, chemistry, philosophy, anatomy, and pharmacology.

When I was seventeen years old, I finished my formal Sanskrit study, and began to learn the classical texts of Ayurveda, including the *Charaka Samhita* (the text of internal medicine), *Sushruta Samhita* (surgery), *Madhava Nidana* (diagnosis), *Madanapala Nighantu* (botany and pharmacology), and *Rasatarangini* (chemistry). I also paid much attention to my study of Buddhism. At the beginning, I studied Naryakarana, the nine original Mahayana Buddhist texts: *Pragyaparamita, Saddharma Pundarika, Lanka Valara, Dosha Bhumi, Gandavyuha, Samadhiraja, Suvarnaprabha Lahilaristara*, and *Guhya Samaja*. I continued my study of Buddhism and Ayurveda for eight years.

During this time, with the help of my brothers, I was gaining more and more medical practice, dealing with different kinds of patients. In addition, I also had much interest to learn painting and sculpture. I practiced by drawing pictures of herbs, and making clay models of the human body. This helped me to learn anatomy in great detail, and to be able to recognize all the plants we used in our medical practice. Finally, I became free to start my individual medical practice, and to choose further advanced study.

In 1955 I realized that, first of all, I must see all the plants, and how they grow in different climates. So, I spent two years traveling on foot in Nepal and India. During this time, I collected almost all the plants that are mentioned in the classical texts of Ayurveda, and made color paintings of them on the spot.

After returning from my trekking, I began to treat patients without supervision. At first, I was not a success in drawing patients because I had no power to convince patients of my skill. But, in a short time, with the help of my brothers and mother, my reputation began to build. For the next fifteen years, I treated many, many Nepali patients. During this time, I decided to study English, and I began to have contact with international people. I started to study Western medical texts in detail, bringing home books each week to read, and our family now has the tradition of studying Western sciences. My son and many of the children of my brothers have attended college for this purpose. My nephew is an ophthalmologist, my son-in-law is a post-doctoral research associate in the Ohio State University School of Natural

Resources, and my son Madhu Bajra Bajracharya is one of six other physicians working at our clinic in Nepal.

In 1969, I started to teach Buddhism and Ayurveda to Westerners. This teaching activity made me famous in Kathmandu. In 1972 I went to Europe and America, following an invitation from one of my students, to speak at Columbia University on Buddhism. After coming back, I realized that the people of the new young generation liked very much Ayurveda. So, I opened an examining room in my family

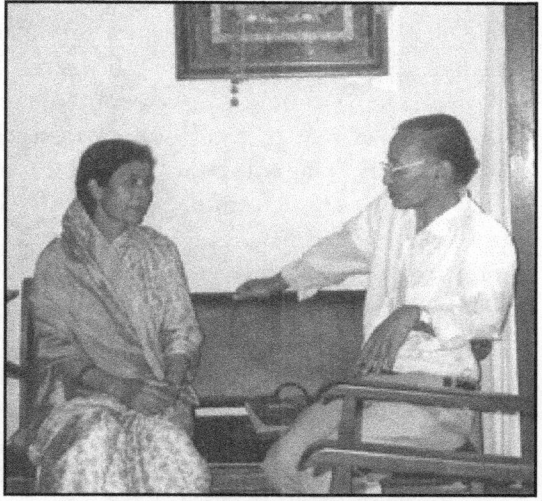

Vaidya Mana Bajra Bajracharya in clinic at Piyushabarshi Aushadhalaya, Kathmandu

clinic, and I concentrated on handling foreign patients. This clinic is named Piyushabarshi Aushadhalaya.

In 1975 I was elected chairman of the Nepal Ayurveda Association, the nation-wide organization of traditional physicians. The main aim of the organization is to help each other for the development of Ayurveda. I have written several books and pamphlets on Buddhism, Ayurveda, and Nepali culture, which are published in the Nepali language. Some are translated into English, such as *Buddhist Mythology of the Kathmandu Valley.*

I continued my work at my clinic for foreigners, and I realized very early the need for writing down all the knowledge of Ayurveda in a form which will preserve it for future generations. I also learned that the way of talking and explaining Ayurveda to patients and foreigners required much thought and practice, and now my Western patients can understand my way of practice when I explain to them. I found out that many diseases that Western medicine has not treatment for can be successfully treated by Ayurveda. I wrote a series of books and pamphlets for my Western patients. Some of the titles are *Eastern Theory of Diet, Hepatitis, An Outline of Ayurveda, Breast Cancer,* and *Ayurvedic Medicinal Plants and General Treatment.*

For many decades I have maintained my practice of four hours study and writing each day, and working in the clinic for five hours in the afternoon. I have completed writing 47 books containing full descriptions of all the different aspects of Ayurveda. The books are in the Nepali and Sanskrit languages. In 1995 I wrote *The Real Facts of Ayurveda Based on Related Ancient Science and Philosophy* in English. This book is a condensed extract briefly covering all the traditional texts of Ayurveda that I have studied, containing short descriptions of each subject.

My dream for many years has been to establish an International Ayurveda Research Center in Kathmandu. This is becoming more important recently, because ecological destruction in Nepal is causing many of our valuable plants to disappear. Some of these plants are essential for formulas which can deal with serious diseases for which there is no medicine in other parts of the world.

To stop this destruction I am attempting to develop a model farm in Kathmandu, as part of the Institute, to teach farmers how to grow and preserve valuable plants. This will improve their incomes, and benefit the Nepali economy. As another part of the Institute, I have decided to translate my books into English so people will realize what Ayurveda really is, and the value it has for mankind. When completed, this will serve as a University level course in Ayurveda. In 1997 I completed the translation of the first of my 47 books into English, entitled *Ophthalmology in Ayurveda*, with the help of my son, Vaidya Madhu Bajra Bajracharya, my senior American student Alan Tillotson Ph.D., and American medical doctor Robert Abel, Jr. I am working very hard these days to realize my dream, and I hope to gather international support to help protect our threatened eco-systems, save our plants, bring our medicines to the world community, and, most importantly, to preserve and strengthen our traditional medicine system in Nepal.

The great sage Vaidya Mana Bajra Bajracharya passed away in January of 2001. His clinic in Kathmandu is now in the hands of his son, Vaidya Madhu Bajra Bajracharya.

Biography of Vaidya Madhu Bajra Bajracharya

Madhu Bajra Bajracharya is the son of the late Vaidya Mana Bajra Bajracharya, studying and refining his knowledge of Ayurveda at his father's side in the traditional gurukula system of education for over 40 years. Born in 1955, Vaidya Madhu also holds a BSc in Zoology, and has been in clinical practice since 1976, specializing in kaya Chikitsa, the branch of Ayurveda that concerns itself with internal medicine. Heir to the tradition of medicine that his family has maintained for almost 800 years, Vaidya Madhu has traveled the world extensively, lecturing on Ayurveda in Europe, SE Asia and North America, training medical

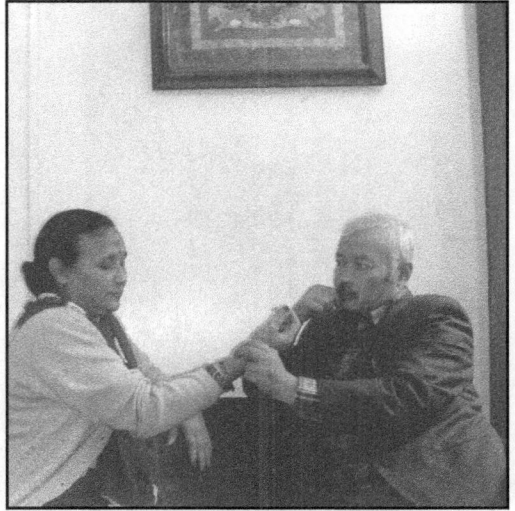

Vaidya Madhu Bajra Bajracharya in clinic, Piyushabarshi Aushadhalaya, Kathmandu

doctors and providing his clinical expertise in Immunity, Cancer, and indigenous Newari medical knowledge. He is Chairman of the Association of Nepal Traditional Ayurvedic Medical Practitioners, and is a proud representative of Newari culture, serving as Vice Chairman of Hapa Guthi, an association of local Newari Culture. He also serves as a consultant for the Himalayan Herbal Preparation Pvt. Ltd., a joint Nepali-Italian venture, and provides his clinical services at his family's ancestral clinic in Kathmandu, Piyushabarshi Aushadhalaya, the oldest Ayurveda clinic in Nepal. For the publication of the present work, Vaidya Madhu has graciously provided the editors with the detailed support required to accurately represent the wealth of knowledge contained in this work.

Foreword by Alan Tillotson, Ph.D., RH (AHG)

In the summer of 1976 I had been travelling in the East, and had contracted severe dysentery in Afghanistan. I had lost almost 80 pounds. My diary from July 10 reads:

Just got out of the hospital today. I've been suffering extreme hypoglycemic reactions for a week now. Though advised by friends and doctors to fly home, I have decided to continue because it would be such a shame to end the trip like this. I must control the diabetes despite the dysentery which is wreaking havoc with me. The lack of drinkable water is the most disturbing thing. Though not happy, I have not been sad either. My decision to continue was hard, because there are people on the bus who do not want the responsibility of my sickness. This is understandable and justifiable, and I hate to be a burden to anyone. I pray I cause no further trouble.

I was travelling in a red Mercedes bus driven by a young American couple named Chris and Mark, who lived in Kathmandu Nepal. Chris came to me after my stint in the hospital and told me that she and Mark had decided it would be better if I flew home as soon as possible – they were afraid I would die by the time we reached Pakistan. Then they told me about a doctor they knew, a miracle doctor in Kathmandu they called

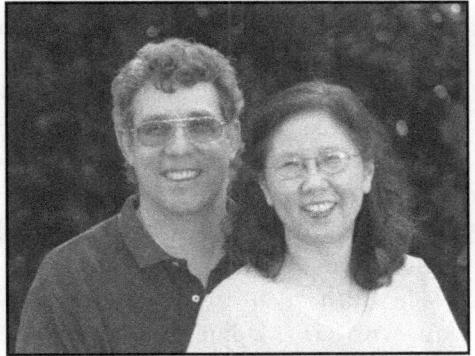

Alan Tillotson and his wife Nai Xin

Dr. Mana. I convinced them to let me continue on to meet this doctor.

When we arrived, I set out for Dr. Mana's clinic. From the (former) King's palace it was only a short walk to Mahaboudha, the concrete Buddhist shrine which lends its name to a small surrounding area. Less than one hundred paces from the shrine was the entrance to Dr. Mana's compound.

I had to stoop down to pass under a brick arch that opened into a flat earthen courtyard. To the right was an open room. I walked up the lone concrete step to enter. To one side were cabinets displaying bottles with Nepalese characters on the labels. I sat down in the small waiting room.

When Dr. Mana entered, I guessed his age to be in the early forties. He was wearing a clean white cotton outfit. His face was angular. There was a small scar barely visible above his mouth. He was wearing brown glasses with square frames that looked as if they had been repaired many times. The forehead was flat, typical of the mountain people of Nepal and Tibet.

He said, "I am Dr. Mana. What can I do for you?"

"I've been having some problems with diarrhea and dysentery, and I am very very weak."

"Your diarrhea is no problem. I also have medicine for energy."

I quickly nodded approval. He led me to a cotton-covered table and checked my stomach. The examination seemed short and precise. He called to an assistant and gave some instructions in Nepalese. In a few minutes I was holding two envelopes formed out of old newspapers. One contained some brown powder and the other crudely formed pills.

Dr. Mana said, "The powder is for diarrhea. You take it in boiled water three times a day before meals. You will be better in four or five days if you are careful about your diet. You must completely avoid greasy, heavy foods and over-ripe fruits. This time of year the fruits are very bad for health. Take the other medicine two times a day, morning and before bed. Come back in five days for a check-up."

I paid a few rupees, said thank you and left. The whole encounter had been surprisingly quick. Within a few weeks I regained most of my strength, and I decide to stay on and study with Dr. Mana, a study I continued by long distance until my dear teacher entered into eternity in January of 2001.

My last in person meeting with Dr. Mana was in 1996. At that time he showed me a large collection of works he had written in Sanskrit. After Dr. Mana died, I made the decision that I would try to work with his son (Dr. Madhu) and translate some of these works into English.

The present manuscript has taken many years to get to its present point. The most difficult part of this has been to change the words so that the resonate with English readers, but do not change the meaning This requires much explanatory detail, which in turn can make the book arcane. After about three years of initial work with Dr. Madhu, I decided to enlist the help of my brilliant young friend Todd Caldecott. Todd took the ball I handed him and ran with it,

There remains a vast library of knowledge still in Kathmandu. Its preservation is vital to the world of medicine. Think of this – a single medical family, with roots going back over 700 years, to this day is running a clinic that has healed tens of thousands of patient of the most serious diseases, including cancer and multiple sclerosis. And that family produced a great sage – Dr. Mana Bajra Bajracharya – who over a period of 40 years wrote down in great detail all his knowledge and all his methods of treating disease.

This first book is but one of the 47 books written by Dr. Mana.

Alan Tillotson
January 9th, 2010
Wilmington DE USA

Foreword by Todd Caldecott, Dip. Cl.H., RH(AHG), CAP(NAMA)

In 2000 I was contacted by Alan Tillotson, who asked me if I might be interested to work with him on a book project, sending over a manuscript written by his teacher Dr. Mana. Honored by Alan's request I readily agreed, fascinated by this opportunity to connect with a tradition of Ayurveda that was totally new to me. Up to that point, my training in Ayurveda was strongly influenced by the Keraliya (Kerala) school of Ayurveda, which itself is based on the Ashta Vaidya medical tradition that arose some time after the 13th century. To my knowledge at the time, there were very few pockets of authentic Ayurveda remaining anywhere on the Indian subcontinent except in the South, which was better insulated against the centuries of foreign invasion and cultural upheaval experienced in the North of India.

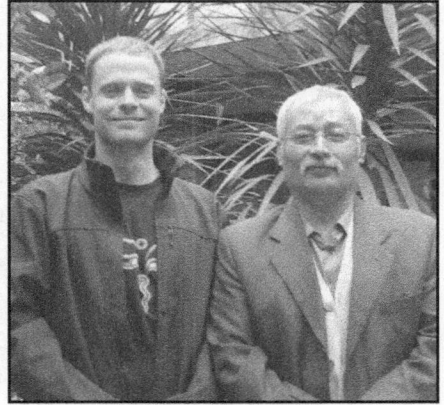

Todd Caldecott with Vaidya Madhu Bajra Bajracharya

As I learned more about the heritage of Dr. Mana, the Newar people, and the history of Kathmandu, it became clear to me that like South India, Nepal is a treasure-trove of ancient Indian culture. Protected by the foothills of the Himalayas, for more than two thousand years the Kathmandu Valley has served as a safe haven for peoples fleeing persecution and war. Immigrants from modern-day India brought with them the language of Sanskrit and their unique cultural practices, integrating with the indigenous population to create a cosmopolitan synthesis that is reflected in traditional Newar society.

Similar to the Ashta Vaidya tradition of Kerala, the Bajracharya lineage of Nepal represents a form of Ayurveda that predates the modern academic model of Ayurveda by many hundreds of years. While the Western model of education has secured a special status in both Nepal and India, the reality is that it might not be the best way to teach Ayurveda. For thousands of years Ayurveda has followed the mentorship or gurukula model of education, a practice that is the basis of both the Ashta Vaidya and Bajracharya traditions. While there will always be the complaint that modernization is necessary, this is not only a false assumption, it can be a dangerous one as well. This is particularly relevant when it comes to the practice of

Rasa Shastra, the alchemical branch of Ayurveda that utilizes toxic minerals such as mercury and arsenic. Ayurveda has come under serious fire as of late because products that intentionally contain these toxic substances are being sold as traditional remedies, when in fact they are not prepared by practitioners that have the authentic knowledge, and nor using the proper techniques.

Despite being a practitioner since 1995, I have long struggled to find a sustainable way for my patients to access the wonderful medicines used in Ayurveda. I have always hesitated to use commercial "Ayurvedic" products because I don't believe them to be authentic nor of sufficient quality. Often these commercial products, which bear traditional names like "Yogaraja Guggulu" or "Chyavanprash," don't even look like the remedies they claim to be, and nor do they contain the same ingredients. It was a revelation then for me to use the artisan-made remedies prepared at Vaidya Madhu's ancestral clinic – not only for their authenticity – but for their efficacy.

Today many of my patients benefit from these medicines, which I only use in more complex conditions. I have over 20 years of successfully using medicinal plants, preparing custom remedies for my patients and developing my own formulations, but my knowledge and expertise pales in comparison to that held by the Bajracharya tradition. Through its intimate connection to the practice of Vajrayana Buddhism, the Newar Bajracharya lineage maintains a practice of Ayurveda that itself was inherited from Nalanda, an ancient center of learning in eastern India that was already a thousand years old before it was destroyed in the 13th century. The depth and sophistication of knowledge expressed within the remedies prepared at Vaidya Madhu's ancestral clinic is a rare thing indeed.

With the publication of this text we are one step closer to manifesting Dr. Mana's dream of establishing a sustainable future for Ayurveda in Nepal. While it might be difficult to imagine given its undaunted survival over the centuries, the reality is that the environmental, economic, and political pressures of modern-day Nepal are threatening the future of the Bajracharya medical tradition. Along with my colleague, Alan Tillotson, we are working hard to publish all of Dr. Mana's texts, with the hope that we can draw others to us and support one of the world's oldest surviving traditions of Ayurveda.

Todd Caldecott
June 13, 2017
Vancouver, BC, Canada

Foreword by James Duke, Ph.D.

I first learned about the extraordinary work of Vaidya Mana Bajra Bajracharya of Nepal from my colleague and his apprentice Dr. Alan Tillotson in the 1980's. I am very glad that Alan was able to engage the help of Dr. Mana's son Madhu Bajracharya in Kathmandu and Todd Caldecott of Canada to translate and edit this text from the original Sanskrit.

This work is important in that it is both a scholarly contribution to ethnomedicine as well as a practical handbook for modern students of Ayurveda. It is extraordinary in that it outlines exact treatments for hundreds of Ayurvedic medical conditions, bringing you into the Kathmandu clinic of Dr. Mana and Dr. Madhu, showing you how they treat different diseases.

It is my earnest hope that the publication of this book in English will stimulate new interest in examining the medical traditions of Ayurveda. It brings to the surface the exact understanding of the ideas and

Dr. Jim Duke, Ph.D.

medicines, developed in a single family tradition spanning several hundreds of years, which have successfully been used to benefits untold tens of thousands of patients.

It is also an urgently needed book for medical researchers, ethnobotanists and even for the peoples of Nepal, because the unique diversity of herbs in Nepal is threatened by deforestation, and the 700 year old tradition of Dr. Mana and his son is being overwhelmed by the advance of modernity.

Some of Dr. Mana's more extraordinary contributions include his development of treatments for the Ayurvedic diseases urustambha, a condition that he correlates with multiple sclerosis, and his treatments for various forms of hepatitis, including chronic hepatitis. Alan Tillotson witnessed dozens of MS and hepatitis patients flying to Nepal for treatment, many with good results. Dr. Mana also describes unique and unknown treatments for various types of cancer, psoriasis, hypertension, asthma, etc.

Some of his insights about common problems show them in a new light, such as his linkages of rheumatoid arthritis with uric acid accumulations and digestive problems.

Dr. Mana was also sensitive to complaints from Westerners that Ayurveda was primitive or unscientific or simple. His many books, well over 30, are his answer to that criticism. I can only hope that more of this work is translated from Sanskrit and made available in coming years.

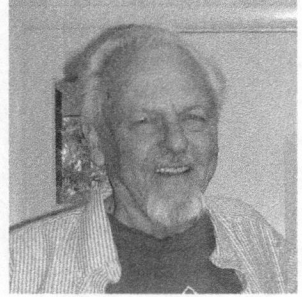

James Duke Ph.D.
April 9, 2010

Knowledge of Ayurveda

Chapter 1: Introduction to Ayurveda

Definition of Ayurveda

Translated into English, the Sanskrit medical word Ayurveda means the 'knowledge of life'. The word Ayus, or 'life', refers to the physical state of being alive, and includes both the mind and the body. It is both the ultimate goal of the mind and its intrinsic nature to pursue happiness and reject suffering. The happiness and suffering experienced by the mind is the result of what happens to the body. The mind rejects suffering because its destination and goal is happiness, and yet the existence of suffering is an inescapable truth. From our first breath, the mind takes upon itself the task of leading the body away from suffering.

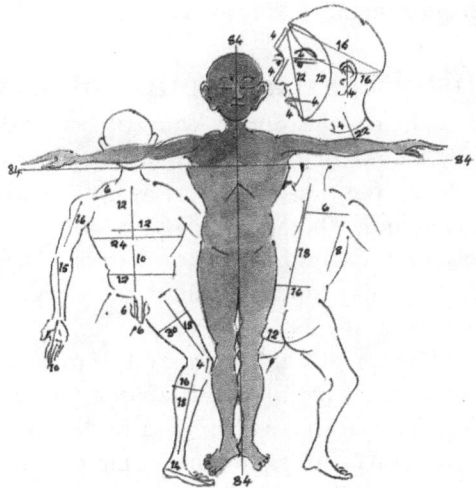

Harmonious ratios of physical proportions, drawing by Dr. Mana Bajracharya

The body and mind are inexorably linked to the physical and metaphysical units of life called Prakriti and Purusha, respectively. The function of these two units and how they mutually coordinate their activities is the primary subject of Ayurveda. Ayurveda is concerned with the achievement of happiness through the proper understanding of happiness and suffering. The body is the physical cause of pain and suffering, and is capable of misleading the mind, disturbing its function. When the mind is misled it cannot function in the proper way. That is to say, when the mind is functioning properly, it is focused and will strive to lead the body towards happiness. When the mind loses its control over the body, however, it invariably leads to suffering.

The word suffering, from the perspective of Ayurveda, is simply another word for disease. Disease is that which destroys the physical construction of the body, and is thus a destructive force. Happiness, in the medical sense, is that which strengthens the bodily construction, and is therefore a constructive force. The constructive and destructive forces within the body are the two major factors of life. The constructive force of happiness exists naturally when the body is in balance, encouraging the mind to guide the body towards its proper activities. The destructive force that arises when the body is out of balance awakens the mind, signaling it to be alert and to change its activities, with the goal of restoring balance. A balanced life leads to health, whereas life's imbalances are the fundamental cause of sickness. This is true not only for individuals, but also for one's progeny and for society as a whole.

The knowledge of how to live a balanced life is the primary subject of Ayurveda, which as a practice has been continuously maintained for thousands of years. In this respect Ayurveda is a 'science' based upon empirical observation, encompassing a spectrum that includes both the good and the bad of life. It teaches us to understand both the happy life and the unhappy life, and the differences between them, seeking always to restore life to its proper balance.

Historical Background of Ayurveda

The true history of Ayurveda begins during the time of the Vedas, the ancient Holy Books of the Aryans ('noble ones'). Hindu mythology tells us that Lord Brahma, the creator of the world, transmitted the knowledge of Ayurveda to humankind. The four Vedas are called the *Rig Veda, Yajur Veda, Sama Veda,* and *Atharva Veda,* and are believed to have been compiled several thousand years ago. All the Vedas contain medical knowledge but especially the *Atharva Veda* contains the basic elements of Ayurveda.

During this ancient period, learned sages and saints called Rishis and Munis devoted their life to understanding the realities of the world. These noble persons lived in Aryavarta, a term used to denote the land of the Aryans, which covers the entire Himalayan region, including the modern countries of Nepal, India, Pakistan, Bhutan, and Bangladesh.

The ancient civilization of this region was strongly influenced by the unique intellectual contributions of the Rishis and Munis, the wise seers and holy sages that lived in Aryavarta. The hymns, liturgical formulations, and medical knowledge found in the Vedas are the primary contributions of the Rishis and Munis. These ancient sages realized that sickness was a major impediment in the search for spiritual liberation, and so many of them became Vaidyas to remove this obstruction and illuminate the path to self-knowledge. The term Vaidya is the Sanskrit word for 'physician', and is derived from the root word Vidya, meaning 'wisdom'.

Thousands of years ago there lived a Rishi named Bharadwaja who was renown in the land of Aryavarta as a highly skilled Vaidya. There are many stories about him and his medical skills, and he is considered to be the first medical teacher of all subsequent Rishis and Munis. Bharadwaja learned Ayurveda directly from Lord Indra, the king of the gods, who in turn learned this teaching from the Ashwini Kumaras, the twin Celestial Physicians. The Ashwini Kumaras received their knowledge from Prajapati, who in turn learned Ayurveda from Lord Brahma.

Modern historians cannot fully understand who these god-like characters actually were. The Vedas describes characters such as Indra, the Ashwini Kumaras, and Prajapati, and give many details about their exploits and personalities. From a historical perspective, however, their roles can never be totally clear, because there is no authentic proof that they ever existed. Nonetheless, the implications of these stories that describe Ayurveda's spiritual beginnings and the transmission of knowledge are thought provoking, because the writers of that time describe these events as the result of direct communication between the Devas and the holy sages.

The Great Medical Conference

The historical record of Ayurveda begins with a medical conference held thousands of years ago in the Himalayan mountains. An account of this event is described in a 'collection' (Samhita) of medical writings called the *Charaka Samhita*. In this text, a sage named Atreya Punarvasu recounts that a large and well-attended medical conference of venerable Rishis and Munis was held under the guidance of Bharadwaja. The primary aim of the conference was to share medical knowledge and compile this information as a text, which up until this point had only been transmitted as part of an oral tradition. While all the participants held Ayurveda to be eternal, the lack of authentic and complete texts available for study made it more difficult to share and preserve. Hence, the compilation of this knowledge as a series of texts became the focus of the conference.

This medical conference was a major undertaking in the history of Ayurveda, made difficult because many scholars conversant in the various aspects of Ayurveda lived far away in different regions. Despite these challenges, the participants of the conference overcame them, and travelled great distances to come together. The conference is estimated to have lasted about three years, during which time the participants engaged in long and complex discussions and debates, forming committees to compile comprehensive texts on the different subjects of Ayurveda. From these scholars, passed down and redacted over time, we have the most important texts of Ayurveda, including the *Charaka Samhita*, the primary text on internal medicine; the *Sushruta Samhita*, the primary text on surgery; and the *Kashyapa Samhita*, the primary text on pediatrics.

Eight Limbs of Ayurveda

During the Great Medical Conference the teachings of Ayurveda were formally organized into 'eight' (Asht) 'branches' (Angas) collectively referred to as Ashtanga Ayurveda. A founding sage was chosen at the conference to head a committee representing each branch of Ayurveda, tasked with creating a defining text on the subject. All the texts were written in Sanskrit, the language of the Aryans, and each formed the basis for the different schools and traditions that evolved over the ensuing centuries. While names of each sage that headed each branch of Ayurveda are still known, most of the texts compiled during this time have been lost, with knowledge of them coming by reference in later texts.

The eight branches of Ayurveda are:

1. Internal medicine: Kaya Chikitsa Tantra.
2. Surgery: Shalya Tantra.

3. Ears, Eyes, Nose, and Throat: Shalakya Tantra.
4. Pediatrics: Kaumarabhritya Tantra.
5. Toxicology: Agada Tantra.
6. Purification of the sex organs: Vajikarana Tantra.
7. Health and Longevity: Rasayana Tantra.
8. Spiritual Healing: Bhuta Vidya.

Internal Medicine

Kaya Chikitsa Tantra is the branch of Ayurveda that deals with the subject of internal medicine, and the general 'treatment' (Chikitsa) of the 'body' (Kaya). Kaya Chikitsa is the most well developed branch of Ayurveda, and includes common diseases such as fever, diarrhea, and tuberculosis. The school of internal medicine was established by Lord Atreya Punarvasu, who was assigned this lineage by his teacher Bharadwaja. Lord Atreya lived in a place called Punchanada, located in the Punjab region of modern-day India, and had six devoted and highly advanced disciples named Agnivesha, Bheda, Jatukarna, Parasara, Harita, and Ksharapani. Lord Atreya encouraged each of them to write their own unique books on internal medicine. As a result of this assignment, each wrote a book that was subsequently named after them, e.g. the *Agnivesha Samhita*, *Bheda Samhita*, *Harita Samhita*, etc. Of these, the *Agnivesha Samhita* was judged by the doctors of the time to be the best, most authentic, and most complete text on internal medicine. All the original copies of this text have since been lost, but Charaka, a famous scholar of Ayurveda who lived during the 1st century CE, redacted this book from an original. Thus the text of Agnivesha is now known by the name of *Charaka Samhita*, which presents in detail the results of the Great Medical Conference. The other texts written by the disciples of Atreya Punarvasu, except for the much smaller *Harita Samhita*, as well as portions of the *Bheda Samhita*, have never been found.

Lord Atreya's school of internal medicine continues to exist, and remains the basis of the traditional medical practices found throughout the entire subcontinent of India, including Nepal, India, and Tibet. Throughout the centuries, there have been many famous scholar-physicians that have preserved this unique knowledge, as well as contributed new ideas about different diseases and their treatments. Over the centuries the basic principles of internal medicine in Ayurveda have remained unchanged, even though the various methods and treatments used to treat disease has continued to evolve. In this way, Ayurveda is a system of universal truths that helps us adapt to a constantly changing world.

Surgery

Shalya Tantra is defined as the branch of surgery within Ayurveda, and was founded by Dhanwantari Divodasa. He was a contemporary of Atreya Punarvasu, and the king of Kashi, which is modern-day Varanasi, in India. Dhanwantari Divodasa had many devoted disciples, including Sushruta, Aupadhenava, Vaitarana, Aurabhra, Puskalavati, Karavirya, and Gopurakshita. As with the students of Lord

Atreya, each of these students was asked to write a unique text on surgery. Each of these texts are known by the names of each author, including the *Sushruta Samhita* and the *Aupadhenava Samhita*. All these texts, however, with the exception the *Sushruta Samhita*, have been lost to time.

Sushruta was a son of Kaushika, and lived in the area of Koshi River, in modern-day Nepal. The text of Sushruta is considered to be the best, most authentic and complete text on surgery found within Ayurveda, presenting in detail the fundamental principles and practices of Ayurveda. The *Sushruta Samhita* is the only surviving text that actually dates back to the great medical conference led by Lord Bharadwaja, thousands of years ago. In the 10th century, a famous surgeon named Nagarjuna redacted the *Sushruta Samhita,* and added an appendix called the *Uttara Sthana.*

Today the surgical school of Divodasa is no longer flourishing, and its practice is limited to only minor operations, such as the lancing of boils. While the ancient knowledge of surgery in Ayurveda was well developed during the time of the Rishis and Munis, during the medieval period traditional healers weren't able to preserve this tradition. In part this was due to a long period of war and conflict in India, resulting in the destruction of higher centers of learning, such as the famous Nalanda university. During this period traditional Vaidyas were for the most part general practitioners, trained in all the different subjects of Ayurveda. This general medical training was important for village doctors, but such training without the support of specialists eventually became counter-productive, and led to the loss of the practice surgery and all its complex knowledge and skills.

Eyes, Ears, Nose and Throat

Shalakya Tantra is defined as the branch of otorhinolaryngology (EENT) and ophthalmology in Ayurveda, concerning diseases of the eyes, ears, nose, mouth, and throat. Videhadhipati Janaka, the King of Videha, established the ancient school of Shalakya Tantra, located within what is now known as the district of Janakapura in modern-day Nepal. Like the scholars that were head of the other schools of Ayurveda, Videhadhipati Janaka was charged with compiling the practical knowledge gained by different physicians of his era within the field of Shalakya Tantra. Janaka wrote the first authentic textbook in the field, called the *Videha Tantra,* but this text has been lost. As a contemporary of Janaka, however, Sushruta quoted sections of the *Videha Tantra* his *Sushruta Samhita,* and devotes an entire section to the subject of Shalakya Tantra.

In the following centuries numerous scholars including Janaka, Nimi, Kankayana, Gargya, Shataki, Saunaka, and Chakshusya all contributed their unique knowledge to the practice of Shalakya Tantra, but many of these texts have been lost to time. Our knowledge of their work mostly comes from references to their texts in existing works such as the *Madhava Nidana,* written by Madhava in the 13th century. The *Atankadarpana* written by Sri Kanthadatta in the 15th century also contains many commentaries on Shalakya Tantra. This branch of Ayurveda, however, has not been fully preserved, and only a few of its practices are still used by general practitioners.

Pediatrics

Kaumarabhritya Tantra is the branch of Ayurveda that concerns the subject of health and disease in children, or pediatrics. The school of pediatrics was established by Maricha Kashyapa, a contemporary of Atreya Punarvasu. He lived in Gangadwara in the area of Haridwara, India, and had many disciples including Vriddha Jivaka. Under the guidance of Maricha Kashyapa, Vriddha Jivaka wrote a text called the *Kashyapa Samhita* , also known as the *Vriddha Jivaka Tantra* ,. Although it has since been lost, this text was redacted by Vatsya, a famous pediatrician from the 5th century. Within the field of Kaumarabhritya Tantra the names of Parvataka, Bandhaka, and Hiranyaksa are well-known as important specialists and contributors in this field, and while their texts are no longer available, references to them can be found in existing commentaries.

The school of pediatrics has been preserved by our family tradition of Buddhist physicians for hundreds of years. Traditionally, we are well-known in our community as spiritual healers. It is believed that almost all diseases of children have to be treated with the basic theory of spiritual healing, using specific religious practices as a form of treatment.

Toxicology

Agada Tantra refers to the practice of toxicology in Ayurveda, and the treatment of poisoning from various sources, including plants, animals, insects, and food. The school of toxicology was established by Kashyapa, also known as Vriddhakashyapa, who was another contemporary of Atreya Punarvasu. Kashyapa lived in Takshashila, located in modern-day Pakistan, and wrote a text was called the *Kashyapa Samhita*. Although the same name, this text is different from the *Kashyapa Samhita* used in pediatric medicine. Kashyapa's text is no longer available now but references to it can be found in different commentaries. Likewise, other texts on toxicology written by specialists including Alambayana, Ushana, Saunaka, and Latyayana were known to exist, but are no longer available.

The traditional practice of toxicology is still practiced by different families of Vishavaidyas ('poison doctors') who claim to be specialists in toxicology. While their knowledge is quite limited compared to earlier physicians, people in living in rural areas still benefit from the practice of Vishavaidyas, and their ability to effectively treat poisonous animal bites. In ancient times, it was the job of Vishavaidyas to protect members of the royal family from being poisoned, as well to poison the enemies of the kings. One method was to use Vishakanyas, or 'poison girls'. These were women destined to become courtesans, who took poisons in small doses starting in childhood, eventually developing immunity just as snake handlers and beekeepers do now. Just the kiss or bite of a Vishakanya could be enough to paralyze or kill.

Purification of the Semen and Uterus

Vajikarana Tantra is branch of Ayurveda that concerns the purification and rejuvenation of the male and female sexual organs. The primary aim of this branch is to provide proper knowledge about sexual relations, and to provide techniques and practices that are important to secure healthy progeny. The study and practice of this subject has no specific text or school of specialists, and is included as a part of general internal medicine in Ayurveda. For example, the chapter on Vajikarana Tantra found in the *Charaka Samhita* is very comprehensive on the subject, as are the relevant sections found in other texts by commentators such as Sushruta and Vagbhata.

Good Health and Longevity

Rasayana Tantra is defined as the branch of Ayurveda that concerns the promotion of long life and good health. It deals with the problems of premature aging and poor immunity. As with Vajikarana Tantra, the subject of Rasayana Tantra is not found in any specific text or tradition of specialists. The unique knowledge gained by the Rishis and Munis in this field of medicine is recorded in the texts of internal medicine. The prestige and success of internal medicine in Ayurveda is largely dependent upon the success of Rasayana Tantra. The medicines used within this branch of Ayurveda can be very effective, and have a wide range of therapeutic application.

In the medieval period there were many renowned Siddhas who claimed to have the power to control death. These Siddhas were not doctors, but religious philosophers and practitioners, but less advanced spiritually than the legendary Rishis and Munis. The Siddhas were interested in long life and the possibility of immortality, and so were drawn to the practice of Rasayana Tantra. As a result of their interest and investigations, the Siddhas developed practices that drew upon the use of purified heavy metals combined with other unique and often very potent medicinal substances. The Siddhas brought to light many new remedies that could be used for rejuvenation, and sparked a revolution that led to development a new branch within Ayurveda called Rasa Shastra, or 'Indian alchemy'. Many of these alchemical medicines are poisonous in their pure form, and are often illegal for use outside India and Nepal. Traditional physicians maintain that the methods of purification used in Rasa Shastra remove the toxicity of these substances, and in our tradition we have safely used these remedies for hundreds of years.

In the history of Ayurveda, the practice of alchemy was traditionally separated into a Hindu and Buddhist school. The head of Hindu school was the physician Adinatha Siddha, whereas the head of the Buddhist school was the physician Nagarjuna. In the lineage of both these schools are the names of many famous Siddhas who all contributed to the development of Rasa Shastra.

Spiritual Healing

Bhuta Vidya is the branch of Ayurveda that concerns the subject of spiritual healing. Bhuta Vidya deals primarily with mental disease, children's disease, and diseases that do not follow the theory of Tridosha. This subject does not have a specific text, but rather, is linked to the ancient *Atharva Veda* as well as other religious texts. In general, the theory of spiritual healing is based upon chanting, called Mantra in Sanskrit. Mantras are composed using specific vowels and consonants that are associated with certain deities or spiritual properties. Hindu and Buddhist religious practitioners believe that the repetition of these Mantras yield supernatural powers that can be used to cure many diseases. Almost all religious texts and many texts of Ayurveda contain a great variety of Mantras traditionally attributed to the Rishis, Munis, and Siddhas. During special ceremonies, invested priests transmit these Mantras to their devoted disciples, and today this tradition can still be found in our hereditary tradition, a practice that has remained unbroken for hundreds of years.

Tridosha Siddhanta: The Theory of Balance

Tridosha Siddhanta is the central concept of Ayurveda, the 'theory' (Siddhanta) that health exists when there is a balance between three fundamental bodily substances called 'Vata, Pitta, and Kapha' (Tridosha). Traditional Vaidyas firmly believe that this ancient theory explains the dynamics of physical reality, and allows the physician to gain a holistic understanding of homeostatic principles and interactions.

To gain a practical understanding of Ayurveda it is necessary to explore the associations between the philosophy of Tridosha Siddhanta and the physiological realities it represents. As a medical concept it can difficult to grasp, as it embraces the full spectrum of medicine and disease. To fully comprehend this concept, Tridosha Siddhanta must be understood from several perspectives, and then applied within the context of the practice of medicine. It is especially important to understand that when this text describes Vata, Pitta, and Kapha from these different perspectives, that each term has a holistic basis that embraces many aspects, and cannot be limited to a narrow definition of its meaning.

Vital Regulators of Bodily Function

Prithvi (Earth), Ap (Water), Tejas (Fire), Vayu (Air), and Akasha (Space) are the primal substances, called the Pancha Buthas (Five Elements), from which the material substance of the universe arises. Each of these word-symbols refers to substantive forces, found in both bodily and medicinal substances, that have different properties and material actions that can be discerned by the mind. As the primary regulators of bodily activities in sentient beings, the various properties and functions of Vata, Pitta, and Kapha are in turn derived from the interaction of the Five Elements.

Vata literally means the substance called 'wind' or 'air', and relates to Vayu, the element of Air. Once Vayu enters into the body it becomes a vital force, moving throughout as the cause of physical sensation, vibration, and movement. In this way, the element of Air is necessary to mobilize the function of the nervous system.

Pitta literally refers to the substance called 'bile', and relates to the element of Tejas, or Fire. The bile produced by the liver is a vital substance that carries the waste products of metabolism to elimination. After being excreted by the liver into the small intestine, the bile contributes to digestion in the gut. During this process, some of the bile is partially reabsorbed, entering into the venous system and is carried back to the liver. Bile is thus both a metabolic and digestive product that regulates the bodily heat, mobilizing the function of the venous system.

Kapha literally means 'mucus', and is related primarily to the element of Ap, or Water. Mucus is a clear, viscid secretion of the mucous membranes that plays a vital role in maintaining homeostasis. The secretions of the mucous membranes that line the gastrointestinal tract function to trap and absorb the nutrients that are eventually distributed to the rest of the body by the arterial system. Thus mucus serves as both a carrier of nutrients, and to mobilize the function of the arterial system.

Inter-relationship of Vata, Pitta, and Kapha

The sensations, movements, and vibrations generated by Vata and expressed through the nervous system control and regulate the supply of the energy released by Kapha, traveling within the arterial system. In turn, the supply of Kapha controls and regulates sensation, movement, and vibration within the nervous system. In this way, the substances of Vata and Kapha control and regulate each other.

Vata and Kapha work as a team to regulate Pitta. The nutrient energy carried by the arterial system along with sensations and vibrations of the nervous system combine to control and regulate the heat generated by Pitta. As the metabolic energy within the liver and venous system, Pitta controls and regulates both Vata and Kapha.

The vital energy of the body, its regulatory flow, and the nutrients that supply it are important considerations. The energy and heat of life, expressed by Pitta, cannot come into being without the nutrient supply of Kapha, and the mobilizing force of Vata. Thus for life to exist and to express it's natural functions, the activities of Vata, Pitta, and Kapha must be coordinated in the proper way, and balanced in their activities.

Vata Defined

As the mobilizing agent for the bodily energy, Vata must be identified in the proper way so that the physician can understand its role within the complexities of health and disease. This is accomplished in Ayurveda by defining the physical properties of Vata that affect the body, comprised of Ruksha, Shita, Laghu, Sukshma, Chala, Vishada, and Khara. Each property of Vata is defined as follows:

1. Ruksha means 'dry', and dry counteracts greasy.
2. Shita means 'cold', and cold counteracts heat.
3. Laghu means 'light', and light counteracts heaviness.
4. Sukshma means 'micro-fine', and micro-fine counteracts density.
5. Chala means 'vibratory', and vibration counteract stillness.
6. Vishada means 'non-sticky', and non-sticky counteracts stickiness.
7. Khara means 'rough', and roughness counteracts smoothness.

The presence of Vata can be identified within any form or any object by the expression of these physical properties. Among these seven physical properties, the property of Ruksha ('dry') is most important physical property of Vata, and its expression allows the physician to correlate this with an increase in the Vata substance.

For example, if the body is exposed to the blowing wind, the resulting sensations of dry, light, cold, and vibration all indicate that the blowing wind is a Vattik substance. Likewise, the gas produced in the colon contains the same properties and effects as the atmospheric wind, and is also regarded as a Vattik substance. Foods and herbs that are bitter, pungent, or astringent in taste also contain some of these same properties, promoting the sensation of dryness in the body, and are thus regarded as Vattik substances.

Pitta Defined

As the agent of energy and heat in the body, Pitta is identified by five physical properties called Sneha, Ushna, Tikshna, Drava, and Sara:

1. Sneha means 'greasy', and greasy counteracts dryness.
2. Ushna means 'hot', and heat counteracts cold.
3. Tikshna means strong or 'sharp', and counteracts dullness.
4. Drava means 'liquid', and liquid counteract solid.
5. Sara means 'movable', and mobility counteracts stability.

The presence of Pitta can be identified within any form or any object by the expression of these physical properties. Among these five properties, the property of Ushna ('heat') is most important physical property of Pitta, and its expression allows the physician to correlate this with an increase in the Pitta substance.

For example, if the body is exposed to the intense rays of the sun, the resulting sensations of heat and burning indicate that it is a Paittika substance. As a by-product of red blood cell metabolism, bile contains all the properties described for Pitta, and thus bile is a Paittika substance. Foods and herbs that are sour, salty, or pungent in taste also contain some of these same properties, and are thus regarded as Paittika substances, promoting the sensation of heat within the body.

Kapha Defined

As the agent responsible for the nutrition of the body, Kapha is identified by six physical properties called Guru, Shita, Mridu, Snigdha, Sthira, and Picchila:

1.   Guru means 'heavy', and heaviness counteracts lightness.
2.   Shita means 'cold', and coldness counteracts heat.
3.   Mridu means 'soft', and softness counteracts hardness.
4.   Snigdha means 'greasy', and greasy counteracts dryness.
5.   Sthira means 'stable', and stability counteracts instability.
6.   Picchila means 'sticky', and sticky counteracts non-sticky.

The presence of Kapha can be identified within any form or any object by the expression of these physical properties. Among these six properties, the property of Guru ('heavy') is most important physical property of Kapha, and its expression allows the physician to correlate this with an increase in the Kapha substance.

For example, if the body is exposed to high humidity, the resulting sensation of heaviness, greasiness, and stickiness indicates that this moist air is a Shlaishmika substance (meaning 'pertaining to Kapha'). Likewise, the bodily mucus contains all the properties described for Kapha, and thus mucus is a Shlaishmika substance as well. Foods and herbs that are sweet, sour or salty in taste also contain some of these same properties, and are thus regarded as Shlaishmika substances that promote the sensation of heaviness within the body.

Understanding Physical Properties in Ayurveda

From these definitions of Vata, Pitta, and Kapha, it should be clear that the proper discernment of these three fundamental principles is based upon the expression of their physical properties. While exerting an influence, a physical property simultaneously decreases the power of its opposite property. For example, the intake or application of a greasy substance will increase the property of greasiness in an organism, while simultaneously decreasing the expression of dryness.

When these properties are expressed in tandem, as each element, Dosha, or combination of Doshas, they in turn exert a limiting influence on their counterparts. For example, all of the physical properties of the element of Air and Vata Dosha – with the exception of cold – counteract the physical properties of Water and Kapha. Due to their opposition, whenever the power or strength expressed by the Air Element and Vata increases, the power or strength of the Water Element and Kapha decreases. In the same way, whenever the power or strength expressed by the Water Element and Kapha is increased, the power or strength expressed by the Air Element and Vata decreases.

The predominant physical property expressed when both the Air and Water Elements come together is Shita ('cold'), which counteracts the predominant physical property of the Fire Element and Pitta Dosha. An increase in cold will suppress the power of the Fire Element and Pitta Dosha, and likewise, an increase in the physical property of Ushna ('heat') will suppress both the Air and Water Elements.

According to Ayurveda, health is defined as the balance of the physical properties, whereas ill health relates to their relative increase or decrease. In order to maintain the equilibrium of Vata, Pitta, and Kapha, their individual physical properties and their opposing actions must be equalized and maintained.

Important Textbooks of Ayurveda

The following is an overview of some of the most important textbooks used by traditional physicians.

1. Charaka Samhita

The *Charaka Samhita* is the oldest and most important text, dealing primarily with internal medicine. It was originally written about 2,500 years ago by Atreya Punarvasu, the devoted student of Bharadwaja, and later preserved and enlarged by the physician Charaka. It is very comprehensive, with sections on fundamental principles, diagnosis, dietetics, physiology, longevity and therapeutics.

2. Sushruta Samhita

The *Sushruta Samhita* was written by the physician Sushruta at the time of the great conference circa 2,500 years ago. It is devoted to the field of surgery, but also contains very comprehensive information on each of the eight branches of Ayurveda, adding much new information not found in *Charaka*, such as treatment of eye diseases.

3. Harita Samhita

The *Harita Samhita* was written by the physician Harita at the same time as the *Charaka Samhita* and the *Sushruta Samhita*. This book deals in internal medicine, is much smaller than either of those two. The existing copy was believed written in the 13th century CE, copied from earlier works.

4. Ashtanga Hridaya

The *Ashtanga Hridaya* was written by a Buddhist physician named Vagbhata circa 500-600 CE. This textbook deals primarily with therapeutics and adds some new herbs, new formulas and advanced information on the use of metals and minerals.

5. Ashtanga Sangraha

The *Ashtanga Sangraha* was also written by the Buddhist physician Vagbhata circa 500-600 CE, and deals with therapeutics.

6. Madhava Nidana

The *Madhava Nidana* was written around 700 CE by the physician Madhava. It deals primarily with disease classification, and gives detailed description of hundreds of diseases with their characteristic signs and symptoms.

7. Siddhayoga

The text *Siddhayoga* was written by the physician Virinda about 800 CE. It gives explanations about the actions of and reasoning behind many formulas.

8. Chakradatta

The *Chakradatta* was written by the physician Chakrapanidatta circa 1060 CE. It is a comprehensive text on pharmacy with many important formulations. It describes for the first time many important alchemical (purified mercury-based) and mineral medicines.

9. Gada Nigraha

The *Gada Nigraha* was written by Gadadhara in the 13 century CE. This book is a compendium. The author is not a original writer but simply compiles information for earlier classics and puts it into simpler language.

10. Sharangadhara Samhita

The *Sharangadhara Samhita* was written by the physician Sharangadhara in the 14th century CE. This text details the practice of pharmacy in Ayurveda, including the methods to prepare many important formulas in Ayurveda, including alchemical preparations.

11. Rasaratna Samucchaya

The *Rasaratna Samucchaya* was written by a physician named Vagbhata in the 14 century CE. This book contains knowledge of internal medicine, aphrodisiacs, rejuvenatives, and alchemical medications.

12. Bhavaprakasha Samhita

The *Bhavaprakasha Samhita* was written by the physician Bhavamisra, a scholar from northwest India, around the 15th century CE It is well written, simple and clear, and deals with diagnosis and formulas.

13. Rasaratnakara

The *Rasaratnakara* was written by the physician Nityanatha in the 15 century CE. It deals with minerals and Bhasmas, especially aphrodisiac medicines and medicines for rejuvenation.

14. Rasavatara

The *Rasavatara* was written by Mandabya in the 15the century CE. This book gives valuable details about diagnosis and proper prescription of medicines and formulas.

15. Satmya Darpana Samhita

The *Satmya Darpana Samhita* was written by the physician Viswanath in the 16th century CE. It deals with the uses of plants and formulas.

16. Bhavaprakasha Nighantu

The *Bhavaprakasha Nighantu* was written by Biswonatha in the 16th century CE. It deals primarily with materia medica and plants.

17. Bhaishajya Ratnavali

The *Bhaishajya Ratnavali* was written by the physician Binoda Lala Sen Gupta in the 18th century CE. It is primarily a book of formulas.

18. Dhanvantari Nighantu

The *Dhanvantari Nighantu* was written in the 18th century by Dhanwantari. It deals with individual plants.

19. Rasatarangini

The *Rasatarangini* was written by the physician Sadananda Sharma in the 19th century CE, and is primarily concerned with formulations.

Chapter 2: Different Aspects of Vata

The concept of Vata in Ayurveda is very broad in meaning. It encompasses many seemingly disparate elements, and in order to be understood, identified and used for therapeutic purposes, must be investigated in detail to understand its different manifestations. In this chapter, eight different perspectives on Vata are described:

1. **Vata as Air**.
2. **Vata and Taste**.
3. **Vata and the Nervous system**.
4. **Vata and Health**.
5. **Vata and Disease**.
6. **Vata as Aggravating Agent**.
7. **Vata in Diagnosis**.
8. **Vata in Treatment**.

Vata as Air

The theory of matter in Ayurveda states that all objects are composed of different proportions of the Five Elements. The Five Elements are metaphysical entities called Prithvi (Earth), Ap (Water), Tejas (Fire), Vayu (Air), and Akasha (Space).

The atmospheric air is an expression of the metaphysical Element called Vayu (Air). While the atmospheric air can be easily observed when the wind blows, however, the element of Air itself cannot be directly perceived. This is because in the constitution of things, including the physical body, the element of Air exists in subtle form. Ayurveda states that the properties of both the element of Air and the atmospheric air are shared by the biological wind called Vata, and that in turn, the physical properties of Vata are very similar to the gaseous excretions of the body. The physical properties of both Vata and these bodily gases are Ruksha ('dry'), Shita ('cold'), Laghu ('light'), Sukshma ('micro-fine'), Chala ('vibration'), Vishada ('non-sticky'), and Khara ('rough'). In this way, the metaphysical element of Air, the atmospheric air, Vata, and the gaseous excretions of the body, are all related by their shared physical properties.

As with the effect of atmospheric air, an increase in the proportion of Vayu counteracts greasiness and increases dryness. The evaporation of moisture occurs because the air is inherently dry. The ventilation of air acts to reduce the moisture of an object, and when something becomes dried, it is rough and less sticky. Thus the physical properties of Ruksha ('dry'), Vishada ('non-sticky'), and Khara ('rough') are all associated as properties of Air.

The weight or heaviness of an object depends largely upon the proportion of moisture it contains. An object affected by air is by nature reduced in water and so becomes Laghu ('light') in nature. When an object affected by air is reduced in its proportion of moisture, the space held by that moisture is filled up by air. The interior structure of an object in which Vayu increases thus becomes hollow and less dense. Its density is broken into minute forms that escape into the air. This condition is the physical property or state called Sukshma ('microfine'). Thus the quality of Sukshma ('microfine') counteracts the quality of Sthula ('density').

When an object affected by air loses its moisture, this water is initially is evaporated into the atmosphere. A person affected by this process during exercise and the generation of Ushna ('bodily heat') feels this as a sensation of Shita ('coldness').

Vayu is everywhere, and the incessant movement of air likewise results in the quality of Chala ('vibration'). When Vata is increased, the quality of Chala diminishes the quality of Sthira ('steadiness').

The Five Vital Airs

Ayurveda states that Vata has five different roles, each with a different name that describes a specific range of functions within the body. These Five Vital Airs are called Prana, Udana, Samana, Vyana, and Apana:

1. Prana is the aspect of Vata that is inhaled during respiration. Prana plays a major role for the proper function of the heart.
2. Udana is the aspect of Vata that is exhaled during respiration. Udana plays a major role in the function of the throat and lungs when mobilizing strength.
3. Samana is the aspect of Vata that is active in the stomach and small intestine. It is involved in helping the digestive system to assimilate the essence of food.
4. Vyana is the aspect of Vata that is active in the entire blood circulation (including the lymphatic duct system) for the proper filtration and flow of blood.
5. Apana is the aspect of Vata that is active in the excretory organs (especially the colon) for the proper excretion of stool, gas, urine, semen, menses, etc.

These Vital Airs, although they have different functions, are not different in the sense of their fundamental substance, all expressing the same physical properties as the element of Air. According to Ayurveda, however, for the proper function of the body, these Vital Airs should not mix or interfere with each other, as this can be the cause of many physical disorders.

Vata and Taste

All foods, herbs or medicines have a 'taste' (Rasa), a natural sensation experienced by all living beings. Ayurveda enumerates six tastes in all, including sweet, sour, salty, bitter, pungent, and astringent. Foods or medications with a sweet, sour and salty taste generally express properties related to the Water Element, such as greasy and heavy. The bitter, pungent and astringent tastes contain much less of the Water Element, and are thus generally dry and light in nature. The sour, pungent and salty tastes contain more of the Fire Element, and generally express the property of heat. Sweet, bitter and astringent tastes contain proportionally more of the Air and Water Elements, and are generally cooling in nature.

Substances with bitter, pungent and astringent tastes that increase the strength and power of Air Element in the body are called Vatala, meaning 'an agent that increases Vata'. The proper use of foods or medicines with bitter, pungent and astringent tastes promotes the balance of the Vata substance, whereas excessive use of them results in an increase of Vata, and problems such as nervousness and shakiness. Sweet, sour and salty tastes that contain more of the Water Element counteract the properties of bitter, pungent and astringent tastes. In this way, the excessive use of sweet, sour and salty taste causes a direct decrease and weakness of the Vata substance.

Vata and the Nervous System

According to Ayurveda, Vata relates to the sense of touch because it is only by the presence of Air Element and the property of emptiness that is touch realized. It is the sense of touch which creates sensations such as hot and cold, greasy or dry, and pleasant or unpleasant. These sensations result in physical vibrations, and in turn the mobilization of the nervous system. The word Vata is derived from a Sanskrit root word which means 'to move', and hence, Vata relates to the mobilizing function of the nervous system. Any disease (Roga) caused by a functional disorder of the nervous system is called a Vata roga. Examples include spasm and pain, which are general symptoms of a Vata increase, as well as the classical disease of Pakshavata ('paralysis').

The nervous system is one of the three major regulatory systems of the body, and along with the venous and arterial systems, is connected to all the different organs and tissues of the body. The nervous system controls and regulates the function of the arterial system, and the arterial system controls and regulates the function of the nervous system. Likewise, the nervous and the arterial systems collectively control and regulate the function of the venous system, whereas the venous system controls and regulates both the nervous and arterial systems.

The proper use of bitter or pungent or astringent tasting foods or medicines stimulates and maintains the nervous system. In turn, the properly stimulated nervous system controls and regulates the function of the arterial system. The excessive use of bitter, pungent or astringent tasting foods or medicines results in the over-stimulation of the nervous system and a loss of regulatory control, whereas excessive use of sweet, sour and salty tasting foods or medicines suppress the function of the nervous system.

Vata in Health

In Ayurveda, health is defined as the balance of Vata, Pitta, and Kapha, which includes the three primary regulatory systems of the body, i.e. the nervous system, the venous system, and the arterial system. To maintain this balance, the Vata substance requires proper food, medicine, and lifestyle behaviors. The bitter, pungent, and astringent tastes contain more Air in comparison to the other tastes. Intake of these tastes in the proper amount is necessary to maintain the balance of Air in the bodily construction, and to counteract the effects of the other tastes. The balance of Air in the body results in the proper function of the nervous system, which mobilizes the activity of the venous and arterial systems.

As described earlier, the element of Air is classified within the body according to five significant activities described earlier: inhalation (Prana), exhalation (Udana), assimilation (Samana), circulation (Vyana), and excretion (Apana). The proper function of these components is called Anulomana, and in order to maintain health, it is very important that these different aspects of Vata, as well as the associated substances that are carried with or propelled by this flow of Air – moves in, through, and out of the body in the proper way. As the inhaled aspect of Vata, Prana is very important for the proper function of the heart and brain. The exhaled aspect of Vata, or Udana, is very important for the proper function of the throat and lungs. The aspect of Vata that relates to assimilation, or Samana, plays an important role for the proper digestion and assimilation of nutrients in the stomach and small intestine. The aspect of Vata that relates to circulation, or Vyana, is very important for the proper function of the circulatory system including the liver, spleen, and lymphatic system. The aspect of Vata that regulates excretion, called Apana, is very important for the proper function of the colon, urinary system, and reproductive organs. The reversed function of these different aspects of Vata is called Udavarta, which is a disease entity that is the cause of many physical disorders (see page 162).

Vata in Disease

A decrease of the Vata substance is called Vata Kshaya, whereas an increase is called Vata Vriddhi or Kruddha Vata. With the exception of short term problems, any decrease or increase of the Vata substance, as well as interference with or reversed function of its five components, will promote diseases related to the nervous system. These imbalances can also affect the opposing forces of energy (Pitta) and the sources of energy (Kapha).

The decrease of Vata substance means that Air and its physical properties have either become less in their natural proportion within the body, or else they have become less active. The increased Vata substance means the element of Air and its physical properties have become too great in their natural proportion within the body, or they have become overactive. Whenever the physical properties of Air decrease in relative proportion, the nervous system by nature becomes less active. Likewise, when there is an increase in the physical properties of Air, the nervous system becomes overactive.

The under-activity and over-activity of the nervous system – in the body as a whole, or in a specific tissue or organ – results in many physical disorders. For example, the under-activity of Vata results in sensations of weakness, impaired function, irregular function, or inactivity in the affected tissue or organ. Sadness and a lack of desire to talk are usually the most prominent symptoms of this decrease, but may include general symptoms of dryness, weight loss, loss of attachment, poor circulation, dislocation, prolapse, dilation, breakage, fatigue, shaking, tremor, atrophy, colic pain, strong pain, contraction, retraction, numbness, paralysis, spasm, jerking, and a weak pulse.

Vata Vikara / Diseases of the Vata system

The following diseases are those most commonly described for Vata within the classical texts of Ayurveda, but it is by no means an exhaustive list:

1.   Breaking of the nails.
2.   Cracking or fissures of the sole.
3.   Pain in the sole.
4.   Loss of balance when walking.
5.   Numbness of the feet.
6.   Swelling of the ankles from gout.
7.   Calf spasms.
8.   Sciatica.
9.   Swelling of the knee.
10.   Dislocation of the knee.
11.   Paralysis of the thigh.
12.   Pain in the thigh.
13.   Lameness of one leg.
14.   Lameness affecting both legs.
15.   Anal prolapse.
16.   Arm pain.
17.   Upward contraction of the testicle.
18.   Paralysis of the penis.
19.   Distention of the bladder.
20.   Swelling of the hip.
21.   Diarrhea.
22.   Neurasthenia.
23.   Dwarfism.
24.   Lumbago.
25.   Back pain.
26.   Spondylitis.

27. Diaphragm spasm.
28. Spasm of the belly.
29. Heart palpitations.
30. Pain of the chest.
31. Contraction of the chest.
32. Atrophy of the arm.
33. Paralysis of the neck.
34. Wryneck (torticollis).
35. Voice defects.
36. Lockjaw.
37. Cracking of the lips.
38. Breaking of the teeth.
39. Loose teeth.
40. Aphasia.
41. Stuttering.
42. Difficulty with speech.
43. Astringent taste in the mouth.
44. Loss of sense of smell.
45. Ear pain.
46. Tinnitus.
47. Loud hearing.
48. Deafness.
49. Paralysis of the eyebrow.
50. Contraction of the eyebrow.
51. Blurred vision.
52. Eye pain.
53. Deformation of the eyes.
54. Deformation of the eyebrow.
55. Temporal pain.
56. Pain of the forehead.
57. Headache.
58. Cracking of the skin on the head.
59. Facial paralysis.
60. Hemiplegia (some forms).
61. Tetanus.
62. Convulsion.
63. Spasm.
64. Arthritis (most forms).

Symptoms of Vata Dysfunction

Beyond the previous list of diseases, there are some signs and symptoms that are specifically linked to Vata. These include:

1. Dryness.
2. Pink/pale or blue color appearing on the face or affected area.
3. Pink/pale color of the nail, conjunctiva of the eyes, or mucous membrane under the tongue.
4. Pink/pale coloration in urine, stool or skin.
5. Pain or symptoms worse while food is transiting the colon.
6. Relief sensation when pressing on the painful area.
7. Symptoms worse in the evening, at dawn or during the rainy season.
8. Exhaustion, depression, restlessness, or insomnia.
9. Strong pain or colic pain.
10. Crawling (slow, weak) pulses.
11. Symptoms worse with use of bitter, pungent or astringent tasting foods or medications.
12. Symptoms worse in cold weather or cold climate.
13. Symptoms worse with constrictitory food or medications that causes poor blood circulation.
14. Symptoms worse in Vata 'constitution' (Prakriti).
15. Symptoms worse with stress and emotional tension.

Reversed Action of the Five Vital Airs

In addition to the problems of decrease or increase, there also are some complications of Vata that are caused by the interference with or reversed action of the Five Vital Airs.

1. If the 'inhalation air' (Prana) interferes with 'circulatory air' (Vyana), it affects the brain and the sense organs of the head. Poor or faulty inhalation (Prana) can inhibit air supply to the head area (Vyana). This can lead to paralysis or fainting as in sudden low blood pressure or shock.
2. If the 'circulatory air' (Vyana) interferes with the 'inhalation air' (Prana), this can cause excessive sweating and numbness.
3. If the 'inhalation air' (Prana) interferes with the 'assimilation air' (Samana), it causes aphasia, stuttering, and stiffness or paresis.
4. If the 'assimilation air' (Samana) interferes with the 'excretory air' (Apana), it causes diarrhea, liver or spleen pain, and colic pain of the stomach.
5. If the 'inhalation air' (Prana) interferes with the 'exhalation air' (Udana), it causes choking, headache, coldness, difficulty in breathing, dry mouth, and heart diseases. For example, this can occur if someone inhales toxic gas and cannot exhale it fully.
6. If the 'exhalation air' (Udana) interferes with the 'inhalation air' (Prana) it results in deafness, collapse and possibly even death.
7. If the 'exhalation air' (Udana) interferes with the 'excretory air' (Apana), it causes vomiting and asthma.

8. If the 'excretory air' (Apana) interferes with the 'exhalation air' (Udana), it causes delusion, weak digestion and diarrhea.

9. If the 'circulatory air' (Vyana) interferes with the 'excretory air' (Apana), it causes vomiting, tympanitis, neurasthenia, abdominal tumor and rectal colic.

10. If the 'excretory air' (Apana) interferes with the 'circulatory air' (Vyana), it causes diarrhea, polyuria and semenuria.

11. If the 'assimilation air' (Samana) interferes with the 'circulatory air' (Vyana), it causes fainting, drowsiness, delirium, body ache, weak digestion and collapse.

12. If the 'exhalation air' (Udana) interferes with the 'circulatory air' (Vyana), it causes stiffness or paresis, weak digestion, lack of sweating, motionlessness and inability to keep the eyes open.

If the Pitta substance or the Kapha substance interferes with the Vital Airs they can become the cause of various heath problems. For example:

1. If 'bile' (Pitta) interferes with the 'inhalation air' (Prana), it causes fainting, hot sensations, dizziness, colic pain, and sour vomiting.

2. If 'mucus' (Kapha) interferes with the 'inhalation air' (Prana), it causes sneezing, belching, difficulty in breathing, vomiting, and loss of appetite.

3. If 'bile' (Pitta) interferes with the 'exhalation air' (Udana), it causes fainting, hot sensation, a gradual decline of the lungs, asthma, and collapse.

4. If 'mucus' (Kapha) interferes with the 'exhalation air' (Udana), it causes paleness of the complexion, hoarseness, difficulty in speaking, weakness,, a loss of appetite, and heaviness of the body.

5. If 'mucus' (Kapha) interferes with the 'assimilation air' (Samana), it causes a low body temperature, lack of sweating, indigestion, and goose pimples.

6. If 'bile' (Pitta) interferes with the 'assimilation air' (Samana), it causes excess sweating, thirst, hot sensation, fainting, and a loss of appetite.

7. If 'bile' (Pitta) interferes with the 'circulatory air' (Vyana), it causes a hot sensation, fatigue, jerking or spasmodic movements, paralysis, body ache, and headache.

8. If 'mucus' (Kapha) interferes with 'circulatory air' (Vyana), it causes heaviness of the body, joint pain, and sluggishness within the organs.

9. If mucus (Pitta) interferes with the 'excretory air' (Apana), it causes dark yellow-colored urine and stool, a burning sensation of the penis and anus, or menorrhagia.

10. If 'mucus' (Kapha) interferes with the 'excretory air' (Apana), it causes mucus colitis and urinary diseases associated with excess mucus secretion.

Vata as Aggravating Agent

The nervous system can become overactive or increased by Vata aggravating agents. These are influences, substances or behaviors that either express or otherwise increase the physical properties of the element of Air. These include:

1. Excessive or daily use of any of food or medication that is bitter, pungent or astringent in taste, used alone or in combination.
2. Hemorrhage or loss of blood.
3. Fasting, irregular meal times, or too little food.
4. Mental anxiety, distress, or excessive thinking.
5. Heavy exercise or excessive labor.
6. Sleeping or sitting for a long time in cramped or otherwise bad positions.
7. Withholding natural urges, e.g. stool, urine, gas, etc.
8. Travel in vehicles that cause constant vibration of the body, or exposure to strong vibrations.
9. Misuse of laxatives (page 174), enema and emetic medications (page 175).
10. Improper practice of Yoga or exercise, using unnatural body positions.
11. Over-indulgence in sex.
12. Trauma of any sort.
13. Excess cold, such as cold weather or living in a cold climate.
14. Excessive use of cold foods, or behaviors that have a cooling (constrictitory) effect within the capillaries.
15. The effect of the rainy season or excess humidity.

Vata in Diagnosis

Ayurveda classifies almost all disease according to each Dosha (i.e. Vata, Pitta, Kapha) or combination of the Doshas (i.e. Vata-Pitta, Vata-Kapha, Pitta-Kapha, Vata-Pitta-Kapha). For the proper diagnosis of a Vata disease, there are certain tests used in Ayurveda that may to be carried out to gain more information. These include:

1. **Touch Test**. If a painful area becomes less painful from gentle pressure, this is positive for Vata causation.
2. **Color Test**. The presence of a blue, black or pink/pale color in the affected tissue, as well as the general complexion, or within the nails, stool, or urine, is positive for Vata causation.
3. **Colon activity test**. If the symptoms of a disease become worse when the colon is active during digestion of food (about 6-8 hours after food intake), it is positive for Vata causation.
4. **Time Test**. If the symptoms of disease worsen in the evening and/or dawn, it is positive for Vata causation.
5. **Pulse Test**. If the pulse is crawling (moving weakly and slowly), it is positive for Vata causation.

6. **Seasonal Test**. If the symptoms of disease are worse in the rainy season and/or winter, it is positive for Vata causation.
7. **Taste Test**. If the symptoms of a disease worsen with the daily or excessive use of food or medicine that are bitter, pungent and/or astringent in taste, it is positive for Vata causation. A feeling of an astringent taste in the mouth is also positive for Vata causation.
8. **Climate Test**. If the symptoms of disease worsen with dryness or in an alpine climate, it is positive for Vata causation.
9. **Constrictitory Test**. If the symptoms of disease worsen while using foods or medications that have a constrictitory effect, it is positive for Vata causation.
10. **Nature Test**. If the symptoms of a disease are worse in nervous, thin-natured people (Vata Prakriti) it is positive for Vata causation.
11. **Test of Mind**. If the symptoms of a disease become worse with anxiety, mental distress, excessive thinking, or fear, it is positive for Vata causation.
12. **Skin Test**. If the affected area is dry, it is positive for Vata causation.
13. **Swelling Test**. If the affected area is swollen with gas, like a balloon, it is positive for Vata causation.
14. **Fever Test**. If the body temperature goes up and down sporadically, or for no apparent reason, it is positive for Vata causation.
15. **Preference Test**. If the patient prefers warmth, it is positive for Vata causation.

Vata in Treatment

The fundamental theory of treatment with regard to nervous disorders or any condition classified with the character of Vata is based upon restoring balance to the hyperactive nervous system, and to reduce the physical properties expressed by the element of Air. The colon is the seat of Vata, which contains a gas that is produced normally and excreted during peristaltic motion. Excess gas within the colon and especially putrefactive gas from weak digestion aggravates the nervous system, because the physical properties of this gas are similar to the properties expressed by the element of Air. As such, a number of methods of utilized to balance the Vata substance, including oil massage, steam bath, medicated enema, breathing exercises, medicated snuff, diet, and medication.

Oil massage and steam bath

The therapeutic application of a medicated oil is called Abhyanga, whereas a steam bath that is typically applied after an oil massage is called Swedana. The primary purpose of an oil massage is to reduce Vata, and counter the properties expressed by the Air element. Following this, a steam bath is applied to stimulate perspiration, increase the circulation of blood, and promote the absorption of the applied oil. In general, when the skin is nourished by grease and stimulated by heat, the properties of the Air Element are reduced in the body. The use of these measures is particularly important prior to the application of enema therapy (Vasti) to prevent the accumulation of Air in the body during treatment.

Therapeutic enema

An important teaching of Ayurveda is that in order to restore balance to the nervous system in any part of the body, it is essential to first balance Vata within the colon by the use of a 'medicated enema' (Vasti). Medicated enemas in Ayurveda contain ingredients such as milk and/or oil, prepared with a decoction of medicinal plants, that counteract the physical properties of the Air element. Medicated enemas are very effective to reduce the aggravation of Vata by excess or toxic gasses that are generated when the nervous system is hyperactive.

The application of medical enema is effective for cleansing the colon, but in order to make the treatment more efficacious and to avoid side effects, it should be applied a short time after the consumption of greasy foods, and the external application of oil (Abhyanga), followed by a hot 'steam bath' (Swedana). In general, stimulating the evacuation of the colon causes more gas to accumulate, causing it to become hyperactive and dry, which in turn, can be the cause of other problems such as diseases of the heart. To avoid these problems, the application of greasy food such as oil, Ghee, butter, or fat is prescribed before taking an enema. This same principle is applied when the nasal passages are cleaned with salt water (i.e. Neti), in which medicated oils are inhaled into the nose (i.e. Nasya) to restore balance, nourish, and moisturize.

Breathing Exercise and Medicated Snuff

The health of the nervous system depends on proper respiration, and clean, healthy air. When properly applied, yogic breathing exercises called Pranayama have great value to restore balance to the nervous system.

In Ayurveda, the nose is a viewed as a passageway to cleanse and restore the structure and function of the entire head, including the nose, sinuses, throat, ears, and even the brain. In some disorders of the head classified with the character of Vata such as paralysis, the use of a medicated 'nasal snuff' (Nasya) made from carminative herbs (page 175) is prescribed. This medicated nasal snuff causes dilatation of the capillaries of the nose, and the strong sensation results in sneezing, initiating a process of nasal cleansing.

Tastes which benefit Vata

Sweet, sour, and salty tasting foods and medicines are generally nourishing and stimulating to the activity of the arterial system. A well-nourished and stimulated arterial system counteracts the hyper-function of the nervous system because sweet, sour and salty tastes counteract the bitter, pungent and astringent tastes that aggravate the function of the nervous system. Foods, beverages, and medications that are sweet, sour, and/or salty are thus prescribed to restore balance to the nervous system. In order for the sweet, sour and salty tastes to be effective in this regard, they must also be greasy and heavy in their physical properties, otherwise, they cannot restore the balance.

Aromatic herbs that are pungent in taste, i.e. carminatives (page 175), cause a heating or dilatory effect in the body. These medications are important because the heat they generate expands and forces the accumulated gas from the colon. In this sense, carminative and spicy-tasting herbs play an important tool to restore balance to the nervous system.

Fats and oils, as well as oily foods, beverages, and medications, no matter what their taste, also have medicinal value to restore balance to the nervous system. This is because the physical properties of grease or oil counteracts dryness, which is one of the most important and powerful physical properties of Vata.

Herbs and Formulas to Treat Vata

Some common herbs used to treat Vata include:

1. **Ashwagandha root** (*Convolvulus arvensis / Withania somnifera*).
2. **Gokshura fruit** (*Tribulus terrestris*).
3. **Shatavari root** (wild asparagus / *Asparagus racemosus*).
4. **Vacha rhizome** (acorus / *Acorus calamus*).
5. **Bilwa fruit** (*Aegle marmelos*).
6. **Nagaram rhizome** (Indian cyperus / *Cyperus pertenuis*).
7. **Vidari tuber** (*Ipomea paniculata*).
8. **Atasi oil** (flaxseed / *Linum usitatissimum*).
9. **Amalaki fruit** (Indian gooseberry / amla / *Phyllanthus emblica*).
10. **Rasna shrub** (*Vanda roxburghii*).

Any non-poisonous plant that is sweet, sour, or salty in taste, dilatory in action, or greasy and heavy in property, will have general value to subdue the hyperactivity of the nervous system, as well as to restore balance to a weakened nervous system. Likewise, formulas that contain these tastes and physical properties can be used as nerve restoratives. One such example is the formula **Maha Yogaraja Guggulu Vati** found in the classic texts. Similar to **Maha Yogaraja Guggulu** but without the purified minerals is **Yogaraja Guggulu Vati**. The standard dose for either remedy is 1-2 grams, twice daily. A medicated oil called **Narayana Taila** is also very useful for Vata disorders.

In summation, general measures to reduce and balance Vata include the use of:

1. Oil massage.
2. Steam bath.
3. Medicated enema.
4. Breathing exercises.
5. Nasal snuff.

6. Sweet, sour, and salty tasting foods, beverages, and medications.
7. Aromatic (carminative) herbs.
8. Oils, fats, and oily herbs.

Chapter 3: Different Aspects of Pitta

Similar to the term Vata, the concept of Pitta in Ayurveda is a very broad in its meaning and application. In order to be properly understood, identified, and applied for therapeutic purposes, it must be investigated in detail with regard to its different manifestations. In this chapter, eight different perspectives on Pitta are presented:

1. **Pitta as Bile**.
2. **Pitta and Taste**.
3. **Pitta and the Venous System**.
4. **Pitta in Health**.
5. **Pitta in Disease**.
6. **Pitta as Aggravating Agent**.
7. **Pitta in Diagnosis**.
8. **Pitta in Treatment**.

Pitta as Bile

A burning fire is an expression of Tejas, the metaphysical element of Fire, but while a physical fire is easy to perceive, the element of Fire is not. This is because in the constitution of objects, including the physical body, the element of Fire exists in subtle form, and can only be identified indirectly by its physical properties. Within the body, the expression of Tejas manifests as the biological fire, called Pitta. Ayurveda states how the properties of both Tejas and a physical fire are very similar to that of the biological fire called Pitta, which in turn, shares the same physical properties as bile. The physical properties of both Pitta and bile are Ushna ('heat'), Tikshna ('strong sensation'), Drava ('liquid'), Sara ('movable'), and Sneha ('greasy'). In this way, the metaphysical element of Fire, a physical fire, Pitta, and the bile, are all related to each other by virtue of their shared physical properties.

'Heat' (Ushna) is the primary expression and signifier of Fire. When an object is heated, it counteracts the quality of cold. This counteraction of cold by heat diminishes the proportion of the Water and Air elements within a physical structure. The coldness of the Water and Air elements is naturally antagonistic the heat of the element of Fire. If the heat is strong enough, Water and Air cannot stand against Fire, and try to escape. It is the nature of heat to try to make Air and Water come under its control. This is seen when any object affected by heat becomes hotter, drier, and smaller. Bile is designated by Ayurveda to be the major representative of Fire within the body. The heat of bile counteracts the bodily representatives of the Water and Air elements, and as bile or when its properties increase proportionally, more heat sensations and inflammation are experienced.

Any object affected by heat or fire can be identified by a 'sharp' or 'strong' sensation called Tikshna. This sensation is the result of the stability of Water being undermined by the activity and power of heat. For example, when water reacts against a sudden, powerful heat source, it results in an explosion. The effect created by the explosion is similar to the sensation of Tikshna. According to Ayurveda, Tikshna counteracts Manda, which is the 'dull' or 'mild' state of Water when not disturbed by heat.

When the elements of an object are affected by heat they begin to decompose. During this process, the 'liquid' (Drava) property of water first separates itself from the physical construct of the object. Functioning as a kind of solvent, the Water element carries the other elements away in the process, causing it to become highly concentrated. Among the decomposed elements, the presence of Fire causes the Water element to move about and become active, expressing the physical property of Sara, or 'mobility'. In this way, the decomposed Fire within the Water element gives it a kind of moving, liquid energy. This dynamic represents the origin and activity of the bile produced by the liver, which is a liquid by-product derived from the decomposition of blood. This process of decomposition is driven by the bodily fire, and bile itself is viewed as form of Fire in liquid form.

The elements are in constant interaction in the universe. To exist without being destroyed by Fire, the Water Element must protect by itself by releasing its greasy components. Grease counteracts the dryness that Fire promotes. Thus within the body, the bile must contain some grease (Sneha) to counteract dryness of Fire.

The Five Biles

Ayurveda states that Pitta has five different roles, each with a different name that describes a specific range of functions within the body. They are called Pachaka, Ranjaka, Sadhaka, Alochaka, and Bhrajaka.

1. Pachaka is an aspect of Pitta that is located within the gall bladder and its duct system. Pachaka is the main source of the other forms of Vital Bile, and its main function is to digest food.
2. Ranjaka is an aspect of Pitta that is located in the liver and spleen. Its main function is to maintain the healthy red color of the blood.
3. Sadhaka is an aspect of Pitta that is active in the heart. The main function of Sadhaka is to stimulate the activity of the mind and brain.
4. Alochaka is an aspect of Pitta located in the eyes. The main function of Alochaka is to provide the power of vision.
5. Bhrajaka is an aspect of Pitta located in the surface of the body, where it stimulates and regulates the function of the skin.

Although these different types of Pitta have different functions, they are all composed of the same fundamental substance, and share the identical same five physical properties, i.e. Ushna ('heat'), Tikshna ('sharp'), Drava ('liquid'), Sara ('movable'), and Sneha ('greasy').

Pitta and Taste

Foods, beverages, and medications with sour, pungent and salty tastes contain a greater proportion of the Fire element, and thus are considered to strengthen the power of Fire and Pitta in the body. Anything that strengthens the power of Fire is called Pittala, meaning 'that which causes more heat or bile'. The proper use of sour, pungent, and salty tasting foods, herbs or medications promotes the balance of the Pitta substance. Excessive use or daily use of these same tastes results in the increase of the Pitta substance. Balance of the Pitta substance is necessary to supply regular heat in the body. An increase of Pitta means to have an excess of heat or inflammation, which is destructive to the bodily constitution.

Sweet, bitter, and astringent tastes generally impart a cooling sensation. This 'cooling' (Shita) influence indicates that these tastes contain a greater proportion of Water, Earth, and Air elements, and counteract sour, pungent, and salty tastes that exert a heating influence. The excessive use of sweet, bitter, and astringent tastes in the diet or as medicine causes a decrease in the Pitta substance, and a general reduction in body temperature and metabolic activity.

Pitta and the Venous System

Pitta represents the bodily heat, and this heat depends upon the circulation of blood for its distribution throughout the body. The blood itself is one of the five types of Pitta in the body called Ranjaka, carried by the arteries and veins. While both arteries and veins contain blood, the blood within the arteries is "sweeter" than the blood in the veins, because the arterial blood contains more of the sweet-tasting blood plasma (Rasa) that is the essence of the digested food. In comparison, the venous blood contains less blood plasma and more pungent and sour tasting by-products, making it similar to bile. As a result, the venous system generates more heat in the body than the arterial system, and thus the venous system is regarded as a place in the body where Pitta concentrates. Ayurveda states that diseases of Pitta can be subdued by taking blood from the veins, which is the basis of the therapeutic practice of 'venesection' (Rakta Mokshana – see page 92).

The venous system controls and regulates the functions of the nervous and arterial systems, and the venous system itself is controlled and regulated by nervous and arterial systems. For example, sour, pungent and salty tastes generate heat and activate the venous system, which in turn controls and limits the function of the nervous and arterial systems. A deficiency of sour, pungent and salty tastes fails to properly activate the venous system, which in turn cannot control and regulate the functions of the nervous and arterial systems. Among these tastes, pungent specifically helps to regulate the arterial system, whereas sour and salty tastes help regulate the nervous system. Overuse of these Pittala tastes, however, results in the hyperactivity of the venous system. Likewise, the excess use of sweet, bitter, and astringent taste promotes a decrease in the Pitta substance, whereas their proper use restores balance.

Pitta and Health

As previously stated, health is defined as the balance of Vata, Pitta, and Kapha, and their balance maintains the proper proportion of the Five Elements in the body. Generally, Pitta symbolizes the element of Fire of the body, generating the energy that signifies the activity of life.

Energy is everywhere, found in the ethereal atmosphere and in the constitution of solid objects. Just as heat of the sun generates the energy of the biosphere, sour, pungent, and salty tastes stimulate the generation of energy within the body. This is because foods and herbs with these tastes contain proportionally more of the Fire element compared to the other elements. For the maintenance of health, it is necessary to keep the Fire element in proper balance. Exposure to the heat of the sun or a fire must be regulated in the proper way and in the proper amount. In the same way, the heat-generating properties of certain foods or herbs must also be regulated. This regulation is necessary to balance opposing climactic effects (such as heat, cold, or damp) as well as the opposing effect of different types of foods in the diet. Any food, beverage or medication that causes heat or has a strong sensation on the tongue is considered to contain Fire, regardless of its taste.

The maintenance of the Fire element in its proper proportion results in the optimal function of the venous system, and the balance of the Pitta substance. In turn, the balanced Pitta substance maintains proper metabolic function, and thus plays a key role in the maintenance of health.

Pitta and Disease

A decrease or increase of the Pitta substance promotes diseases related to the venous system, altering the energy and heat of the body. A decrease of the Pitta substance is called Pitta Kshaya, whereas its increase is called Pitta Vriddhi or Kruddha Pitta. A decrease of the Pitta substance indicates that the element of Fire and its physical properties have become diminished. In contrast, an increase of the Pitta substance indicates that Fire and its physical properties have become greater in their natural proportion within the bodily construction.

In general, the Pitta substance should be bitter and pungent in nature. When in an increased state, the Pitta substance becomes excessively sour in taste. Likewise, when the physical properties of the Fire element decrease in proportion, the venous system by nature becomes less active or even inactive, along with a decrease in the sour taste.

Over-activity or under-activity of the venous system in any organ or part of the body causes many physical disorders. Inactivity of the venous system in any tissue or organ will cause weak digestion, poor circulation, reduced temperature, and weak metabolism. Over-activity within the venous system results in excessive blood flow, increased heat, perspiration, discharge, burning sensations, inflammation, infection, and decay or rot.

Pitta Vikara / Diseases of the Pitta System

The following diseases listed here are those most commonly described for Pitta within the classical texts of Ayurveda, but it is by no means an exhaustive list:

1. Hot sensations (whether inside the body or outside, for the entire body or only a local area).
2. Acid burping.
3. Heartburn.
4. Excess perspiration.
5. Bad smelling sweat.
6. Ulcers.
7. Lesions or breaks in the skin or tissue.
8. Areas of red, raw tissue.
9. Hematorrhea.
10. Herpes zoster.
11. Blue cataract.
12. Hepatitis.
13. Stomatitis.
14. Bitter taste in the mouth.
15. Increased thirst.
16. Inflammation of the mouth, throat, eyes, anus or penis.
17. Blurred vision.
18. Fevers.

Symptoms of Pitta Dysfunction

Besides the various conditions and diseases that are associated with Pitta and an overactive venous system, there are several symptoms that point towards an overactive venous system:

1. Yellow, green or red color appearing on the face or over the affected area.
2. Slight greasy condition in the affected area.
3. Yellowness seen in the urine, stool, skin, color of the nails, conjunctive of the eyes, or mucous membrane of the mouth.
4. Pain and other related symptoms worse while digesting food (4-5 hours after ingestion).
5. Pain feels worse when pressing the painful area.
6. Symptoms worse at midnight, midday, and summer/autumn season.
7. Irritation.
8. Burning pain.
9. Jumping or bounding pulse.

10. Symptoms are worse with the use of sour, pungent and salty tasting foods beverages, or medications.
11. Symptoms are worse in the heat or a hot climate
12. Symptoms are worse due to the consumption of heat-promoting foods, beverages, or medications.
13. Symptoms are worse in aggressive-type, Pitta-natured persons.
14. Appearance of anger.

Pitta as Aggravating Agent

The venous system can become overactive or increased by Pitta aggravating agents. These are influences, substances, or behaviors that either express or otherwise increase the physical properties of the Fire Element. These include:

1. Excessive or daily use of any kind of food, beverage, or medication that is sour, pungent and/or salty in taste.
2. Hyperactivity of the small intestine while food is still being digested.
3. Overuse or daily use of alkaline tasting foods, beverages or medications, as well as alcoholic beverages, hot tea or coffee, as well as burnt, roasted, or fried foods.
4. Overuse or daily use of soybean products, sesame seed products, leafy green vegetables, rotten or stale food, over-ripe fruits, liquid diet, sugar or oily foods.
5. Working near or exposure to the heat of the sun or fire.
6. Excessive heavy labor or exercises.
7. Over-eating, irregular meal times, or eating at the time of indigestion.
8. Excessive use of foods, beverages, or medications with dilatory effect.
9. The effect of summer, autumn, or living in a hot climate.
10. The natural Pitta-increasing effect experienced during midday and midnight.

If these influences aren't excessive a healthy body can neutralize their effect. If these Pitta-aggravating agents are active in any condition of disease, it will increase the activity of the venous system and manifest as inflammatory symptoms or as symptoms of infection.

Pitta and Diagnosis

There are number of tests that can be used to help diagnose whether or not a disease is Pitta in character, or has a Pitta component. These tests have to be carried out one by one in order to come to a proper diagnosis. These tests include the:

1. **Pain Test**. The presence of burning sensations or pain is positive for Pitta causation.

2. **Touch Test**. If a painful area becomes more painful from gentle pressure, this is positive for Pitta causation.
3. **Color Test**. The presence of a yellow, green, or red color in the affected tissue, as well as the general complexion, or within the nails, stool, or urine, is positive for Pitta causation.
4. **Small intestine activity test**. If the symptoms of disease become worse while the small intestine is active digesting food (4-5 hours after intake), it is positive for Pitta causation.
5. **Time Test**. If the symptoms of disease worsen in the midday and/or midnight, it is positive for Pitta causation.
6. **Pulse Test**. A strong, jumping pulse is positive for Pitta causation.
7. **Seasonal Test**. If the symptoms of disease are worse in summer and/or autumn it is positive for Pitta causation.
8. **Tastes Test**. If the symptoms of disease worsen with the daily or excessive use of food or medications or herbs that are sour, pungent, and/or salty it is positive for Pitta causation. Likewise, sensing a bitter taste in the mouth is also positive for Pitta causation.
9. **Climate Test**. If the symptoms of disease worsen in heat or tropical climates, it is positive for Pitta causation.
10. **Dilatory test**. If the symptoms of disease worsen while using foods, herbs or medications that have a strong dilatory effect, it is positive for Pitta causation.
11. **Nature Test**. If the symptoms of a disease are worse in aggressive, robust people (Pitta Prakriti) it is positive for Pitta causation.
12. **Test of Mind**. If the symptoms of disease become worse with irritation or anger, it is positive for Pitta causation.
13. **Skin Test**. If the affected area is slightly greasy, it is positive for Pitta causation.
14. **Swelling Test**. If a swollen part does not change with pressure, it is positive for Pitta causation.
15. **Fever test**. If the temperature suddenly elevates or remains very high, it is positive for Pitta causation.
16. **Preference Test**. If the patient prefers cold, it is positive for Pitta causation.

Pitta and Treatment

The treatment of diseases or conditions classified with the character of Pitta consist of practices that restore balance to the hyperactive venous system, or by subduing the excess physical properties of the Fire element. Ayurveda states that in order to restore balance to the venous system – in any part of the body – the small intestine must first be cleaned with laxative or purgative herbs, along with diuretics to flush the urinary system.

The Small Intestine and Bile

The small intestine is the primary location for the secretion of bile, in which the bile plays a key role for proper excretion during defecation and urination. If excess bile in the small intestine is reabsorbed by the digestive tract and into the blood it causes hyperactivity of the venous system.

Cleansing the small intestine means ridding the body of excess bile through defecation and urination. When the bile reabsorbed by the gut slowed or stopped, the body loses heat and the aggravated venous system calms down and returns to normal. Thus, the use of laxative or purgative herbs (page 174) along with diuretics (page 195) has been found to be the most important method of cleansing the small intestine and restoring balance to the venous system. Employing such measures is often the first thing done by the physician of Ayurveda in cases of inflammation.

Fasting and Venesection

Fasting has medicinal value in the treatment of diseases classified with the character of Pitta. This can be done either without any food, with a light amount of food, or with a liquid diet. During fasting, there is less supply of bile from the digestive system, and this creates fewer digestive by-products, reducing the supply of bile that causes heat. In this way, the practice of fasting is beneficial to restore the balance of the venous system and Pitta

The practice of Rakta Mokshana or 'venesection' (page 92) through the application of leeches or puncturing the vein has therapeutic value to restore balance to the venous system. This practice can be applied for general benefit or for local treatment. Unlike the arterial blood, the blood within the veins normally contains a higher proportion of toxic substances that are hot in nature. Ayurveda states that Rakta Mokshana has unique and often powerful effects to subdue the symptoms of diseases classified as Pitta.

Tastes which benefit Pitta

Sweet, bitter, and astringent tasting foods and medicines stimulate the activities of the arterial and nervous systems. These two systems work together to counteract and control the hyperactive function of the venous system. Some substances that are sweet, bitter, or astringent in taste, however, can promote heat and dilate the capillaries. Thus in order to be effective, these tastes used to balance Pitta must also have a cooling (Shita) effect. In the same way, any cooling herb, whatever its taste may be, can be used as a medicine to restore balance to the venous system and Pitta.

Herbs and Formulas to Treat Pitta

Some common herbs and formulas used to treat Pitta include:

1. **Rakta Chandanam wood** (red sandalwood / *Pterocarpus santalinus*).
2. **Chandanam wood** (white sandalwood / *Santalum album*).

3. **Parpata herb** (*Fumaria indica*).
4. **Vasaka leaf** (Malabar nut / *Adhatoda vasica*).
5. **Ushira rhizome** (*Andropogon muricatum*).
6. **Nimba leaf** (neem / *Azadirachta indica*).
7. **Haritaki fruit** (*Terminalia chebula*).
8. **Bibhitaki fruit** (*Terminalia belerica*).
9. **Kiratatiktam plant** (*Swertia chirata*).

A reliable formula for treating Pitta is **Kaishora Guggulu**. Another formula for treating Pitta disease, especially fever, is **Sudarshana Churna**.

In summation, general measures to reduce and balance Pitta include the use of:

1. Laxative or purgative medications along with diuretics.
2. Fasting.
3. Venesection.
4. Sweet, bitter, and astringent tasting foods, beverages, or medications.
5. Foods, herbs or other methods that have a cooling effect.

Chapter 4: Different Aspects of Kapha

Similar to the terms Vata and Pitta, the concept of Kapha in Ayurveda is also very broad with regard to its meaning and application. In order to be understood, identified and used for therapeutic purposes, the concept of Kapha must be investigated in detail to understand its different manifestations. To this end, eight different aspects of Kapha are described:

1. **Kapha as Mucus**.
2. **Kapha and Taste**.
3. **Kapha and the Arterial system**.
4. **Kapha and health**.
5. **Kapha and Disease**.
6. **Kapha as Aggravating Agent**.
7. **Kapha and Diagnosis**.
8. **Kapha and Treatment**.

Kapha as Mucus

A lake or a flowing river is an expression of Ap, the metaphysical element of Water. Similar to both the blowing wind and a burning fire, the nature of flowing water is easy to perceive, but because the element of Water is subtle in nature, it can only be identified indirectly through the expression of its physical properties.

Within the body, the expression of Water manifests as the biological water, called Kapha, which shares the same physical properties as mucus. The physical properties of both Kapha and mucus are Guru ('heavy'), Shita ('cold'), Mridu ('soft'), Snigdha ('grease'), Sthira ('stable') and Picchila ('sticky'). Thus the metaphysical element of Water, molecular water, Kapha, and mucus, are all related to each other by virtue of their shared physical properties.

All of the physical properties of Kapha belong solely to the element of Water, with the exception of Sthira ('stable'), which is also expressed by the element of Earth. In a living organism, this property of stability is dependent upon the combined influence of Water and Earth elements, which increases density and weight. Anything that contains more Water and Earth, in comparison to Air, Fire, or Space, is considered to be heavy in nature.

If a light substance absorbs moisture, it becomes 'heavy' (Guru) because this moistness is an expression of the property of the Water Element. The ability to increase weight and density through the accumulation of moisture is an important function of Kapha in the body. This is true for all animals, as well as plants, which use moisture to add weight and density to their tissues.

Any object that contains more water by nature is reduced in temperature, because the nature of water is 'cold' (Shita). The physical property of cold counteracts heat, and as the power of cold increases, the power of heat reduces in turn. Anything that contains more water is naturally cold or imparts a cooling sensation. In this way, the mucus of the body reacting with the bodily heat helps regulate the temperature of the body.

Objects that contain more of the Water element are observed to be 'soft' (Mridu) to the touch. Softness is a sensation created by Water that has the nature of expanding and dissolving components that arise from the different elements. The property of softness increases in objects as they absorb more water. For example, many things that are hard to the touch will swell and become softer after being soaked in water. If a soft object is kept in the sun, it hardens as its moisture evaporates. The softening property of Kapha counteracts hardness to keep the tissues and organs of the body soft and pliable.

Any object that contains moisture, when reacting with heat, will protect itself by releasing some of its 'grease' (Snigdha), one of the properties of Kapha. Grease counteracts dryness, and dryness is the condition that occurs when water is diminished by heat and air. For example, when exposed to the heat of the sun, the greasy quality of Kapha is released as a form of protection, which is why the skin becomes greasy on hot days.

For something to have an adherent property, it must be 'sticky' (Picchila) in nature, a property expressed by the element of Water. Water plays a key role in physical contact and attachment by virtue of the sticky or viscous property of Picchila. When this property is condensed by the presence of the Earth element it becomes more viscous and sticky. This relates to an increase in the property of Sthira, and when it is fully condensed nothing can move, because 'stability' (Sthira) is counteractive to motion. In a state of health, the sweet-tasting bodily fluids contribute to the stability and solidity of the body.

Although Kapha relates to the role of mucus, the term also includes other expressions of the Water element within the body. Similar to the Five Vital Airs of Vata and the Five Biles of Pitta, there are five aspects of Kapha, each of which has different roles to play in the function of the body.

The Five Types of Mucus

As the biological water of the body, Ayurveda states that Kapha has five different forms that encompass its complete function, called Kledaka, Avalambaka, Bodhaka, Tarpaka, and Shlesaka.

1. Kledaka is the aspect of Kapha that is active in the stomach. This Kapha is the main source of other biological waters of the body, and its primary function is to dissolve and capture food for proper digestion.
2. Avalambaka is the aspect of Kapha that is active in the chest. Its primary function is to give stability and power to the arteries, veins and pericardium in the chest that both protects and keeps the heart suspended in place.

3. Bodhaka is the aspect of Kapha that is active in the tongue, necessary to properly distinguish the six tastes.
4. Tarpaka is the aspect of Kapha that is active in the brain, necessary for proper function of the sense organs.
5. Shlesaka is the aspect of Kapha that is located in the joints, necessary for the proper function and lubrication of the joints.

Although these five aspects of Kapha have different names and functions, they are all identical with respect to their physical properties, i.e. Guru ('heavy'), Shita ('cold'), Mridu ('soft'), Snigdha ('grease'), Sthira ('stable'), and Picchila ('sticky').

Kapha and Taste

The sweet, sour, and salty tastes found in foods, beverages, and medicines are collectively called Shleshmala, a term used to refer to ingested or applied substances that cause the accumulation of either mucus or weight in the body. Shleshmala substances contain more Water Element in their physical construction. In this way, the proper use of sweet, sour and salty taste promotes the balance of the mucus substance (Kapha), which in turn regulates the function of the arterial system. The excessive use or daily use of Shleshmala substances results in the increase of the mucus substance and hyperactivity of the arterial system. The proper balance of the mucus substance results in a regular and healthy supply of biological water within the body, used for the purpose of fueling energy. An increase of the mucus substance reflects the excess accumulation of biological water in the body, causing congestion and weight gain.

Bitter, pungent, and astringent tastes contain a greater proportion of Air, Fire and Earth Elements compared to the other tastes, and all promote dryness. The excessive use of these tastes results in decrease of the mucus substance, causing a reduction in the function of the arterial system. A decrease of the mucus substance indicates that the proportion of the biological water in the body has diminished.

Kapha and the Arterial System

The blood plays a key role in the maintenance of health, delivering vital nutrients obtained from digestion to the tissues and organs of the body. This role is an expression of the Water Element, and relates specifically to the blood plasma, called Rasa. This watery fluid of the blood is cooling in nature, and helps to control the bodily heat generated from digestion and metabolism. Compared to the venous blood, the blood of the arterial system contains more Rasa, due to its role in supplying nutrition to the tissues of the body. In this way, the arterial system is a primary expression of Kapha in the body.

The arterial system controls and regulates the function of the nervous system, and in turn, the nervous system controls and regulates the function of the arterial system. Although opposite in nature, their proper function expresses a mutual coordination. When a combination of sweet, sour, and salty tastes are used in the proper way and amount, it activates the function of the arterial system. Properly activated, the arterial system in turn regulates the function of the nervous system. A deficiency of sweet, sour, and salty tastes results in a weakness of arterial function, and an inability to properly regulate the nervous system, causing an increase in Vata. In a similar fashion, the excessive use of these tastes promotes hyperactivity of the arterial system, causing the nervous system to become weak. This is why eating too much greasy and heavy food can make a person feel sluggish and dull.

Kapha and Health

Health is signified in Ayurveda by the balance of Vata, Pitta, and Kapha. Each Dosha has its own role to play, and for Kapha one primary function is to provide the fuel required to produce bodily energy. The source of energy is the nourishment of the body tissues, or Dhatus (see page 253). This nourishment has to be supplied in the proper way and in the proper amount for health. Without the proper supply of nourishment the energy within any living system begins to diminish.

There are sources of energy everywhere, in the surrounding atmosphere, as well as in the foods, beverages, and medications we ingest. The capacity to feel energized or refreshed relates to the element of Water, and hence water from natural, clean sources is an important source of nourishment. Within the atmosphere the expression of this energy can be seen as the morning dew, a nutritive moisture that condenses on plants during the coolness of the night.

The energy contained within various foods and herbs is related to presence of sweet, sour, and salty tastes, all of which contain a greater proportion of the Water Element. To maintain health, the Water Element obtained from various physical sources, supplied in proper way and in the proper amount. This is a general rule necessary for maintaining the proper function of the arterial system and the balance of Kapha, which in turn, provides for the proper nourishment of the body.

Kapha and Disease

The imbalance, decrease, or increase of Kapha results in the arising of specific types of disease. The decrease of the Kapha substance, called Kapha Kshaya, occurs when Kapha substance does not have enough nourishing substances within its composition. This decrease of the Kapha substance indicates that the Water Element and its physical properties have likewise decreased. An increase of the Kapha substance is called Kaphavriddhi or Kruddha Kapha. In general, the nourishing Kapha substance should be sweet in taste, but when increase occurs, the toxic Kapha substance that forms is termed 'salty mucus' or Kapha Dosha. The increase of the Kapha substance indicates that the Water element and its physical properties have increased.

When the physical properties of the Water Element decrease in proportion, the arterial system becomes less active, or even inactive. Under-activity of the arterial system causes poor circulation, dryness, burning sensations, malnourishment, and insomnia. When the physical properties of the Water Element increase proportionally, the arterial system becomes over-active, resulting in the excess exudation and accumulation of this 'salty' or 'toxic' mucus in the affected area. In this condition, cold sensations, heaviness, edema, itching pain, numbness, paralysis, and various forms of blockage are characteristic signs and symptoms. The under or over-activity of the arterial system – in any tissue or organ – is the cause of many physical disorders.

Kapha Vikara / Diseases of the Kapha System

The following diseases listed here are those most commonly described for Kapha within the classical texts of Ayurveda, but it is by no means an exhaustive list:

1. Drowsiness.
2. Laziness, sluggishness or excess need for sleep.
3. Watery mouth.
4. Excess phlegm, urine or stool.
5. Thickening of the artery walls.
6. Goiter.
7. Obesity.
8. Weak digestive power.
9. Urticaria.
10. Heavy sensation in the heart.
11. Sweet taste in the mouth.

Symptoms of Kapha Dysfunction

Beyond the conditions described above, there are some general signs and symptoms that indicate a dysfunction of Kapha and the hyperactivity of the arterial system. These include:

1. Diseases where symptoms develop very slowly with mild complications.
2. The appearance of a white or pale color on the face or affected area.
3. Greasiness in any affected area of the body.
4. White or pale color of the nail, stool, urine, or in conjunctiva of the eyes or mucus membrane of the mouth.
5. Obesity.
6. Patients with a dull or sluggish character.

Kapha as Aggravating Agent

The arterial system becomes hyperactive due to an increase in the Kapha substance, or due to an increase in the physical properties associated with the Water Element. Factors that increase Kapha include:

1. The excessive or daily use of any kind of food or medication that is either sweet, sour, and/or salty in taste, including greasy food, dairy products

(except old cheese), pork, beef, fish, buffalo, mutton, or new rice (eaten soon after harvesting).

2. Sleeping during the day, especially after meals.
3. Lack of exercise, over-eating, or not bathing.
4. A cold climate, cold foods, and cooling medications.
5. Heavy food that is hard to digest.
6. Starchy foods with sticky properties.
7. Expressing overconfidence or excessive joy.
8. The effect of winter and spring.
9. Physical exercise and exertion immediately after eating.
10. The natural effect of early morning (after sunrise) and early evening (after sunset).

Agents that aggravate Kapha applied in a Kapha-type disease will naturally result in the hyperactive function of the arterial system, which will typically worsen the symptoms of any disease related to Kapha.

Kapha and Diagnosis

In order to diagnose diseases classified as Kapha, or to ascertain the presence of Kapha in any disease, there are certain unique tests that are undertaken to yield key information. These include the following tests:

1. **Pain test**. The presence of an itching or dull pain is positive for Kapha causation.
2. **Touch Test**. If a painful area or the area affected with disease gets no better or worse from having gentle pressure applied, it is positive for Kapha causation.
3. **Color Test**. A pale or white color of the affected area, as well as the complexion, nail, stool or urine is positive for Kapha causation.
4. **Stomach activity Test**. If the symptoms of a disease become worse while the stomach is active digesting food (within two hours after food intake), it is positive for Kapha.
5. **Time Test**. If the symptoms of disease become worse in the early morning and or early evening, it is positive for Kapha causation.
6. **Pulse Test**. If the pulse is felt to move around up and down with a strong sensation, almost like double pulses, it is positive for Kapha causation.
7. **Seasonal test:** If the symptoms of disease worsen in winter or spring, it is positive for Kapha causation.
8. **Taste Test**. If the symptoms of disease worsen from the daily or excessive use of foods, beverages, or medications that are sweet, sour, and/or salty in taste, it is positive for Kapha causation. A sweet taste of the mouth is also positive for Kapha causation.

9. **Climate Test**. If the symptoms of disease worsen in humid and/or cold climate, it is positive for Kapha causation.
10. **Constrictitory Test**. If the symptoms of disease worsen while using foods, beverages, or medications with constrictitory effects, it is positive for Kapha causation.
11. **Nature Test**. If the symptoms of disease are worse in a person that exhibits the properties of slow, dull and heavy (Kapha Prakriti), it is positive for Kapha causation.
12. **Mind Test**. If the symptoms of disease worsen when the mind is over-confident or overjoyed, it is positive for Kapha causation.
13. **Skin test**. If the affected area is greasy, it is positive for Kapha causation.
14. **Swelling Test**. If a swollen area goes down when pressed and does not immediately restore its shape, it is positive for Kapha causation.
15. **Fever Test**. A mild body temperature is positive for Kapha causation.
16. **Preference Test**. A desire for heat or a preference for hot foods is positive for Kapha causation.

Kapha and Treatment

The fundamental theory of treatment concerning diseases and disorders classified with the character of Kapha is based upon restoring balance to the hyperactive arterial system, and to reduce the physical properties associated with the Water Element. Ayurveda emphasizes that to restore balance within the arterial system in any part of the body, the stomach should be cleaned first with emetic medications (see page 175).

The stomach is the primary source of the mucus substance in the body. It is secreted during gastric digestion, and as it is mixed with the ingested food, it receives the nutrients of digestion. Now containing the essence of the food dissolved within it, the mucus substance is released into the blood, where it activates the arterial system and the circulation of the nutritive blood plasma. In this way, emetic medications that expel excess mucus are used by traditional physicians to inhibit the exudation and circulation of mucus, and to reduce the Watery Element within the arterial system. Before using emetic medications, however, it is important to apply a therapeutic steam bath (Swedana). The application of heat during a steam bath promotes sweating and the purification of the lymphatic system, improving glandular filtration, breaking up blockages caused by excess exudation.

When bitter, pungent, and astringent tastes are taken in the diet or as medicine their 'dry' (Ruksha) and 'light' (Laghu) properties stimulate the activities of the nervous system. These tastes counteract the properties of sweet, sour, and salty tastes that aggravate the function of the arterial system. Bitter, pungent, and astringent tasting foods, beverages, and medications that are dry and light property are thus prescribed to restore balance to the Kapha substance.

Fasting, Nasal Snuff, and Exercise

Fasting has medicinal value in the treatment of diseases or conditions associated with Kapha. During periods of fasting there is less supply of the watery mucus normally secreted by the stomach, which in turn, reduces the activity of the arterial system.

The practice of cleaning the sinus with a medicated 'nasal snuff' (Nasya) has particular therapeutic value to restore balance to the cerebral arterial system, because the nose is the passageway to purify the head. A medicated nasal snuff will usually promote the dilation of the nasal capillaries, and when applied, the patient will open their eyes wide and sneeze, causing the discharge of excess mucus.

Physical exercise (Vyayama) also has therapeutic value in the treatment of an increase in Kapha. The primary purpose of exercise is to increase blood circulation, and to loosen and warm the body. The heat dilates the capillaries and increases lymphatic flow, initiating a natural cleansing process that occurs through increased lymphatic filtration and perspiration.

Herbs and Formulas to Treat

Some common herbs and formulas used to treat Kapha are:

1. **Vidanga seeds** (*Embelia ribes*).
2. **Guduchi stem** (*Tinospora cordifolia*).
3. **Chitraka root** (*Plumbago zeylanica*).
4. **Maricham** (black pepper / *Piper nigrum*).
5. **Pippali fruit** (long pepper / *Piper longum*).
6. **Gajapippali fruit** (*Piper chaba*).
7. **Shatapushpa seed** (anise / *Pimpinella anisum*).
8. **Bibhitaki fruit** (*Terminalia belerica*).
9. **Yavani seed** (wild omum / *Trachyspermum ammi*).

A reliable formula for treating Kapha to aid digestion and reduce mucus is **Trikatu**. For Kapha with swelling and/or solid accumulations the formula **Kanchanara Guggulu** can be used.

In summation, general measures to reduce and balance Kapha and the arterial system include the use of:

1. Steam bath.
2. Emetics.
3. Fasting.
4. Medicated nasal snuff.
5. Physical exercise.
6. Bitter, pungent, and astringent tasting foods, beverages, or medications.
7. Foods or medications that increase heat.

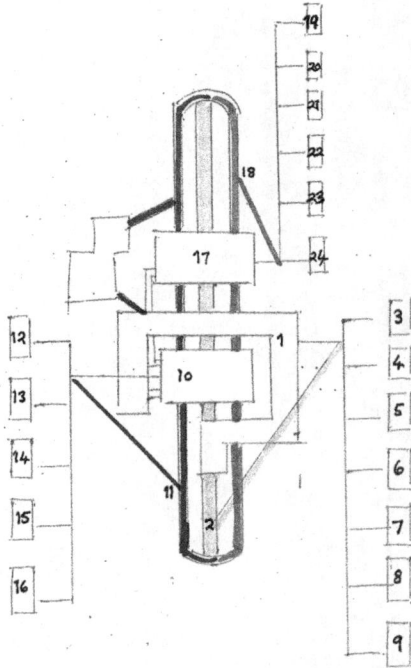

A diagram of the three Doshas and their associated properties, drawing by Dr. Mana

Chapter 5: Diseases Involving Two or More Systems

Many diseases involve two or more systems out of balance. In such cases, the treatment differs based upon the combination of factors. Knowing how to treat such disease processes properly is very important for two reasons. First, such combinations are the rule rather than the exception in clinical practice; and second, the methods derived from a purely theoretical analysis can appear to be contradictory. Fortunately, the empirical evidence gathered by Ayurveda over the centuries has shown the most effective ways to deal with such complex diseases.

Diseases Caused by Vata-Pitta

When the functions of the nervous and venous systems become increased together in any disease state, it is classified as having the character of Vata-Pitta. In such cases, the disease will have combined symptoms of the increased nervous system (Vata) and the increased venous system (Pitta). The aggravating agents of either the Vata substance or the Pitta substance will cause worsening of symptoms. This kind of condition or disease has to be diagnosed following the different diagnostic tests mentioned in the Vata and Pitta sections of this text. While treating this sort of condition, the emphasis should be on herbal medications that are both sweet and nourishing, which balance both Vata and Pitta.

Diseases Caused by Vata-Kapha

If the functions of the nervous and arterial system together are increased in the same disease process, it is classified as a Vata-Kapha condition. The disease will display the combined symptoms of an increase of nervous (Vata) and arterial (Kapha) systems. The symptoms of such a disease are by nature much stronger than when a single Dosha is out of balance, because it is susceptible to the aggravating agents for both Vata and Kapha. For diagnosis, the tests mentioned in the sections of Vata and Kapha have to be carried out side by side and compared. The treatment should be based on the principle of balance. Using foods and medications with a with sweet, bitter, and astringent tastes has been found to have the strongest medicinal value. The sweet taste calms the Vata, while the bitter and astringent tastes control Kapha.

Disease Caused by Pitta-Kapha

When the functions of the venous and arterial system are out of balance together in same disease, it is classified as Pitta-Kapha. The aggravating agents for either Pitta or Kapha substance will worsen the symptoms. For diagnosis the different tests mentioned in the section of Pitta and Kapha have to be applied side by side and compared. A Pitta-Kapha condition expresses the contradictory natures of both hot and cold, and at the outset of treatment, it should be determined which aspect is stronger. Treatment is then applied to this aspect first, and only after it is controlled is the other aspect then treated.

Diseases Caused by Vata-Pitta-Kapha (Sannipata)

Diseases classified with the combined characteristics of Vata, Pitta, and Kapha are called Tridoshaja or Sannipataja. This occurs if the functions of the nervous system, venous, and arterial systems are all out of control at the same time. In general, any Tridoshaja disease is considered very serious and complicated, sometimes malignant, and always difficult to cure. These complex diseases usually have no fixed symptoms, and any number of symptoms can be prominent at one time or another. During the malignant stage of disease, the combined symptoms of Vata, Pitta, and Kapha begin to appear simultaneously, and any aggravating agent will causes a worsening of symptoms.

In some Sannipataja cases, certain symptoms of one system can be subdued, but this often causes a worsening of symptoms in another system. For diagnosis, none of the tests used to diagnose Vata, Pitta, and Kapha are reliable, and thus in such situations, a careful analysis of the symptoms and symptoms, as well as the nature of the pathology and its complications, provide hints for proper diagnosis and treatment. Traditional physicians in Ayurveda have paid a great deal of attention to carefully and exactly detailing the unique symptoms of different disease states that express the character of Sannipataja.

The treatment against such complicated diseases usually does not have any miraculous effect. However, the method of first controlling only one of the increased systems has often been found to be beneficial. For example, although severe forms of Jwara ('fever') are classified as Sannipataja, they can be treated first by controlling the increased arterial system (Kapha). Once the increased arterial system is under control, the other systems can be controlled one by one. The disease of Rajayakshma, or tuberculosis, is another where all the systems are out of control, and is treated using symptomatic measures, with an emphasis placed upon ensuring the health of the digestive system.

Chapter 6: Theory of Spiritual Healing

The ancient scholars of Ayurveda enumerated and analyzed all the known physical and mental diseases one by one. In so doing, they discovered that there are certain diseases that do not follow the theory of Tridosha Siddhanta. These diseases are classified into three groups:

1. Mental diseases caused by the Bhuta (invisible atmospheric personalities).
2. Children's diseases caused by the Graha.
3. Diseases that are caused partly by the Bhuta, and partly by an imbalance in Vata, Pitta, and/or Kapha.

The ancient way of identifying spiritual diseases was based upon the observation that the sudden emergence of drastic symptoms could sometimes occur prior to any morbid change in anatomy. This is the reverse of the usual process, in which physiological changes typically precede the onset of symptoms. It was further found that in such cases the regular medicines applied on the basis of Tridosha Siddhanta could not be prescribed because they caused a worsening of symptoms. In such critical situations, the use of spiritual treatments was found to be beneficial to control this sort of disease, at least to some extent.

These spiritual treatments can be broken down into five categories, each related to one of the five sense organs:

1. Sound therapy.
2. Figure therapy.
3. Odor therapy.
4. Taste therapy.
5. Contact therapy.

Mental Diseases Caused by the Bhuta

Mental diseases caused by the Bhuta are called Bhutonmada or Agantuja-unmada. In these cases, a powerful change of personality is the primary symptom, and are not the result of factors that aggravate Vata, Pitta, and/or Kapha.

This unseen mental personality or Bhuta has both negative and positive characteristics. In the negative sense, the Bhuta can be the cause of certain diseases that do not follow the theory of balance. In a positive sense, however, the Bhuta can also be a remedy for the same set of diseases.

Normally, all the bodily systems function in a coordinated fashion with the mind. When the Bhuta affects the patient, the mind can be become persistently obsessed by unusual or extraordinary memories that exist outside the patient's normal life experience. Sometimes this affliction results in a complete change of personality, such that it seems like the patient becomes a different person. The Sanskrit word Bhuta is used to define these unseen biological entities, each of which is classified on the basis of characteristic personality changes that occur in the patient. These different entities include Deva, Rishi, Pitri, Gandharva, Yaksha, Rakshasa, and Pishacha. It is thought that these biological forces are active in the atmosphere, but cannot be seen with the naked eye. Generally, these invisible entities are not harmful to humans, but when people violate the disciplines of society, breaking the social order, the Bhutas can bring harm by causing mental disorders and certain types of physical illness.

Physical Diseases Caused by the Bhuta

Apart from mental illness the Bhuta can also cause physical diseases that involve the theory of balance. These diseases are characterized by the sudden onset of symptoms prior to any morbid anatomical change. For a disease to have real symptoms there first should be some kind of anatomical change, and only after this change do the real symptoms of a particular disease appear. In diseases caused by the Bhuta, however, the symptoms appear first and only after some time are they followed by anatomical changes. Severe disease in patients with no signs of prior imbalance, such as the sudden symptoms that occur in malaria, or that occur with an improper diet or lifestyle are included in this group.

Children's Diseases caused by the Graha

Children's diseases caused by the Graha are called Bala-Graha. The word Graha is similar to the word Bhuta, but the Grahas only affect children. For treatment of children's diseases caused by the Grahas, spiritual healers within Ayurveda utilize word-symbols such as Skanda, Skandapasmara, Shakuni, Revati, Putana, Andhaputana, Shitaputana, Mukhamandika, and Naigameya. These word-symbols are synonyms for the various types of Grahas, each of which exhibits particular characteristics and behaviors in the patient. According to traditional belief, Grahas can cause healthy children to suddenly develop serious symptoms of gastro-intestinal disease, accompanied by great fear and alternations in perception. The Grahas are usually not as harmful as the Bhutas, but under conditions of poor sanitation or a violation of the social order, they can enter the mind of children and cause many complicated diseases that cannot be cured using the principles of Tridosha Siddhanta.

Sound Therapy

Among the different measures to treat afflictions of the Bhuta and Graha is Mantra Chikitsa, or 'sound therapy', related to the sense of hearing. Mantras are composed of specific vowels and consonants uttered in Sanskrit. Vowels and consonants join together to form words, and these words in turn have a symbolic meaning, which are required by higher functions of the mind in order to function.

Traditional mantras such as Swastivachana, Mangalacharana, and Dharani are compositions of auspicious words, or words that have spiritual significance. For example, the Mangalacharana mantra is used to bring a sense of auspiciousness to the beginning of any activity, including religious ritual. If someone was starting a new job or preparing to travel, the Mangalacharana mantra could be chanted to create a positive result. The Swastivachana mantra has more or less the same effect, but also specific properties as well, such as reducing the chance that a bad event will happen, protecting oneself from negative influences, and removing psychological problems such as fear and confusion.

Mantras are pronounced with silent vocalization, whereas Dharanis are chanted out loud with melodious vocalization. It is clear that meaningful sounds, whether pronounced in silence or out loud, have a direct effect on the operation of the mind. Positive sounds stimulate the mind via the sense organs to connect with the body. The mind-body connection is very important for physical and mental health, and negative sounds mislead the mind, disturbing both the mind and body. Positive sounds are generally pronounced with an emphasis upon the consonants, whereas the negative sounds are pronounced with an emphasis on the vowels. Based upon this consideration, Mantras and Dharanis are composed to emphasize various unique methods of projecting the sounds of either vowels or consonants to create specific effects.

Mantra Chikitsa is part of the spiritual healing branch of Ayurveda. There are many Mantras and Dharanis composed by the different Rishis and Munis. A particular Mantra is often associated with a specific religious path. Religion itself is the discipline that seeks to find the reality of the universe beyond the physical. Without such discipline, it is not possible to concentrate one's mind enough to understand universal truths. The recitation of Mantras or Dharanis is one of the most important religious disciplines, and a very powerful method for concentrating the mind in a positive way, which is beneficial to health.

Mantras developed for treatment are written down in both the religious and spiritual healing texts used in Ayurveda. Anyone can read and recite them, but their effect depends upon the 'mental confidence' of the recipient. This 'confidence' is defined by the Sanskrit word Siddhi, which is synonymous with the highest stage of confidence and mental focus a human being can attain. A person who has developed this Siddhi can strongly focus the mind and mobilize the nature of desire. With this power, the practitioner can fix their attention on the patient's disturbed mind/body, and using the positive vibrations emanating from their mind, or spoken aloud, restore the patient back to normal.

Figure Therapy

Image therapy is called Rupa Chikitsa or Murti Chikitsa. Rupa means 'form', 'shape' or 'figure', and is related to vision, and the apprehension of visual objects. Rupa Chikitsa consists of using colorful images of deities, images of spiritual persons, and special diagrams called Mandalas. These figures play a major role in influencing the disturbed mind and body in a positive way. Beautifully drawn or carved figures of deities that are symbols of a deeper spiritual reality can positively affect a disturbed mind, and draw it back to civility. A civil or polite mind is one with a restored sense of what is right and wrong. In the same way, the use of Mandalas, which are considered to be abodes of different deities, can similarly affect a disturbed mind/body and return it to normal.

There is great power in the personality of those who have accomplished spiritual mastery, great learning, physical ability, or great wealth. The mental power of such persons can be an aid to bringing the wayward mind back under control. A strong mind naturally holds sway over a weak one, causing the weaker mind to become considerate and polite in the presence of an acknowledged superior. Accomplished spiritual healers and priests thus play a major role in the ritualistic of figure therapy.

Odor Therapy

Odor therapy is called Gandha Chikitsa, and is related to the sense of smell. For this type of therapy, many kinds of incense are made from medicinal plants, animal products, and minerals. The nose is considered by Ayurveda to be a direct passageway to the brain that in turn is connected to all the sense organs. Medications such as incense thus have a direct effect upon the brain, and the disturbed mind can be awakened to reality by the smell of incense. Over the centuries, practitioners of Ayurveda have discovered certain types of incense that have extraordinary powers to awaken and draw the disturbed mind back to reality. Only a mind awakened to reality can properly distinguish right from wrong.

In addition to this general concept, another valuable aspect of Odor Therapy concerns the negative effect of a polluted atmosphere. Polluted air is the cause of many physical and mental diseases. Ayurveda has clearly pointed out that the disease-causing effects of air pollution are related to a defilement of Bhutas and Grahas. Although the naked eye cannot see this defilement, it can nonetheless bring harm to human beings, and cause conditions such as 'insanity' (Unmada). The use of incense that spreads quickly through the atmosphere has been found to be very effective in clearing out the defilement caused by Bhutas and Grahas. This kind of medicinal incense, made from specific herbs, has two general effects. The first is that it cleans the atmosphere and helps dissipate the polluting elements. Secondly, medicinal incense also helps to cleanse the body as it is inhaled, stimulating a physical response the blood to remove pollutants, toxins, and wastes. Smelling a medicinal incense also affects the mind by stimulating its positive functions.

Taste Therapy

Taste therapy is called Rasa Chikitsa, and is related to the sense of taste. Rasa Chikitsa is also known by the term Bali, which refers to a food that is offered to different deities. In Rasa Chikitsa, special foods are prepared to tempt the desire of the patient, who then offers it to their favorite deity as Bali. If the patient can resist the temptation to eat the Bali, the disturbed mind can be restored to normal. The general concept of Taste Therapy is to fix the disturbed mind on the this act offering, to give it something to focus on that is positive.

Perhaps the most interesting aspect of Bali is how each Bhuta and Graha can be tempted by a particular food. When this food desired by a Bhuta or Graha is presented to the patient, they will attempt to control the patient's mind and get them to eat it. At this moment the Bhuta or Graha becomes concentrated in the food itself, but instead of eating it, the patient offers it to their chosen deity. After the ceremony, the Bali is then thrown away in a restricted area, such as the bank of river, the cemetery grounds, or at a crossroads. The Bali that has been offered to a deity is not allowed to be eaten by anyone, because it now contains Bhutas or Grahas.

Among traditional physicians in Nepal, the term Bali also refers to the practice of animal sacrifice, and is concerned with killing the unseen Bhuta. In this practice, a spiritual healer who is devoted to wrathful deities performs a special ritual ceremony in which an animal is killed. During this ritual, the sacrificial animal is transformed into a living being that is now inhabited by the Bhuta. Sacrificing this animal is believed to be a spiritual way of killing the Bhuta that is causing the physical or mental problems of the patient. It is the experience of spiritual healers within my family's tradition that this method can eliminate certain types of mental and physical illness.

Contact Therapy

Contact therapy is called Sparsha Chikitsa, and is concerned with the sense of 'touch' (Sparsha). In Sparsha Chikitsa various objects including jewels, unique animal products, minerals, or plants are touched or handled to exert their medicinal properties. These types of objects have been observed by traditional physicians to have the power to relieve mental and physical problems caused by the Bhutas or Grahas. Called Mani or Divyousadhi, these objects are considered to have miraculous powers.

The sense of touch is the foundation of the five sense organs, because without 'contact' (Sparsha) no sense organ can perceive. Perception itself, however, also requires the understanding of the mental faculties. Traditional healers discovered that by touching and holding Mani, patients experiencing a disturbance of the mind/body could be returned to normal. These spiritual healers also found that the effect of the Mani did not operate according the laws of Tridosha, and therefore they classified their actions to the Divine, because no one understood why and how they worked. There are many stories and legends in the literature of Ayurveda about the miraculous effects of Mani. To this day there are some spiritual healers who claim to have powerful Mani passed down to them from generation to generation.

Chapter 7: The Principles of Surgery

The principles of surgery in Ayurveda are generally based upon the theory of balance, but the application of this theory is different from internal medicine. Surgical treatment is separated into two basic stages. The first stage, or preparatory stage of treatment, is concerned with subduing existing inflammation. The second stage of treatment includes the actual operation as well as post-surgical methods to promote healing. To subdue inflammation prior to surgery, Ayurveda describes eleven different practices, each of which are used depending on the circumstance. The surgical operations and post-surgical healing practices constitute forty-nine different techniques that are similarly chosen and applied as required in different situations. In total, surgical treatments in Ayurveda are comprised of 60 basic techniques, described below.

General Principles of Wound Healing

Wound healing in surgery is a complex subject. Prior to, during, and after surgery the wound has to be cleaned. The choice of which medications are to be used depends upon the expression of Vata, Pitta, and Kapha.

There are many external medicines that can be used to speed wound healing. For complex (Sannipata) wound and sores, a reliable medicine for direct application is a paste made from **Tila oil** (sesame seed / *Sesamum indicum*), **Haridra root** (turmeric / *Curcuma longa*), **Trivrit root** (Indian rhubarb /*Operculina turpethum*), **Ghrita** (Ghee / clarified milk), **Nimba leaf** (neem / *Azadirachta indica)* and **Madhu** (honey). Another formula used to heal complicated sores and wounds is **Kaishora Guggulu**.

Other wound-healing remedies include:

1. **Arjuna bark** *(Terminalia arjuna).*
2. **Daruharidra bark/extract** (barberry / *Berberis aristata* / *B. nepalensis).*
3. **Kovidara bark/flower** *(Bauhinia variegata).*
4. **Nimba leaf** (neem / *Azadirachta indica).*
5. **Tila oil** (sesame seed / *Sesamum indicum).*

In addition to the use of these applications prior to surgery, all surgical procedures have to be followed by proper post-surgical treatment based upon the condition and needs of the patient. While treating patients who have undergone surgery due to trauma, the use of treatments to reduce Vata such as medicated incense is important to keep the nervous system balanced, in addition to techniques such as stitching, bandaging, and the use of wound-healing medications.

Surgical Preparatory Practices

The following is a list of preparatory practices used in surgery to promote wound healing:

1. The application of fasting to subdue the inflammation at the beginning stage.
2. The application of anti-inflammatory plasters.
3. The application of anti-inflammatory liquid medicines.
4. The application of medicated oils for massage.
5. The application of steam or fomentation to cleanse the duct systems.
6. The application of pressure by any means including massage to soften hard swellings.
7. The application of poultices made of anti-inflammatory herbs.
8. The practice of venesection to relieve pain and inflammation (page 92).
9. The intake of greasy foods for Vata related problems.
10. The intake of emetic medications for Kapha related problems (page 175).
11. The intake of laxative medications for Pitta related problems (page 174).

Surgical Practices

The following is a list of surgical practices to promote wound healing:

1. The application of poultices which concentrate pus for easier operation.
2. Operations that include simple opening, draining and/or cutting of the affected area.
3. Complex operations using more advanced surgical technology and instruments.
4. The application of alkaline medications to break open boils.
5. The use of specialized instruments or medicines to scrape out abnormal growths.
6. The application of instruments or use of finger to open and thoroughly drain the sinus.
7. The application of instruments or use of the finger to remove foreign attached objects inside the body.
8. The application of instruments to puncture the vein (venesection).
9. The stitching of wounds.
10. The application of wound-healing herbs.
11. The application of herbs or medications that astringe and squeeze out pus.
12. The application of herbal medications that stop bleeding.
13. The application of cooling medications to prevent infection.
14. The application of poultices to grow muscle and speed wound-healing.

15. The application of herbal decoctions to sterilize and cleanse the wound.
16. The application of tablets that slowly dissolve and cleanse the wound.
17. The application of herbal powders mixed with water to cleanse the wound.
18. The application of medical Ghee preparations to cleanse the wound.
19. The application of prepared minerals (Bhasmas) to cleanse the wound.
20. The application of dry plant powders sprinkled over wounds to heal.
21. The application of medical plasters to increase muscular growth.
22. The application of herbal powders to decrease abnormal muscular growth.
23. The application of Vata based treatments to soften wounds for quicker healing.
24. The application of astringent herbal powders to harden wounds.
25. The application of alkaline herbal medications to cleanse chronic wounds.
26. The application heated instrument to cauterize wounds to stop bleeding and discharge.
27. The application of plasters made of fruit seed oil to remove white scars.
28. The application of herbal medications to remove black scars.
29. The application medications to remove scars with abnormal growth (cancerous or pre-cancerous).
30. The application of herbal medications to stimulate the hair follicles.
31. The application of medications to remove hair.
32. The use of enemas to subdue Vata aggravations.
33. The application of enemas applied through the uterus or the bladder.
34. The application of bandages to throat wounds for quick healing.
35. The application of green plant leaves to wrap wounds for healing.
36. The application of anthelmintic medications to counteract maggots carried by flies.
37. The application of medications that increase weight.
38. The application of anti-toxin medications.
39. The application of medicated 'nasal snuffs' (Nasya) to induce nasal discharge to cleanse head wounds.
40. The application of medicated nasal snuffs to induce sneezing to cleanse head wounds.
41. The application of herbal mouthwashes to clean and heal mouth wounds.
42. Smoking herbal medications for healing head wounds with the character of Vata or Kapha.
43. The application of honey and Ghee for healing traumatic wounds.
44. The knowledge of the proper use of different surgical instruments.
45. The application of a proper diet.
46. The application of spiritual healing practices to protect against the Bhuta and Graha.

Venesection

Venesection (Rakta Mokshana) is a surgical operation that involved the puncturing of veins near the site of the disease to carefully remove pathogenic blood containing the Dosha. During venesection, maintaining moderate atmospheric temperature is very important and cold, wind, and heat must be avoided. Before the operation, the patient is fed a diet of rice gruel. Circulation to the area around the vein to be punctured should be stimulated with a steaming poultice application. If this is done, after the vein punctured, the bleeding should stop automatically. This is the proper way to perform venesection. Immediately after the properly performed procedure, the patient will feel much better, and is relieved of the severe pain caused by the disease.

SECTION TWO

Pharmacology and Materia Medica

Chapter 8: Pharmacology in Ayurveda

In this section we will review some of the most commonly used medicinal remedies in Ayurveda. To understand the descriptions for each, it is important to first review how these medications are classified and organized.

The analysis of medicines and their activities is the subject of pharmacology in Ayurveda, called Dravyaguna Vignana. Remedies are analyzed on the basis of their stable tastes, potency, physical properties, unstable tastes, and unique powers. In Ayurveda, these qualities are the active components of the medicine. There is no separation between the action of a medicine and its elemental components. If a medicine has a warming action then is comprised of a greater proportion of the Fire element. Likewise, if a medication is greasy in property, then it contains an abundance of the Water Element. Understanding the correlation between the physical properties of a medication and its elemental constitution allows the physician to understand the therapeutic value of the medicine.

Analysis of Stable Tastes (Rasa Pariksha)

The actions of a medicine can be analyzed based upon taste. Rasa or 'taste' is divided into two categories: stable and unstable. A medicine is said to have a stable taste if that taste and its related properties persist after digestion. This statement is of course a generalization, and actions can vary in the case of specific medicinal agents.

In most cases, sweet-tasting medicines exert the physical properties of greasiness and heaviness, and so directly nourish the Dhatus ('tissues') of the body. Such medications also strengthen physical energy, increase weight and lifespan, counteract toxins, and help to heal injuries. Sweet-tasting medications are indicated in diseases of 'bile' (Pitta) and 'wind' (Vata), but are contraindicated in diseases of 'mucus' (Kapha).

Sour-tasting medicines tend to be greasy and heating, and because of this stimulates digestive function, increases peristaltic movement, regulates the heart, and moisten and stoutens the body. Sour medicines are useful for diseases of 'wind' (Vata), but are contraindicated in diseases of 'mucus' (Kapha) and 'bile' (Pitta).

Salty-tasting medicines increase both fluid and heat, and so stimulate appetite, promote digestion, moisten the body, open blockages, stimulate glandular secretion, and promote the circulation of blood. Salty medicines are useful for diseases of 'wind' (Vata), but are contraindicated in diseases of 'mucus' (Kapha) and 'bile' (Pitta).

Pungent-tasting medicines are hot in nature and so stimulate the senses, promote appetite, and purify the blood (by "burning away" toxins). Pungent medicines are useful for diseases of 'mucus' (Kapha), but are contraindicated in diseases of 'wind' (Vata) and 'bile' (Pitta).

Bitter-tasting medicines tend to be dry and light in property, and so promote appetite and digestion, counteract toxins, kill parasites, purify breast milk, strengthen the skin and muscles, and cause a decrease in weight, mucus secretion and perspiration. Bitter medicines are useful for diseases of 'mucus' (Kapha) and 'bile' (Pitta), but are contraindicated in diseases of 'wind' (Vata).

Astringent-tasting medicines tend to be dry, heavy and hard digest, constricting the capillaries and suppressing the excretion of feces and urine. Astringent remedies also help promote the healing of injuries, by reducing heat and inflammation, and drawing the edges of a wound together. Astringent medicines are useful for diseases of 'mucus' (Kapha) and 'bile' (Pitta), but are contraindicated in diseases of 'wind' (Vata).

There is an additional taste referred to as alkaline, that is not one of the six classical tastes described by Ayurveda. Many of the purified mineral medicines (Bhasmas) are described as being alkaline in taste. According to the alchemical tradition of Rasa Shastra, the alkaline taste is actually a combination of several tastes, and in particular pungent (Katu) and salty (Lavana), which acts to neutralize the effect of acid and Pitta.

Analysis of Potency (Virya Pariksha)

The potency or efficacy of a medicine depends upon its dilatory (heating) and constricting (cooling) effects. Medicines are classified according to those that dilate and generate heat, and those that constrict and cause a cooling sensation. Medications that are warming counteract the pathogenic properties of mucus (Kapha Dosha) and wind (Vata Dosha), whereas medications that are cooling counteract the pathogenic properties of bile (Pitta Dosha). In general, sour, salty, and pungent tasting medications generate heat, whereas sweet, bitter, and astringent medications exert a cooling effect.

Analysis of Physical Properties

Ayurveda defines twenty physical properties, called the Gurvadi Guna:

1. Heavy (Guru) and Light (Laghu).
2. Dull (Manda) and Sharp (Tikshna).
3. Cold (Shita) and Hot (Ushna).
4. Greasy (Snigdha) and Dry (Ruksha).
5. Smooth (Slakshana) and Rough (Khara).
6. Solid (Sandra) and Liquid (Drava).
7. Soft (Mridu) and Hard (Kathina).
8. Stable (Sthira) and Unstable/Mobile (Sara).
9. Microfine (Sukshma) and Dense/Bulky (Sthula).
10. Non-Sticky (Vishada) and Sticky (Picchila).

In diet and medicine, these physical properties manifest as specific tastes. A dietary article or medicine that follows convention exhibits properties that are aligned with its taste. For example, a food or medicine that is sweet in taste is usually heavy in property, meaning that it is both heavy to digest, and makes the body heavier if ingested over time.

If the physical properties of a medicine are different than predicted by the taste, however, that medicine becomes more powerful in counteracting the physical properties of pathogenic wind, bile, or mucus. For example, if a sweet medicine also has a warming in property, it has a more powerful effect to control neurological (Vata) problems.

Analysis of Unstable Tastes (Vipaka Pariksha)

Ayurveda states that the tastes of certain foods or medications can change after digestion, and this modifies its action upon the body, and the bowel in particular. Such changes make the medicine more powerful than the effect predicted by its taste alone. Medicines that become sweet after digestion help moisten the bowel (increase mucus) and increase vitality. Medicines that become sour after digestion help stimulate the evacuation of stool and urine, and increase bile secretion. Medicines that become pungent after digestion dry the stool (causing constipation) and increase gas.

Analysis of Unique Power (Prabhava Pariksha)

The unique and powerful components of a medicine can create extraordinary effects that are specific to it, called Prabhava. Such effects do not follow the rules of the stable tastes (Rasa), physical properties (Guna), unstable tastes (Vipaka), or potency (Virya). These unique powers are often correlated with a specific action, such as laxatives, emetics, intoxicants, and Rasayanas (longevity promotion), or are related to specific benefits in a particular tissue or organ. Knowledge of Prabhava adds a greater degree of sophistication to Dravyaguna, and is the result of the direct experience of many different physicians over a long period of time.

Chapter 9: Materia Medica of Ayurveda

This chapter is a review of the most commonly used medicines in Ayurveda, including individual herbal extracts, minerals, and certain formulas. Altogether, this review represents less than 25% of the entire materia medica of Ayurveda.

Herbal and Food extracts

Agaru or Aguru wood (eaglewood / krishnagaru / *Aquilaria agallocha*)
Agaru is a tropical and sub-tropical, fragrant evergreen tree. The wood is very heavy, and sinks in water. The wood is bitter in taste, hot in action, and used in asthma. It has a second variety, black in color, called krishnagaru. It reduces Vata and Kapha. It is also an alterative used for rejuvenation (Rasayana), and is a specific for Vata spasmodic asthma. It is also used in brain defects, and for eye, ear and skin diseases. For any disease resulting from cold it is used in the form of incense to create heat in the body, especially in the chest and head areas.

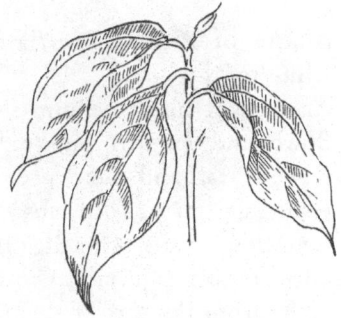

अगरू

Agaru (*Aquilaria agallocha*)

Agnimantha bark/root/leaf (*Premna integrifolia*)
Agnimantha is a tropical and sub-tropical thorny tree with aromatic leaf, found in the mountains. There are two varieties used, large and small. The bark and root are bitter and pungent in taste, and used for edema, urinary diseases, neurasthenia, and to reduce Vata. The alkali extracted from the ash of the bark is used in ascites. It is a strong digestive medicine.

Aila or Ela fruit/seed (greater cardamom / *Amomum subulatum*)
Aila is an annual tuberous plant cultivated in temperate and sub-tropical valleys. The seed (fruit) is pungent in taste, light and dry in property aromatic, and has a cooling sensation. It reduces Kapha and Pitta defects. It is carminative, appetizing, sedative and an aid in digestion. It is used as a mild anti-poison in body for aches, coughs, and vomiting. It is also good for mouth diseases and nausea. Aila is a good spice for bean and meat preparations, and can be used after meals for its pleasant aroma.

Ajamoda seed (wild celery / *Carum roxburghianum*)
Ajamoda is a biennial herb that grows everywhere. The seed is pungent in taste. It aids in rheumatism and gout by reducing pain (Vata) and swelling (Kapha). It is a strong digestive aid, used as part of the classic **Hingwastaka Churna** digestive formula. The whole seeds can be chewed to stimulate Agni, the digestive fire. Because of its strength, the dose is very small when used alone or in combinations. Ajamoda has a stimulating action on the respiratory system and acts as a decongestant and expectorant. Ajamoda is used for colds, flu, laryngitis, bronchitis, asthma, cough, colic, indigestion, edema, and arthritis. Also used for bladder pain and abdominal colic.

Alarka or Arka flower/latex/leaf/stem (milkweed / arka / *Calotropis gigantia*, white/red)
Alarka is a stout medium size shrub that comes in two varieties, one with white flower and one with pink-red flower. Both flowers have an alkaline taste. The white flower, leaf and stem are used for leprosy, itching, detoxification of poisons (especially rat poison), abscess, worms, tumors and liver and spleen diseases. The pink flower is used for digestion, nausea, asthma, and hemorrhoid. The latex that is salty and bitter in taste, is used for constipation, tumor, and hemorrhoid. The salt made from the leaf of this plant is used for constipation and for liver and spleen diseases.

Amalaki or Amalakam fruit (Indian gooseberry / amla / *Phyllanthus emblica*)
Amalaki is a tropical and sub-tropical middle sized tree that grows in dry areas. The fruit is sour, sweet and astringent in taste, and cooling in action. It is a heart restorative, and a Rasayana when used over a long period of time. It is used in bronchitis, cough, fever, alcoholism, and hemorrhage. It reduces Vata, Pitta, and Kapha. It is also used for anemia, asthma, burning sensation, lung disease, and cancer. It is part of Triphala, where it is mildly laxative. It is tridoshaghna, an agent that stimulates the brain to subdue the increased body systems.

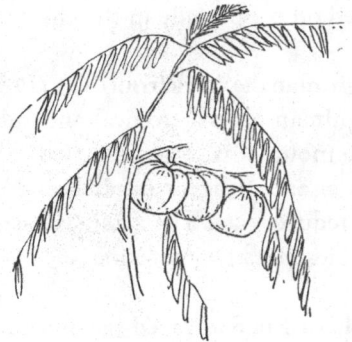

आमलकी

Amalaki (Phyllanthus emblica

Amlavetasa rhizome/fruit (rhubarb / *Rheum emodi*)
Amlavetasa is an annual alpine plant. Its rhizome and stem are sour in taste and warming in action. It is strong, light to digest and dry in property. It reduces Vata and Kapha. It is a laxative. It is used for cirrhosis of liver, alcoholism, neurasthenia, gas, asthma and for cleaning the ducts. The fruit is sour in taste and used as a heart

restorative, for urinary diseases and tympanitis, and strong enough to help in the digestion of the fat of sheep, wild boar or pigs. Because of its strong sour taste, it is used only in small amount, and overdose can cause blood defects and Pitta and Kapha defects.

Apamarga herb/root/seed/ash *(Achyranthes aspera)*
Apamarga is a temperate annual small herb that grows in shady areas. The whole plant, root, seed and ash are used. It comes in two varieties, green and red. Apamarga is bitter and pungent in taste, light to digest, strong and dry in property, warming in action (green), and reduces Kapha and Vata. It can be used as a medicated nasal snuff to reduce mucus and relieve headache. The alkaline ash is used in eardrops (ash and water boiled with sesame oil) for otitis media as well as nosebleeds. Apamarga is emetic in large doses. Based on the principles of Tridosha, green Apamarga is good for Kapha and Vata disease, while red Apamarga can exert an opposite effect because it has a cooling action. Both varieties are good for defects of fatty tissue, skin diseases, and stomach diseases. The seed of red Apamarga is good for hemorrhage (Raktapitta).

Adrakam root (ginger / Shunthi / *Zingiber officinalis)*
Ginger root is an erect cultivated perennial spicy plant with thick tubers. It is very pungent (hot) in taste, carminative and an aid to digestion. It is cooling in action. It is light to digest and strong in property. It reduces Kapha and Vata. It is used for urticaria, common cold, allergies, asthma, cough and rheumatism. It is also a heart restorative. Its post-digestive action is sweet (Madhura), increasing its nourishing qualities and creating a mild aphrodisiac effect as well as aiding in peristaltic movement. It is a good spice for everyone (all body types), though excessive use is not good in micturia, Pitta diseases, ulcer, fever, or during the summer or autumn seasons. Dried ginger is called Shunthi.

Arjuna bark *(Terminalia arjuna)*
Arjuna is a large perennial tree that grows in the mountains of temperate climate. The bark is astringent in taste, and cooling. It reduces Kapha and Pitta defects. It is a strong heart restorative, an anti-poison, and has medicinal value for healing wounds. It is also used for lymph swelling.

Ashwagandha root *(Convolvulus arvensis / Withania somnifera)*
There are two different plants which are called by the Sanskrit name Ashwagandha. Both are effective. *Convolvulus arvensis* is a perennial bushy plant with white roots that grows in tropical areas. *Withania somnifera* is a small to middle-sized shrub that flowers throughout the year. The root of both plants is bitter in taste, and a powerful Rasayana. It is aphrodisiac and reduces Vata and Kapha. It is used for any Vata (nervous system) disease, and to increase weight. It increases mother's milk

production. It is used for nervous exhaustion, poor memory, weakness of muscles and impotence. Used as a nerve restorative when combined with Gokshura fruit.

Ashoka bark/leaf/flower (Ashoka tree / *Saraca indica*)
Ashoka is an evergreen tree that grows tropical and sub-tropical areas. The bark is astringent and bitter in taste, and constrictitory in action. It reduces Pitta. It is used for menorrhagia and bleeding, especially uterine bleeding.

Atibala plant *(Sida rhombifolia)*
Atibala is an annual bushy plant with yellow flowers. All parts are sweet in taste. It is part of the **Bala group**. It reduces Vata and is used for nervous system diseases.

Ativisha tuber, purified (aconite / *Aconitum heterophyllum*)
Ativisha is an alpine tuberous herb. It is very toxic and must be purified before use by steaming in cow or goat's milk for three hours. Purified Ativisha tuber is bitter and pungent in taste, light and dry in property, and heating in property. It is used as an anti-poison for fever, diarrhea, toxemia, and dysentery. Single dosage in an adult should not exceed 10 mg.

Bala plant (country mallow / *Sida cordifolia*)
Bala is an annual small plant with yellow flowers that grows in dry areas. It is part of the **Bala group**. All parts of the plant are sweet in taste, hot in action (Virya), Balyam (restores tone and increases energy) and Rasayana to promote long life and good health. It reduces Vata. Bala has a generalized activating effect on the nervous system by increasing both blood circulation and nourishment. It has medicinal value in treating neuropathy related with any organ. It is also used for tuberculosis for healing the lung, as well as chronic bronchitis and hemoptisis. It can be mixed into oil and used as a massage useful for muscle stiffness caused by Vata.

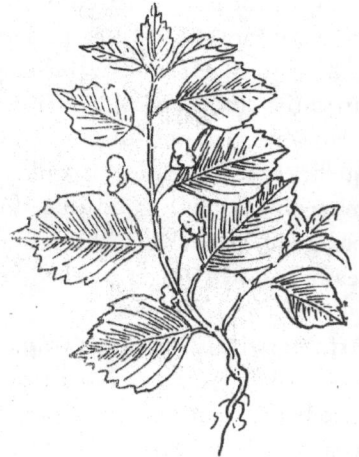

Bala *(Sida cordifolia)*

Bhringaraj *(Eclipta alba)*
Bhringaraj is a small annual cultivated vegetable that also grows wild in moist areas and during the rainy season. It has two varieties, one with white flowers, and one with yellow flowers. All parts of the plant are pungent and bitter in taste, light to digest and dry in property, and hot in action. It reduces Vata and Kapha Dosha and is a Rasayana. Used as a medicated nasal snuff it can be applied in the treatment of sinusitis, migraine, and diseases of the head, eye, nose, throat and ear. For these purposes it is usually added to sesame oil and dropped in the nose. The leaf juice is a

rejuvenative and deobstructant of the liver used in liver and spleen enlargements, fevers, dropsy, anemia and skin diseases. To make the hair black and luxuriant, boil the leaf juice with sesame or coconut oil and apply externally. A paste of the plant mixed with sesame oil is used over glandular swellings, elephantitis, and skin diseases.

Bhutakeshi herb *(Valeriana wallichii)*
Bhutakeshi is an alpine and sub-alpine small strong smelling herb that grows in shady areas. All parts of the plant are bitter in taste. It is an anti-poison used in throat defects (such as swelling in the throat and mouth) and malaria. It is used as an anti-poison in swelling caused by toxins or gout and in malaria. It is also used as a calmative in formulas for high blood pressure, epilepsy and insomnia. It is used as an antispasmodic incense in asthma, hiccough, and cough and to calm the mind and brain. In high doses it is emetic.

Bibhitaki fruit *(Terminalia belerica)*
Bibhitaki is a large tree that grows in sub-tropical mountainous climes. The fruit is sour and astringent in taste, and mildly laxative. It reduces Kapha and Pitta, and is used in cough and fever. It is a Rasayana and part of **Triphala**, the three fruits compound.

Vijaya flower (marijuana / bhang / *Cannabis sativa*)
Vijaya is an annual plant with a tough fibrous inner bark. All parts of the plant are bitter and pungent in taste, and hot in action. Used as a pain killer, antispasmodic and aphrodisiac. It helps in diarrhea and summer colds. It is vyavayi, an intoxicating agent that first starts to affect the body, and then later strengthens digestion.

Bilwa fruit/root/leaf/root bark (bael / vilwa / *Aegle marmelos*)
Bilwa is a tropical and sub-tropical middle sized thorny tree that fruits in all seasons. Bilwa is warming in effect, carminative and it reduces Vata Dosha. The raw unripe fruit is sweet and astringent in taste, and is used especially in diarrhea, dysentery, chronic sprue, and amoebic dysentery. The root and leaf are bitter and astringent in taste. The root bark is bitter in taste and is used in nerve disorders to reduce pain. It is a very good digestive restorative.

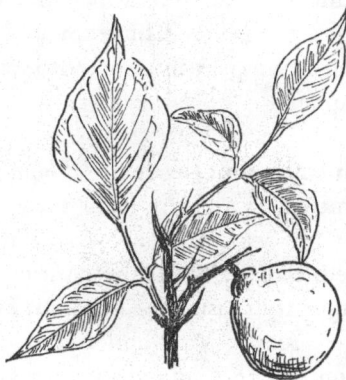

बिल्व
Bilwa (Aegle marmelos)

Brahmi leaf/root (gotu kola / *Hydrocotyle asiatica* / *Centella asiatica*)
Brahmi is an annual (perennial) small spreading plant that grows near rivers and ponds. All parts of the plant are bitter in taste and cooling in action (Virya). It is used in epilepsy, to improve memory and concentration and to prevent miscarriage. It is also an anti-poison and good for throat hoarseness.

Brihati shrub (vrihati / *Solanum indicum*)
Brihati is an annual thorny plant that grows in the plains areas. All parts of the plant are sweet in taste. Used in fever, typhoid fever, throat defects, coughs and edema. It is an anti-poison.

Chakramarda seed/leaf (taper / *Cassia tora*)
Chakramarda is a perennial bush that grows in temperate climates. The seed is pungent in taste, warming in action, light to digest and dry in property. It is germicidal, and is used for ringworm and skin diseases. The leaf is sour in taste, hot in action, and used as an external plaster for ringworm. For skin eruptions or itching, grind the leaf or seed with sour buttermilk or lime juice.

Chandana wood (white sandalwood / *Santalum album*)
White sandalwood is a tropical tree with aromatic wood. The wood is bitter in taste, and cold in action. Used as a refrigerant to reduce Pitta, effective for fever, dizziness, heat sensations, menopausal hot flashes. It also works as an anti-poison (Vishaghna) in the case of various types of poisoning.

Chavyam fruit/stem *(Piper chaba)*
Chavyam is a sub-tropical creeper that grows in the shade in forests. The stem is pungent in taste, and appetizing. Used in asthma, coughs, abdominal colic and to reduce Kapha. It is dipanam, an agent that increases appetite, but does not aid digestion. Note: **Chavyam** is the whole plant, and **Gajapippali** is the fruit. The fruit is pungent in taste, hot in action, appetizing and digestive. It reduces Vata and Kapha.

Chitraka root (leadwort/ *Plumbago zeylanica*)
Chitraka is a bushy plant that grows in temperate and sub-tropical climates. There are two varieties, one with white flower and another with blue flower. Both are used, but the blue flower variety is considered more potent. The root and stem are pungent in taste, hot in action (Virya), digestive and appetizing (dipana-pachanam). They reduce Vata and Kapha. It is used for worms, abdominal colic, abdominal tumor, edema, anemia, hemorrhoids without bleeding, and obesity.

Dadima rind/fruit (pomegranate / *Punica granatum)*
Dadima is a small cultivated tree. Pomegranates come in two varieties: sweet-astringent, and sour-astringent. The rind is astringent in taste, and cool in action (Virya). It is used as a rejuvenative for anemia. It increases mother's milk production. The fruit is easy to digest, carminative, nourishing to the heart and is helpful to digestion. The sweet-astringent variety has medicinal value in treating diarrhea, alcoholism, indigestion and heart problems. The sour-astringent variety is more effective in treating indigestion and alcoholism.

Danti seed/root *(Baliospermum montanum)*
Danti is a small-sized evergreen tree that grows in the tropical climate. Danti is pungent in taste and a strong purgative. It is used in hemorrhage, and is good for any stomach disease.

Daruharidra bark/extract (barberry / *Berberis aristata* / *B. nepalensis)*
Daruharidra is a perennial spiny shrub *(B. aristata)* or small tree *(B. nepalensis)* with thorny leaves and yellow wood. It grows in the sub-alpine to temperate mountainous climates. The root bark, often made into a condensed extract called **Rasanjana**, is bitter and astringent in taste, light to digest and dry in property, and hot in action. Its post-digestive action is pungent (Katu), causing a drying effect in the colon. It reduces Kapha and Pitta. The condensed paste is boiled in water and used as eyewash for conjunctivitis, as a gargle for mouth sores or infections, and as drops for infections of the nose and ears. Also used as a vaginal wash for leucorrhea. Externally the paste can be used for skin fungus, sores and to speed wound healing. Taken internally it is used in urinary diseases with pus and for infections.

Devadaru bark (Himalayan cedar / *Cedrus deodara)*
Devadaru is an alpine and sub-alpine evergreen with aromatic bark. Devadaru bark is bitter in taste, aromatic, and warming in action. It is used for fever and constipation, and to reduce Vata and Kapha. It is also used for bloated stomach, sinusitis, and urinary diseases.

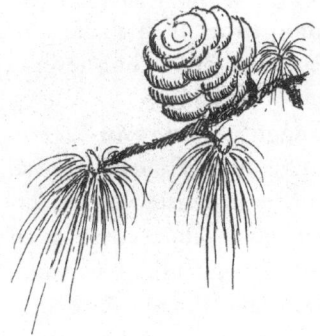

Devadaru
(Cedrus deodara)

Dhanyakam seed (coriander / *Coriandrum sativum)*
Dhanyakam seed is pungent in taste, carminative, digestive and refrigerant. It is pachanam, a digestive agent that increases digestive power, but does not increase appetite. It is good for thirstiness, burning sensation, nausea and worms. The green vegetable form is especially good for Pitta disorders.

Duralambha bush *(Fragonia cretica)*
Duralambha is an alpine and sub-alpine thorny bush. All parts of Duralambha are bitter, sweet and astringent in taste, and cooling in action. Used in fever, hay fever, bronchitis, intoxication and dizziness. It reduces Pittaja blood defects. It has another variety that grows in the desert, called **Yasa** *(Alhagi maurorum)*.

Ghrita (Ghee / clarified butter)
Ghrita is made by heating butter and discarding the curds that fall to the bottom. It is considered to be the best of all oily foods, and is used to cure disturbances in Pitta and Vata. It enhances quantity and quality of Ojas (vital fluid) and strengthens digestion (Agni) while reducing Pitta. Ghee also promotes memory and intelligence by nourishing the brain as well as the subtle tissues of the body. It is used as a preferred carrier (Anupanum) for herbs used to reduce Pitta.

Gokshura fruit *(Tribulus terrestris)*
Gokshura is an annual spreading small herb with thorny seeds. The fruit is sweet in taste and hot in action (Virya). It reduces Vata (nervousness) and is a Rasayana good for energy and long life. It is especially good for urinary diseases (Mutraroga), and is used for edema, cystitis, cough, kidney and bladder stones and fever. It becomes a nerve rejuvenative when combined with **Ashwagandha root**.

Guduchi stem *(Tinospora cordifolia)*
Guduchi is a long creeper that grows in temperate and sub-tropical forests. The stem is bitter in taste and warming in action. It is a Rasayana, for good health and longevity, as well as being an anti-toxin. It reduces Vata and Pitta. It is used for fever due to cold, including malaria fever, as well as to remove toxins in hepatitis, gout, toxemia, and urinary diseases. It is diuretic and aphrodisiac, useful in impotence. It has the Prabhava ('special power') called samanam, meaning it restores balance, but never causes increase.

Guggulu gum resin *(Commiphora wightii)*
Guggulu is a small tropical, thorny tree with aromatic gum. The gum is bitter-pungent in taste, hot in action and alterative. It is also a Rasayana for long life and health. It reduces Kapha and Vata. It is used for abnormal growth, tumors, cysts, arthritis, glandular swelling, cancer, and inflammation. It is frequently used with **Triphala** (three fruits compound) and/or **Guduchi stem**.

Haridra root (turmeric / *Curcuma longa*)
Haridra root is a common cultivated spice. It is bitter, pungent and hot in taste, warm in action (dilates capillaries), and light to digest and dry in property. It reduces Kapha and Pitta. As a spice it is beneficial for all food preparations, used specifically to prevent food poisoning. Used for skin and urinary diseases, for liver diseases (including hepatitis), and for inflammation with swelling (including sinus).

Used externally for skin diseases and as a plaster for swelling. It has an especially beneficial effect upon Kapha energy.

Haritaki fruit (chebulic myrobalan / *Terminalia chebula*)
Haritaki is a sub-tropical middle-sized mountain tree. The fruit is sweet, sour, astringent, pungent, and bitter in taste, and hot in action. It contains all tastes except for salty. It is a Rasayana, good for long life. It reduces Vata and Pitta, and is part of **Triphala** (three fruits combination). It is a 'mild laxative that aids digestion' (anulomanum), and due to its rejuvenative properties is a good laxative for weak or elderly patients. It is used both internally and externally to nourish heart, liver, kidney and eye. It is especially and extensively used in urinary diseases.

Hastikarnapalasa seeds/root (bastard teak / *Butea monosperma*)
Hastikarnapalasha is a sub-tropical annual bush with large leaves and a thick root. The seed is bitter in taste and used as an anthelmintic, especially effective in roundworm. The root is used in goiter.

Hingu gum (asafoetida / *Ferula narthex*)
Hingu is a tropical, thorny bush with a strong aromatic gum. The gum resin is bitter in taste, carminative and an appetite stimulant. It is an agent that helps neutralize gas-forming properties of beans (Vataghna), and is used in flatus and colic pain.

Hriverum plant (*Pavonia odorata*)
Hriverum is a temperate annual plant with aromatic leaves that grows on the shady side of hills. All parts of the plant are bitter in taste, and used in fever, hemorrhage, alcoholism, bacillary dysentery, enteritis, and piles. It reduces Pitta.

Jatamansi rhizome (spikenard / *Valeriana jatamansi* / *Nardostachys jatamansi*)
Jatamansi is an alpine annual plant with an aromatic rhizome. It is bitter, astringent and sweet in taste, strong and greasy in property, and cooling in action. It reduces Vata, Pitta, and Kapha Dosha (defects). Its post-digestive action is pungent (Katu), causing a drying effect in the colon. It is used as an anti-poison in swelling caused by toxins or gout and in malaria. It is also used as a calmative in formulas for high blood pressure, epilepsy and insomnia. It can be used for swelling in the throat and mouth. It is used as antispasmodic incense in asthma, hiccough, and cough and to calm the mind and brain. Overdose is emetic.

Jirakam seed (cumin / *Cuminum cyminum*)
Jirakam is a tropical spicy plant cultivated in plains areas. There are three varieties, small, large and black, all of which are used. Jirakam seed is pungent in taste, aromatic, dilatory (warming) in action, carminative and digestive, and used to purify the uterus. It is good in all food preparations, and helps to balance Vata

energy. It is Grahi, a digestive and appetizing agent that causes heat and tightens the stool.

Jatiphalam seed (nutmeg / *Myristica fragrans*)
Jatiphalam is a tropical tree with aromatic nuts that grows in the south of India. It is bitter in taste, light to digest and greasy in property, and warm in action. It is carminative and stimulates digestion. It is used in diarrhea, nerve diseases, neuropathy, and throat defects. Externally used for skin disease. It can be used for bad breath and also plastered on sore gums.

Jivaka bulb (wild garlic / *Allium wallichii*, small)
Jivaka is an alpine bulbous herb that grows in the mountains. There are two varieties, small and large. The bulb is sweet in taste, rejuvenative, aphrodisiac, and is used in hemorrhage and to reduce Vata and Pitta.It is also used for rejuvenating effects and longevity. It is a frequently used herb in many internal and external applications. In Ghee form, the bulb is used for traumatic eye injuries.

Kanchanara bark (mountain ebony / *Bauhinia tomentosa*)
Kanchanara is a sub-tropical, medium-sized tree. Its bark is astringent in taste and cold in action. It is sansodhanum, a body and blood purifying agent that excretes defective bile, mucus and gas. It is used in diarrhea, leprosy, glandular swelling and ulcers.

Kankola (long pepper, large / *Piper cubeba*)
Kankola is a sub-tropical and tropical creeper that grows in the forest, and is also cultivated. The aromatic fruit is bitter and pungent in taste, and heat producing in nature. It is good for Vata and Kapha diseases. It is used for heart diseases, mouth odor (halitosis) and is especially good used internally for eye diseases that cause blindness.

Kantakari herb (black nightshade / *Solanum xanthocarpum*)
Kantakari is an annual thorny plant. It has three varieties, with yellow, white, and red flowers. All are good medicine. All parts of the plant are bitter and astringent in taste and neutral in action. It is a diuretic, and is used in bronchitis, fever, colds, edema, chronic fever, anemia and hiccough. It is especially used for body pain. It reduces Vata and Kapha. The fruit and root are used in anemia.

Kapikacchu seeds (cowhage / *Mucuna pruriens*)
Kapikacchu is a tropical and sub-tropical climber with poisonous hairs on the pods. The seed is sweet and slightly bitter in taste, heavy to digest, rejuvenative and aphrodisiac (Vajikarana). It is used for impotence, for nerve disorders (Vata), and to help gain weight.

Karanja bark/seed oil (Indian beech / *Pongamia pinnata*)
Karanja is a tropical and sub-tropical tree that grows everywhere. Both bark and seed oil, taken internally, are good for nerve (Vata) disorders. The bark is pungent in taste, and is used in neurasthenia, abdominal tumor and worms. The seed oil is applied in skin diseases, in scabies, sores, herpes and eczema.

Karpura leaf/extract (camphor / *Cinnamomum camphora*)
Karpura is a perennial evergreen that grows to 100 feet. The crystallized extract of the leaf is bitter in taste, cold and refrigerant in action. It is used in mouth and throat diseases. It stimulates the bladder and skin in both internal and external uses.

Karchura tuber/seed (zedoary / *Curcuma zedoaria*)
Karchura grows on the shady sides of mountains in temperate climates. The tuber and seed are bitter-pungent in taste, light to digest and strong in property, and warming in action. They reduce Vata and Kapha. Both tuber and seed are carminative and digestive, and used in asthma and hiccough. The tuber is used for hemorrhoids, enteritis, swelling, typhoid fever, and coughs.

Karkatashringi fruit gall (*Pistacia intergerrima* insect gall)
Karkatashringi is an "insect house" secretion attached to the Pistachio nut tree. It is pungent in taste, and hot in action. It reduces Kapha (mucus). It is a major herb in Ayurveda used for lung problems, asthma, tuberculosis, bronchitis and pleurisy. Also used for allergy, hay fever and neuralgic eye pain.

Kashmari bark/root/fruit (kashmarya / *Gmelina arborea*) Kashmari is a tropical and subtropical large trees. When cut it produces a latex that becomes red as it dries. The bark is astringent, bitter, and sweet in taste, and is heat producing in nature. It is good for fever, digestion, blood poisons, and leucorrhea. It increases semen and can be used in any complex (Sannipata) case.

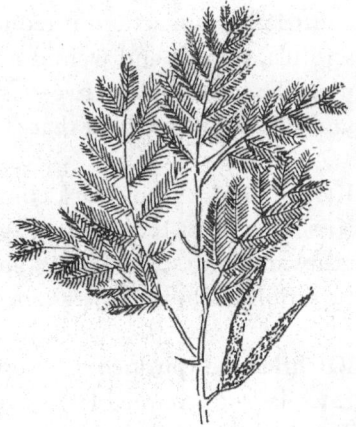

Kashmari (*Gmelina arborea*)

Katuki rhizome (Indian gentian / *Picrorhiza kurroa*)
Katuki is an alpine annual herb. The rhizome is bitter and pungent in taste, and hot in action, as well as being laxative. It reduces Pitta and Kapha. It is a purgative agent that cleans the bowel (Bhedanam). It is very beneficial for fever.

Khadira extract (catechu / *Acacia catechu*, white)
Khadira is a tropical and sub-tropical small tree that grows in sandy areas and near rivers. A condensed extract made from a decoction of the bark, wood, flowering tops and gum. It is bitter and astringent in taste, light to digest and dry in property, and cooling in action. It reduces Kapha, for which it is frequently used. It is used externally as a paste to counteract mucus and swelling for all skin diseases, psoriasis, fungal infections and herpes. It is used for urinary frequency and is especially useful for Kapha urinary diseases. Also used for stomatitis or sore and spongy gums. The flower is used in hemorrhage.

Kinkirata flower (shahachara / *Borlaria prionitis*)
Kinkirata is an annual small plant that grows everywhere. It is bitter and pungent in taste, and good for blood purification and cancerous diseases.

Kiratatiktam plant (*Swertia chirata*)
Kiratatiktam is an alpine and sub-alpine mountainous plant. All parts of the plant are bitter in taste, and cold in action. It is especially good for fevers, for which it is used frequently. It reduces Kapha and Pitta.

Kovidara bark/flower (*Bauhinia variegata*)
Kovidara is a tropical and sub-tropical tree. The bark is astringent in taste and constrictitory in action. It reduces Kapha. It is used for abnormal glandular swelling, scrofula, tumors and wound healing. It is always combined with **Guggulu gum** for use. The flower is sweet-astringent tasting, and used as an emetic. It is samsodhanam, an agent that cleans and excretes defective bile, mucus and gas.

Krishnajiraka seed (black cumin / *Nigella sativa*)
Krishnajirakam is an annual spicy cultivated tropical plant. The seed is pungent in taste, aromatic, carminative, and appetizing. Used in diarrhea and abdominal colic. Its action is similar to **Jirakam** (cumin).

Kuchila seed (purified nux vomica /*Strychnos nux vomica*)
Kuchila is a perennial large tree that grows in the tropical and sub-tropical climate. The seed is bitter in taste, hot in action, and poisonous. Purified seed is rejuvenative and used for indigestion, menorrhagia, back pain, rabies, twitching, lumbago and paralysis (oil form). Purify by first soaking in vinegar and cow urine for three days, then boil until red.

Kumari (Aloe leaf gum extract / *Aloe barbadensis*)
Kumari is a cultivated plant that grows everywhere. The leaf and gum extract is bitter in taste, and cooling (constrictitory) in action. It is sticky, mobile, and heavy to digest in property. It is laxative, and an anti-poison. Used for enlargement of liver and spleen, burns, and amenorrhea.

Kushtha root *(Saussurea lappa)*
Kushtha is a sub-alpine annual bush that grows especially in Kashmir. The root is bitter and pungent in taste, light to digest, dry and strong in property, and warming in action. It reduces Kapha and Vata. It is used for leprosy, gout and all skin diseases as an ointment made from powdered root. It can be used internally for fever, cough and poor appetite. It is also a stimulant, mild rejuvenative and anti-poison (Vishagna).

Kutaja bark/seed/leaf *(Holarrhena antidysenterica)*
Kutaja is a small sub-tropical tree with pods. The name Indrayava refers to the seed. The bark, seed and leaf are bitter in taste, and cold in action. They reduce Pitta and Kapha. Kutaja is an agent that stops motion and bleeding (Stambhanam). It is used to stop dysentery, fever and hemorrhoidal bleeding.

Lavangam seed (clove / *Syzigium aromaticum*)
Lavangam seed is pungent in taste, aromatic, carminative and digestive. The seed can be held in the mouth after meals to refresh and purify the mouth, and also for dental problems. It is good for acid producing diseases. It is beneficial in winter meat preparations.

Madhukam root (licorice / *Glycyrrhiza glabra*)
Madhukam is a perennial climber. The root is sweet in taste, heavy to digest and greasy in property, and cooling in action. It reduces Pitta and Vata. It is a Rasayana, an expectorant and an anti-poison. It promotes good eyesight, clear voice and clean complexion. It is used for sore throat, hypertension and ulcers. Continual use for 2-3 days can reduce pain. It is useful to sweeten herbal formulas.

Mahabala *(Sida cordifolia*, white)
Mahabala is an annual small plant with white flowers that grows in dry areas. Mahabala is sweet in taste, heavy and greasy in quality, and cold in action. It is part of the **bala group**. It reduces Vata and Pitta. It is especially used in urinary disorders.

Mahanimba leaf/flower/seed (Persian lilac / *Melia azadirachta*)
Mahanimba is a medium sized tree. The leaf is bitter in taste and cooling in action, and reduces Kapha and Pitta. It is used to cure malaria fever. The flower is used for pain and headache. The seed is mildly poisonous, and used for leprosy and worms. It is good for any skin disease.

Maricham seed (black pepper / *Piper nigrum*)
Maricham is a tropical climber that grows in the shade. The fruit is pungent in taste, hot in action, appetizing and digestive. It reduces Vata and Kapha. It is used for colic pain, worms, cough, and asthma. It helps to digest minerals. It is

Sukshmam, an agent that enters the micro-tissues. It is chedanam, an expectorant agent that promotes release of mucus attached to the ducts.

Methika seed (fenugreek / *Trigonella foenum-graecum*)
Methika seed is bitter in taste, warming in action, easy to digest and an appetite stimulant. It is useful in cases of fever, blood impurity and cancer. It is anthelmintic (kills worms), and is good for diabetes.

Murva plant/root *(Bauhinia vahlii)*
Murva is a tropical and sub-tropical forest climber. All parts of the plant are bitter and sweet in taste. Used in skin diseases and to reduce Pitta. The root is used in pulmonary tuberculosis.

Musali tuber *(Curculigo orchioides)*
Musali is a tropical and sub-tropical tuberous herb that grows on hills. The tuber is sweet in taste, cooling, restorative and aphrodisiac. It is useful for increasing weight, and is used for its nourishing effects in tuberculosis, atrophy, increased nervous system (Vata), weight loss, atrophy, impotence,

Musta tuber (nut grass / mustaka / *Cyperus rotundus*, large)
Musta is a tuberous grassy plant tuber grows in tropical climates. There are three varieties called musta (large tuber), kasheruka and nagara. The large tuber is bitter and astringent in taste, cooling in action, digestive and appetizing. It is light to digest and dry in property. It reduces Pitta and Kapha. It is used for diarrhea, sprue, dysentery, enteritis, edema, and fever.

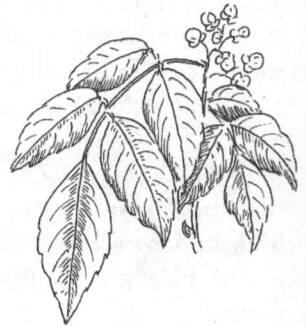

Nagabala *(Sida spinosa*, wild)
Nagabala is an annual plant with yellow flowers. It is sweet in taste and cooling in action. It is part of the **bala group**. Nagabala is used especially for blood defects and also has an aphrodisiac effect. Excessive use causes constipation, bloated stomach, and weight loss.

Nagabala *(Sida spinosa)*

Nagakeshara seed/flower (ironwood tree / *Mesua ferrea*)
Nagakeshara is a middle sized evergreen tree that grows in the sub-alpine climate, especially the eastern Himalayan range. The seed is pungent in taste. Used as an anti-poison in throat defects, hay fever and diseases of the head.

Nagaram rhizome (Indian cyperus / *Cyperus pertenuis*)
Nagaram is a tropical and sub-tropical annual tall grassy plant with tuberous rhizome that grows in swampy areas. There are three varieties called musta, kasheruka and nagara. The rhizome is bitter and pungent in taste, used as a

carminative and digestive in constipation, abdominal colic pain, fever, typhoid fever, liver and spleen defects, and to reduce Vata and Kapha.

Nimba leaf (neem / *Azadirachta indica*)
Nimba is a tropical and sub-tropical small sized tree that grows in plains areas. Neem leaf is bitter in taste, light in property, and cooling in action. The post-digestive action is pungent (Katu), causing a drying effect. It reduces Kapha and Pitta. It is used in all skin diseases, especially to reduce swelling and itching. It is also used for fever, malaria in particular, as well as for leprosy, toxemia, and allergies. It is used internally and externally for all forms of fungal infection. Externally it is used to heal wounds, boils and other skin problems.

Padmam plant/seed (white lotus / *Nelumbo nucifera*) Lotus comes in many varieties: white lotus is **Padmam**, red is **Raktotpalam**, and blue is **Nilotpalam**. The taste is astringent, bitter, and sweet and it is cooling in effect. It causes constipation, increases gas, and is good for Kapha and Pitta. The seed is good for infertility.

Palasha seed/flower/alkali (bastard teak / *Butea frondosa*)
Palasha is a subtropical tree that grows in mountainous areas. The seed is pungent in taste, and used in worms and toxemia. The flower is pungent and astringent in taste and used in hemorrhage. The alkali extracted from the bark ash is used in hemorrhage and menorrhagia.

Parpata herb *(Fumaria indica)*
Parpata is a small annual herb that grows in wheat farms. All parts of the plant are bitter in taste, and cooling in action. It reduces Pitta. It is used for fever and is good for dehydration (increases fluids) it can be combined with **Chandana wood** (white sandalwood / *Santalum album*) to make a basic anti-Pitta formula.

Pashanabheda root (rockfoil / *Bergenia ligulata*)
Pasanbheda is a perennial herb with rhizome that grows in rocky mountainous areas. Its root is bitter and astringent in taste, and warming. It is diuretic and reduces Pitta. Used for kidney and bladder stones, painful urination, dysuria, and urinary system infection.

Patala root/bark *(Stereospermum personatum)*
Patala is a large sub-tropical tree. The root and bark are bitter in taste. It is a rejuvenative and alterative. Used in edema and to reduce Vata.

Patha root *(Stephania hernandifolia)*
Patha is an annual climber with tuber that grows in temperate forests. The tuber is bitter in taste. Used in fever, typhoid fever, diarrhea, chronic diarrhea, hemorrhage, throat defects, and anemia caused by clay-eating. It reduces Vata and Pitta.

Patram leaf *(Cassia cinnamon / Cinnamomum tamala)*
Patram is a temperate and sub-tropical evergreen tree with aromatic leaves. The leaf is bitter and pungent in taste, and an alterative for immunity. Used in respiratory diseases, coughs, hemoptysis, nose defects, gout, edema, toxemia, and skin diseases.

Pippali fruit/root (long pepper / *Piper longum*)
Pippali is a sub-tropical and tropical creeper that grows in the forest, and is also cultivated. It is grouped with **Pippali**, **Gajapippali** and **Chavyam**, all of which share similar effects. The fruit is pungent in taste, appetizing, and digestive. It reduces Vata and Kapha. It is used in bronchitis, asthma, cough and fever. It stimulates the medicinal effects of other herbs, has restorative qualities and is good for long life. The root is pungent in taste, light in quality and aids in food digestion. It is good for stomach diseases, liver and spleen diseases, and tuberculosis.

Punarnava plant/root *(Boerhavia difusa)*
Punarnava is an annual spreading plant that grows well in sub-tropical forests. It has two varieties, one with red stem and one with green stem. All parts of the plant are bitter in taste, constrictitory in action, diuretic and alterative. It reduces Kapha and Pitta. It is used for painful urination (caused by bladder or kidney stone), edema, gout, and anemia. When prepared with bone marrow soup it becomes a Rasayana. It is also used for hemorrhoids, and for bleeding in the lungs and uterus. The plant with red stem is more effectively used in coughs, hemoptysis and menorrhagia.

Rakta Chandanam wood (red sandalwood / *Pterocarpus santalinus*)
Rakta Chandanam is a woody tropical tree. The wood is bitter in taste and constrictitory in action. It is an anti-poison (vishaghna), refrigerant, and anti-toxin used in fevers and to reduce Pitta. Good for dizziness caused by high or low blood pressure. It can be used by itself or combined with **Parpata herb** *(Fumaria indica)* as a basic anti-Pitta formula for up to three months. Combine with **Chandanam wood** (white sandalwood / *Santalum album)* for menopausal hot flashes.

Rasna shrub *(Vanda roxburghii)*
Rasna is a perennial shrub that grows on hills in temperate and sub-tropical hills. All parts of the plant are bitter in taste, heavy to digest, and heat producing in nature. It reduces Vata. Used internally and externally in medicated oils for any kind of Vata disorder.

Rohitaka stem (rhododendron / *Rhododendron arboreum*)
Rohitaka is an alpine and sub-alpine small tree with red flowers. The stem is pungent in taste, and is used in enlargement of liver and spleen. It reduces Pitta. The root is pungent in taste, and used in leucorrhea. It is mildly poisonous.

Sarpagandha root (*Rauwolfia serpentina*)
Sarpagandha is a tropical bushy annual plant, found especially in eastern Nepal. The root is bitter in taste and cool in action. It reduces Vata and Pitta. It is used for hypertension and insomnia. It is not a cure, but causes quick blood pressure reduction over 4 to 6 hours.

Shalaparni plant (*Desmodium gangeticum*)
Shalaparni is a sub-tropical perennial spreading herb that grows on dry hills. All parts of the plant are sweet in taste, with a mild heat-generating property. It is used as a restorative, aphrodisiac and alterative to increase immunity. It has a sedative effect, especially in the brain. It is used in fever, and to reduce Vata, Pitta, and Kapha. It has the unique effect (prabhava) of reducing imbalance without ever causing increase. It is used in difficult to control diseases like typhoid fever and tuberculosis.

Shatavari root (wild asparagus / *Asparagus racemosus*)
Shatavari root is a tropical and sub-tropical, thorny, perennial, and tuberous shrub. The root is sweet and bitter in taste, cooling (refrigerant) in action, and heavy to digest and greasy in property. It reduces Vata and Pitta Dosha. It is used for gout, hemorrhoids, and bleeding in the urine, as well as inflammation or bleeding from the lung, stomach or uterus. In large dose, it can be used to control blood pressure. It is a brain restorative (Vata), used in epilepsy and hypertension. It strengthens the heart and the Ojas (vital water), and is used in inflammatory heart and liver diseases. It promotes fertility and breast milk in women.

Sukshmaila seed (cardamom / *Elettaria cardamomum*)
Sukshmaila seed is a perennial rhizomatous plant cultivated in temperate and sub-tropical valleys. The seed is pungent in taste, aromatic, and has a cooling sensation. It is carminative, appetizing, sedative and an aid to digestion. It is used as a mild anti-poison in body ache, coughs, and vomiting. It is a good spice for bean and meat preparations, and can be used after meals for its pleasant aroma.

Shunthi root (dry ginger / *Zingiber officinalis*)
Shunthi is an erect cultivated perennial spicy plant with thick tubers. It is pungent in taste, carminative, digestive, and aphrodisiac. It is cooling in action. It is light to digest and strong in property. It reduces Kapha and Vata. It is used for urticaria, common cold, allergies and rheumatism. Its post-digestive action is sweet

(Madhura), increasing its nourishing qualities, creating a mild aphrodisiac effect as well as aiding in peristaltic movement. Fresh ginger is called Adrakam.

Shurana tuber *(Amorphophallus campanulatus)*
Surana is an annual tuberous plant that grows in shady forest areas. The tuber is pungent in taste, hot in action, stomachic, carminative and restorative. Used in hemorrhoids and abdominal tumors.

Swarnapatri leaf (senna / *Cassia auriculata*)
Swarnapatri leaf is annual plant with alterate pinnate leaves that grows in tropical climates in plains areas, especially in South India. Its leaf is bitter in taste, and used as a laxative in Pitta increase cases.

Talisam leaf (rhododendron / *Rhododendron setosum*)
Talisam is an alpine small bushy plant with aromatic leaves. The leaf is bitter and sweet in taste. Used in pulmonary tuberculosis, asthma, hay fever and cough, tumor, and anorexia.

Tila seed/oil (sesame / *Sesamum indicum*)
Tila is a cultivated spice. It is pungent, bitter, sweet and astringent in taste. It is very good in Vata diseases, internally or externally, and is especially good for skin problems. The oil benefits the hair and teeth, and can be used for cuts and wounds. It can decrease the force of urine if taken in excess.

Trivrit root (Indian rhubarb / *Operculina turpethum*)
Trivrit is a milky climber that grows in the temperate forest. Its root is pungent in taste and cold in action. It causes liquid stools (Rechanam). It reduces Pitta, and is the best laxative for Pitta conditions. It is used in fevers.

Twak bark (cinnamon / *Cinnamomum zeylanicum*)
Twak is a tropical and sub-tropical evergreen tree with aromatic bark. The bark is sweet and pungent in taste, and warm in action. It has a cooling after-effect in the mouth. It is a carminative and a digestive, a mild anti-poison, and reduces Kapha and Vata. It is used in coughs, heart disease, loss of appetite, rheumatism and sinusitis. It is good in all vegetable preparations.

Ushira rhizome *(Andropogon muricatum)*
Ushira is a tall grassy plant with fragrant rhizome that grows in the sub-tropical swampy forest. The rhizome is bitter in taste, and reduces Pitta. It is used as a refrigerant for fever and thirst.

Vacha rhizome (sweet flag / *Acorus calamus*)
Vacha is a perennial aromatic herb that grows in muddy ponds. The rhizome is pungent and slightly bitter in taste, warming and drying in action, and light to digest and strong in property. It reduces Kapha and Vata. Its special power (Prabhava) is epilepsy, and it is medhya (improves memory and intellect). It is used in epilepsy, insanity, as a brain and longevity restorative, and for loss of memory. It increases the digestive fire (Agni). It is Lekhanam, an agent that causes dryness, and promotes expectoration of mucus. It improves blood circulation to the brain and drains the ducts. In large doses it is an emetic. It can be chewed and sucked for hoarseness.

Vakuchi seed *(Psoralia corylifolia)*
Vakuchi is an annual bushy plant cultivated everywhere. The oily aromatic seed is bitter and pungent in taste, and hot in action. It is used in all skin diseases, eczema, leprosy, psoriasis and leucoderma.

Vamshalochana (bamboo manna / *Bambusa breviflora*)
Vamshalochana is a perennial tree that grows in tropical climates. It contains white manna which is sweet-astringent in taste and which reduces Pitta. It is used in asthma and cough.

Vasaka leaf/root/flower (Malabar nut / *Adhatoda vasica*)
Vasaka is a perennial evergreen bush which grows everywhere in dry areas. The leaf is bitter and astringent in taste, light to digest and dry in property, and cooling in action. Its post-digestive action is pungent (Katu), causing a drying effect in the colon. It reduces Kapha and Pitta. It is used for hemorrhoids, hemoptitis, and blood in the lungs (hemorrhage or tuberculosis), hepatitis, fever, asthma, cough, and chronic bronchitis. Fresh leaf

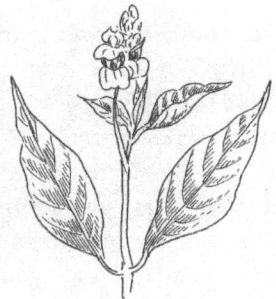

Vasaka
(Adhatoda vasica)

juice with honey and/or ginger can be used for cough. The root and flower are bitter in taste and used in inflammatory abdominal tumor.

Vidanga seeds *(Embelia ribes)*
Vidanga is an evergreen small sized tree that grows in temperate forests. The seed is pungent in taste and hot in action. It reduces Kapha and is used frequently to reduce mucus. It kills parasites (Krimighna), and is used for leprosy, abdominal tumors and sprue.

Yavani seed (wild omum / ajagandha / *Trachyspermum ammi*)
Yavani is a spicy cultivated plant. The seed is bitter and pungent in taste, carminative, digestive and appetizing. It reduces Vata and Kapha. Used in colds, urticaria, heart pain, bladder pain and abdominal colic. Also used in skin diseases. Used extensively for treatment of the common cold in tea form.

Mineral extracts

Abhraka Bhasma (purified mica oxide)
There are four kinds of mica oxide: white, pink, yellow & black. Only the black variety is used as medicine. Within the category of black varieties, there are many additional varieties that reveal themselves when placed in fire. Some separate into layers, some make a hissing sound, some make a popping or cracking sound and some make no changes in color and sound. This last group is called vajrabhraka, and is the one that is used in medicine. Unpurified and unoxidized mica can be a cause of heart disease, anemia, edema, skin diseases, and stones of the gallbladder, kidney and bladder. Purified mica Bhasma, the red powder of mica oxide, is used in heart disease, anemia, impotence, and skin diseases. It is restorative and alterative, and is used for increasing milk in pregnant women, longevity, and for eye diseases. It can be used in any chronic tridoshaja disease.

Gandhaka Bhasma (purified sulfur oxide)
Unpurified sulfur can cause hot sensations, blood defects and mental disorders. Gandhaka Bhasma is used for skin diseases, blood defects, lead poisoning, and mercury poisoning.

Haritala Bhasma (orpiment / purified yellow arsenic trisulphide)
Unpurified orpiment can cause heat, skin diseases, and death. Purified orpiment is used in skin diseases, gout, and blood defects, and also as a Rasayana.

Hingulu Bhasma (cinnabar / purified red cinnabar sulphide)
Unpurified cinnabar can cause urinary diseases, delusions and mental disorders. Cinnabar Bhasma is good for mentality and strongly promotes good blood circulation. It is a Rasayana. It is used in rheumatism, fevers, urinary diseases, and liver and spleen diseases.

Kajjali (mercury powder ground with pure sulphur for purification)
Kajjali is mercury powder ground with pure sulphur until a black powder forms. The mercury is almost completely inert in this form, but still has potential for misuse and must be prescribed by a trained doctor. It is a restorative useful for all three Doshas (Vata, Pitta, and Kapha), and is especially good for increasing Shukra Dhatu (semen).

Lauha Bhasma (purified iron oxide)
Unpurified and unoxidized iron can be the cause of heart disease, leprosy, colic, impotence, constipation and gallbladder, bladder and kidney stones. Purified and oxidized Lauha Bhasma is used in anemia, hepatitis, liver disease, and edema.

Manashila Bhasma (purified realgar)
Realgar is a natural mineral product. Unpurified realgar can cause arsenic poisoning, constipation, dysurea, and skin diseases. Purified realgar is used as a strong anti-toxin and anti-poison, especially used in skin diseases, asthma cough, and chronic fever. It is widely used as an external application for eye diseases for the same reasons.

Mandura Bhasma (purified iron ore oxide)
Mandura Bhasma is astringent and bitter-like in taste, and cooling in action. It is used in splenitis, enlarged spleen (Plihabriddhi), enlarged liver (Yakritvriddhi), hepatitis (Kamala), anemia (Pandu), edema (Shotha), blood loss (Raktakshaya) and itching (Kandu). It is usually given with honey or **Triphala decoction** (three fruits compound). For swelling, it is given with **Punarnava decoction** (*Boerhavia difusa)*.

Rasakarpura (white crystal of mercury sulphide / mineral camphor)
Rasakarpura is made by taking mercury and sulphur and burning in fire. The resultant combination is mixed with mineral salt then heated in a bottle with hot sand until camphor-like white crystals form in the neck of the bottle. It is toxic, and only qualified Vaidyas can prescribe it, and even then only in minute doses. It is illegal to use in many countries. Used for skin diseases, blood defects and worms.

Samudraphenam (sea foam / *Sepia spp.*)
Samudraphenam is the Sanskrit name for the cuttlefish bone that is found floating on sea-water (thus called sea foam), then collected and dried into a layered natural product. It is astringent in taste, and reduces Kapha Dosha. For its drying effect, it is used as a powder in otorrhea, and in pastes for skin diseases, psoriasis, For the same reason it is a major ingredient in external formulas for certain eye diseases.

Sauvarchalam (black salt)
Black salt is made by combining mineral salt (Saindhavam) and sodium bicarbonate (Sarjikshara). It is good for heart disease, indigestion, bloated stomach, tumors, and colic pain.

Sauvira Bhasma (purified antimony sulfide)
Sauvira is a mineral product found in the form of heavy black rock. It has two varieties, sauviranjan and srotoja-anjan. Both are used similarly. It is astringent in taste with a cooling effect. Purified antimony made into a microfine powder is used in hemorrhage, menorrhagia, hiccup, and vomiting. Unpurified, it causes lead

poisoning, colic, arthritis, skin diseases, paralysis, tumors and nerve defects. A collyrium made of the purified powder is used to prevent cataract formation.

Shankha Bhasma (purified conch shell ash, *Turbinella pyrum*)
Shankha Bhasma is the white powder of conch shell oxide. Used in diarrhea, duodenal ulcer and acidity. Externally used as a plaster for acne.

Shilajatu
Shilajatu is 'ejected' out of rocks during hot weather in the Himalayas. It is bitter and slightly pungent in taste, and mildly warming in action. It has the distinct odor of cow urine. Shilajatu strengthens immunity, reduces fatigue, slows aging, tonifies the brain, cleanses the blood, and strengthens the liver and kidneys. It is a Rasayana and an aphrodisiac, given to people suffering from chronic bronchitis, digestive disease, diseases of the nerves, and fractures. Shilajatu is a brain restorative, and is used to purify the urinary tract, kidneys and the genitals. It is anti-fatigue and anti-diabetic, used in diabetes, anemia, aging, bronchitis, skin diseases, liver disease, constipation, dyspepsia, and all urinary diseases. It strengthens the effects of other herbs (yogavaha).

Shukti Bhasma (oyster shell ash /*Ostrea gigas*)
Shukti Bhasma is alkaline in taste. The shell is purified and burnt into ash before use. It is used for gastritis, duodenal ulcer, splenitis, hepatitis, stomach acidity, and kidney stones. It is often added to hypertension formulas. It is diuretic and has medicinal value in the treatment of some types of blurred vision. Used externally as a plaster for erysipelas and blisters.

Soraka (potassium chloride)
Soraka is used as a diuretic and for edema.

Sphutikarika (purified alum)
Sphutikarika is a natural product extracted from Saurastra clay in the form of a crystal. It is astringent and acidic in taste. In general, it is used in the form of a honey paste for gargling or washing, for the purpose of stopping bleeding, or to treat tonsillitis, stomatitis, and prolapses of the anus or uterus. In the case of conjunctivitis, eye drops made of purified alum are very effective. Alum is also used in scabies, ringworm, eczema, erysipelas and freckles.

Tamra Bhasma (purified copper oxide)
Unpurified and unoxidized copper can be a cause of vomiting, dizziness, fainting and diarrhea. Tamra Bhasma is used for vomiting, dizziness, fainting and diarrhea. In general, it reduces Pitta. It can also be used for any cranial disease.

Vanga Bhasma (purified tin oxide)
Vanga Bhasma is the white powder of tin oxide. Unpurified tin oxide causes leprosy, tumors, urinary diseases, anemia, and blood defects. Purified Vanga is salt-like, bitter and astringent in taste, and good for fatty defects, urinary diseases and anemia. It is also a Rasayana and brain restorative.

Yashada Bhasma (purified zinc oxide)
Unpurified and unoxidized zinc can be the cause of tumors, urinary diseases, and debility and skin diseases. Purified and oxidized zinc is used for urinary diseases, especially urinary frequency, for menorrhagia and for Vata imbalance. It has a very constrictitory effect on the mucous membranes.

Yavakshara alkaline ash (barley plant / *Hordeum vulgare*)
Yavakshara is a diuretic medicine made of barley plant ash. It is used for dysuria, painful urination, kidney stones, and cystitis and to flush the kidneys. It is always used with plenty of water to drink. Due to its power, it is used in minute quantities. Overdose can cause nausea.

Compounds and Formulas

There are a great many formulas described in Ayurveda, with many different variations. To avoid confusion, many of the following formulas are listed with reference to the classical text in which they are described. Where no text is mentioned, the formula is unique to the Bajracharya medical tradition.

Abhayarista (*Charaka Samhita* is a herbal wine containing **Haritaki fruit** (*Terminalia chebula*), **Amalaki fruit** (Indian gooseberry / amla / *Phyllanthus emblica*), **Kapittha fruit** (wood apple / *Feronia limonia*), **Indravaruni fruit** (bitter apple / *Citrullus colocynthis*), **Vidanga seed** (*Embelia ribes*), **Pippali fruit** (long pepper / *Piper longum*), **Lodhram bark** (*Symplocos paniculata*), **Maricham seed** (black pepper / *Piper nigrum*), **Ela fruit** (greater cardamon / *Amomum subulatum*), **Kustha root** (*Saussurea lappa*) and **Matsyandika** (molasses).

Ahiphenasava (*Bhaishajya Ratnavali*) is herbal wine prepared with **Ahiphenam seed extract** (poppy / *Papaver somniferum*).

Ajamodadi Churna (*Sharangadhara Samhita*) is a herbal powder containing **Ajamoda seed** (wild celery / *Carum roxburghianum*), **Vidanga seeds** (*Embelia ribes*), **Saindhavam** (mineral salt), **Devadaru wood** (Himalayan cedar / *Cedrus deodara*), **Chitraka root** (leadwort / *Plumbago zeylanica*), **Pippali root** (long pepper / *Piper longum*), **Pippali fruit** (long pepper / *Piper longum*), **Shatapushpa seed** (anise / *Pimpinella anisum*), **Maricham seed** (black pepper / *Piper nigrum*), **Haritaki fruit**

(*Terminalia chebula*), **Bidhara root** (*Gmelina asiatica*), and **Shunthi root** (dry ginger / *Zingiber officinalis*).

Alarasayana contains **Nimba leaf** (neem / *Azadirachta indica*), **Bibhitaki fruit** (*Terminalia belerica*), **Gandhaka Bhasma** (purified sulfur oxide), **Vasaka leaf** (Malabar nut / *Adhatoda vasica*), **Haritala Bhasma** (orpiment / purified yellow arsenic trisulphide), and **Bibhitaki fruit** (*Terminalia belerica*).

Amalakyadi Churna contains **Swarnapatri leaf** (senna / *Cassia auriculata*), **Pippali root** (long pepper / *Piper longum*), **Chitraka root** (leadwort, white flower / *Plumbago zeylanica*), **Amalaki fruit** (Indian gooseberry / amla / *Phyllanthus emblica*), and **Haritaki fruit** (*Terminalia chebula*).

Anandabhairavarasa Vati contains **Vatsanabha** (aconite tuber, purified / *Aconitum palmatum*), **Pippali fruit** (long pepper / *Piper longum*), **Maricham seed** (black pepper / *Piper nigrum*), **Tankana Bhasma** (purified borax) and **Hingulu Bhasma** (cinnabar / purified red cinnabar sulphide).

Apamargakshara Taila (*Bhavaprakasha Samhita*) contains **Achyranthes root ash** (*Achyranthes bidentata*) and **Tila oil** (sesame seed / *Sesamum indicum*).

Arjuna Ghritam (*Chakradatta*) is made from **Arjuna bark** (*Terminalia arjuna*) cooked in **Ghrita** (clarified butter).

Arkalavanam (*Bhaishajya Ratnavali*) contains the fresh leaf of **Arka** (milkweed / *Calotropis gigantean*) cooked with **Saindhavam** (mineral salt).

Ashwattha Kashaya (*Sushruta Samhita*) is a decoction made from **Pippali fruit** (long pepper / *Piper longum*).

Avipattikara Churna *Bhaishajya Ratnavali*) is made primarily from **Trivrit root** (Indian rhubarb / *Operculina turpethum*) and **Lavangam seeds** (clove / *Syzigium aromaticum*), along with **Trikatu** (*Piper longum, Piper nigrum, Zingiber officinalis*), **Triphala** (*Phyllanthus emblica / Terminalia belerica / Terminalia chebula*), **Musta tuber** (*Cyperus rotundus*), **Vidanga seed** (*Embelia ribes*), **Ela fruit** (greater cardamon / *Amomum subulatum*), and **Patram leaf** (Cassia cinnamon / *Cinnamomum tamala*).

Bala Taila (*Sushruta Samhita*) is a medicated oil containing **Bala plant** (country mallow / *Sida cordifolia*), **Atibala plant** (*Sida rhombifolia*), **Vidanga seed** (*Embelia ribes*), **Trikatu** (*Piper longum, Piper nigrum, Zingiber officinalis*), **Punarnava** (*Boerhavia difusa*), and **Tila seed oil** (sesame / *Sesamum indicum*).

Baladyam Ghritam *(Chakradatta)* is a medicated Ghee preparation made from **Nagabala** *(Sida spinosa,* wild), **Bala plant** (country mallow / *Sida cordifolia)*, **Arjuna bark** *(Terminalia arjuna)*, **Madhukam root** (licorice / *Glycyrrhiza glabra)*, and **Mustaka tuber** *(Cyperus rotundus)* based in **Ghrita** (Ghee).

Bhallataka Rasayana *(Rasatarangini)* contains **Shunthi root** (dry ginger / *Zingiber officinalis)*, **Vidanga seed** *(Embelia ribes)*, **Lauha Bhasma** (purified iron oxide), **Bhallataka** (marking nut tree / *Semecarpus anacardium)* taken with **Ghrita** (Ghee) and **Madhu** (honey).

Bilwa Taila *(Bhavaprakasha Samhita)* contains **Bilwa fruit** (bael / *Aegle marmelos)*, **Goumutra** (cow urine), and **Ajakshira** (goat milk), prepared in sesame oil.

Brihatyadigana Churna *(Chakradatta)* contains **Brihati shrub** (vrihati / *Solanum indicum)*, **Kantakari herb** (Black nightshade / *Solanum xanthocarpum)*, **Nilotpalam flower** (blue lotus / *Iris nepalensis)*, **Bhargi root/resin** (Turk's turban / *Clerodendron serratum)*, **Karchura tuber/seed** (zedoary /*Curcuma zedoaria)*, **Karkatashringi fruit gall** *(Pistacia intergerrima* insect gall), **Duralambha bush** *(Fragonia cretica)*, **Indrayava seed** *(Holarrhena antidysenterica)*, **Patola leaf** *(Trichosanthes dioica)* and **Kutki rhizome** (Indian gentian / *Picrorhiza kurroa)*.

Chandanadi Churna is made from **Rakta Chandanam wood** (red sandalwood / *Pterocarpus santalinus)*, **Ela fruit** (greater cardamon / *Amomum subulatum)*, **Musta tuber** *(Cyperus rotundus)*, **Jirakam seed** (cumin / *Cuminum cyminum)*, **Dhanyakam seeds** (coriander / *Coriandrum sativum)*, **Nagakeshara seed** (Ironwood tree / *Mesua ferrea)*, **Pippali fruit** (long pepper / *Piper longum)*, **Twak bark** (Cinnamon / *Cinnamomum zeylanicum)*, **Madhukam root** (licorice / *Glycyrrhiza glabra)*, **Ushira root** (khus khus / *Andropogon muricatum)*, **Chandanam wood** (white sandalwood / *Santalum album)*, and **Maricham seed** (black pepper / *Piper nigrum)*.

Chandraprabha Vati *(Sharangadhara Samhita)* contains **Shilajatu Rasayana** and **Guggulu gum resin** *(Commiphora wightii)*, and a small amount of the very powerful **Karapura leaf** (camphor / *Cinnamomum camphora)*. The formula also contains **Vacha rhizome** (acorus / *Acorus calamus)*, **Musta tuber** (nut grass / *Cyperus rotundus,* big), **Kiratatiktam plant** *(Swertia chirata)*, **Guduchi stem** *(Tinospora cordifolia)*, **Devadaru wood** (Himalayan cedar / *Cedrus deodara)*, **Haridra root** (turmeric / *Curcuma longa)*, **Ativisha tuber, purified** (aconite / *Aconitum heterophyllum)*, **Darvi root** *(Berberis nepalensis)*, **Pippalamulam** (long pepper root / *Piper longum)*, **Chitraka root** (leadwort, white flower / *Plumbago zeylanica)*, **Dhanyakam seeds** (coriander / *Coriandrum sativum)*, **Triphala** *(Phyllanthus emblica / Terminalia belerica / Terminalia chebula)*, **Chavyam stem** *(Piper chaba)*, **Vidanga seed** *(Embelia ribes)*, **Gajapippali fruit** *(Piper chaba)*, **Trikatu** *(Piper longum, Piper* *nigrum, Zingiber officinalis)*, **Makshikam Bhasma** (purified copper/iron pyrite), **Yavakshara alkaline ash** (barley plant / *Hordeum vulgare)*, **Lavanatrayam** (mineral salt, sea salt and **Vidam**, salt made from *Phyllanthus emblica)*, **Trivrit root** (Indian rhubarb /*Operculina turpethum)*, **Danti seed** *(Baliospermum montanum)*, **Patram leaf** (Cassia cinnamon / *Cinnamomum tamala)*, **Twak bark** (Cinnamon / *Cinnamomum zeylanicum)*, **Ela fruit** (greater cardamon / *Amomum subulatum)*, **Vamshalochana** (Bamboo manna / *Bambusa breviflora)*, **Lauha Bhasma** (purified iron oxide) and **Vetasa** (cane sugar / *Saccharum officinarum)*.

Chandrodayavarti *(Chakradatta)* is made from **Haritaki fruit** *(Terminalia chebula)*, **Vacha rhizome** (acorus / *Acorus calamus)*, **Kustha root** *(Saussurea lappa)*, **Pippali fruit** (long pepper / *Piper longum)*, **Maricham seed** (black pepper / *Piper nigrum)*, **Bibhitaki seed pulp** *(Terminalia belerica)*, **Shankha Bhasma** (purified conch shell oxide), and **Manashila Bhasma** (purified realgar) ground with **Ajakshira** (goat milk).

Chaturdasanga Churna is made from **Katphalam bark** (box myrtle / *Myrica nagi)*, **Nilotpalam flower** (blue lotus / *Iris nepalensis)*, **Karkatashringi fruit gall** *(Pistacia intergerrima* insect gall), **Pippali fruit** (long pepper / *Piper longum)*, **Maricham seed** (black pepper / *Piper nigrum)*, **Shunthi root** (dry ginger / *Zingiber officinalis)*, **Duralambha bush** *(Fragonia cretica)*, **Krishnajiraka seed** (black cumin / *Nigella sativa)*, **Musta tuber** *(Cyperus rotundus)*, **Talisham leaf** (rhododendron / *Rhododendron setosum)*, **Twak bark** (Cinnamon / *Cinnamomum zeylanicum)*, **Patram leaf** (Cassia cinnamon / *Cinnamomum tamala)*, **Ela fruit** (greater cardamon / *Amomum subulatum)* and **Nagakeshara seed** (Ironwood tree / *Mesua ferrea)*.

Chhuchhundari Taila is made from **Chhuchhundara** (muskrat meat), water and **Tila oil** (sesame seed / *Sesamum indicum)*.

Chyavanaprasha *(Charaka Samhita)* contains **Amalaki fruit** (Indian gooseberry / amla / *Phyllanthus emblica)* as the main ingredient, along with **Bilwa fruit** (bael / *Aegle marmelos)*, **Agnimantha** *(Premna integrifolia)*, **Shyonaka** (Indian trumpet flower / *Oroxylon indicum)*, **Kashmari** (kashmari / *Gmelina arborea)*, **Patala** *(Stereospermum personatum)*, **Bala plant** (country mallow / *Sida cordifolia)*, **Prishniparni plant** *(Uraria lagopoides)*, **Shalaparni plant** *(Desmodium gangeticum)*, **Masaparni** *(Teramnus labialis)*, **Mudgaparni** *(Phaseolus trilobus)*, **Pippali fruit** (long pepper / *Piper longum)*, **Gokshura fruit** *(Tribulus terrestris)*, **Brihati shrub** (vrihati / *Solanum indicum)*, **Kantakari herb** (Black nightshade / *Solanum xanthocarpum)*, **Karkatashringi fruit gall** *(Pistacia intergerrima* insect gall), **Tamalaki herb** *(Phyllanthus niruni)*, **Draksha fruit** (grape / *Vitis vinifera)*, **Jivanti leaf** *(Leptadenia reticulate)*, **Nilotpalam flower** (blue lotus / *Iris nepalensis)*, **Agaru wood** (eaglewood / *Aquilaria agallocha)*, **Haritaki fruit** *(Terminalia chebula)*, **Guduchi stem** *(Tinospora cordifolia)*, **Vriddhi tuber** *(Paris polyphylla,* big), **Jivaka bulb** (wild garlic

/ *Allium wallichii,* small), **Karchura** (zedoary /*Curcuma zedoaria)*, **Musta tuber** *(Cyperus rotundus)*, **Punarnava plant/root** *(Boerhavia difusa)*, **Ela fruit** (greater cardamon / *Amomum subulatum)*, **Rakta Chandanam wood** (red sandalwood / *Pterocarpus santalinus)*, **Utpala** *(Nymphaea stellate)*, **Vidari tuber** *(Ipomea paniculata)*, **Vasaka leaf** (Malabar nut / *Adhatoda vasica)*, **Kakoli bulb** *(Fritillaria cirrhosa)*, **Kakanasika shrub** *(Leea aquata)*, **Tila seed oil** (sesame / *Sesamum indicum)*, **Ghrita** (Ghee / clarified butter), **Vetasa** (cane sugar, brown / *Saccharum officinarum)*, **Madhu** (honey), **Vamshalochana** (Bamboo manna / *Bambusa breviflora)*, **Pippalamulam** (long pepper root / *Piper longum)*, **Twak bark** (Cinnamon / *Cinnamomum zeylanicum)*, **Sukshmaila seed** (cardamom / *Elettaria cardamomum)*, **Patram leaf** (Cassia cinnamon / *Cinnamomum tamala)* and **Nagakeshara seed/flower** (ironwood tree / *Mesua ferrea)*.

Dadimadi Churna contains **Dadima rind** (pomegranate / *Punica granatum)*, **Dhanyakam seeds** (coriander / *Coriandrum sativum)*, **Chitraka root** (leadwort, white flower / *Plumbago zeylanica)*, **Shunthi root** (dry ginger / *Zingiber officinalis)* and **Maricham seed** (black pepper / *Piper nigrum)*.

Dashamula contains **Bilwa root** (bael / *Aegle marmelos)*, **Shyonaka root** (Indian trumpet flower / *Oroxylon indicum)*, **Kashmari root** (kashmari / *Gmelina arborea)*, **Patala root** *(Stereospermum personatum)*, **Agnimantha root** *(Premna integrifolia)*, **Shalaparni root** *(Desmodium gangeticum)*, **Prishniparni root** *(Uraria lagopoides)*, **Brihati root** *(Solanum indicum)*, **Kantakari root** (Black nightshade / *Solanum xanthocarpum)* and **Gokshura root** *(Tribulus terrestris)*

Dhanwayasa Yoga contains **Duralambha bush** *(Fragonia cretica)*, **Kantakari herb** (Black nightshade / *Solanum xanthocarpum)* and **Brihati shrub** (vrihati / *Solanum indicum)*.

Dhanyapanchakam is made from **Dhanyakam seeds** (coriander / *Coriandrum sativum)*, **Hriverum plant** *(Pavonia odorata)*, **Musta tuber** *(Cyperus rotundus)*, **Bilwa fruit** (bael / *Aegle marmelos)*, **Shunthi root** (dry ginger / *Zingiber officinalis)* and **Saindhavam** (mineral salt from Sindhu).

Drakshyasava *(Sharangadhara Samhita)* contains **Twak bark** (Cinnamon / *Cinnamomum zeylanicum)*, **Sukshmaila seed** (cardamom / *Elettaria cardamomum)*, **Patram leaf** (Cassia cinnamon / *Cinnamomum tamala)*, **Nagakeshara** (ironwood tree / *Mesua ferrea)*, **Priyangu seed** *(Prunus mahaleb)*, **Maricham seed** (black pepper / *Piper nigrum)*, **Pippali fruit** (long pepper / *Piper longum)*, and **Vidanga seed** *(Embelia ribes)* fermented with raisins and brown sugar or molasses.

Gairikadi Anjanam *(Sushruta Samhita)* is made from **Gairika** (red clay / ocre), **Saindhavam** (mineral salt from Sindhu), **Pippali fruit** (long pepper / *Piper longum)*, and **Godantamasi** (charred cow teeth) with honey.

Gandhakarasayana contains **Gandhaka Bhasma** (purified sulfur oxide), **Nimba leaf** (neem / *Azadirachta indica)*, **Bibhitaki fruit** *(Terminalia belerica)*, **Vasaka leaf** (Malabar nut / *Adhatoda vasica)*, **Haritala Bhasma** (orpiment / purified yellow arsenic trisulphide), and **Bibhitaki fruit** *(Terminalia belerica)*.

Gokshuradi Guggulu Vati *(Sharangadhara Samhita)* are made primarily from **Gokshura fruit** *(Tribulus terrestris)* and **Guggulu gum resin** *(Commiphora wightii)*. They also contain **Trikatu** *(Piper longum, Piper nigrum, Zingiber officinalis)*, **Triphala** *(Phyllanthus emblica / Terminalia belerica / Terminalia chebula)* and **Musta tuber** *(Cyperus rotundus)*.

Gomansadi Anjanam *(Sushruta Samhita)* is made from **Gomansa** (beef), **Maricham seed** (black pepper / *Piper nigrum)*, **Shirisha seed** *(Albizzia lebbeck)* and **Manashila Bhasma** (purified realgar) with honey.

Guduchi Chitraka Rasena is the decoction of **Guduchi stem** *(Tinospora cordifolia)*, **Chitraka root** (leadwort, white flower / *Plumbago zeylanica)*, **Kustha root** *(Saussurea lappa)*, **Kutaja bark** *(Holarrhena antidysenterica)*, **Patha root** *(Stephania hernandifolia)*, **Hingu gum** (asafoetida / *Ferula narthex)*, and **Kutaki rhizome** (Indian gentian / *Picrorhiza kurroa)*.

Haridra Amalaki Rasena *(Charaka Samhita)* is the decoction of **Haridra root** (turmeric / *Curcuma longa)* **Amalaki fruit** (Indian gooseberry / amla / *Phyllanthus emblica)*, **Madhu** (honey), **Triphala** *(Phyllanthus emblica / Terminalia belerica / Terminalia chebula)*, **Devadaru wood** (Himalayan cedar / *Cedrus deodara)* and **Mustaka tuber** *(Cyperus rotundus)*.

Haridra Amalirasena *(Charaka Samhita)* is made from **Haridra root** (turmeric / *Curcuma longa)*, **Amalaki fruit** (Indian gooseberry / amla / *Phyllanthus emblica)*, **Haritaki fruit** *(Terminalia chebula)*, **Katphalam bark** (box myrtle / *Myrica nagi)*, **Mustaka tuber** *(Cyperus rotundus)*, **Lodhram bark** *(Symplocos paniculata)*, **Patha root** *(Stephania hernandifolia)*, **Vidanga seed** *(Embelia ribes)*, **Arjuna bark** *(Terminalia arjuna)*, and **Chandanam wood** (white sandalwood / *Santalum album)*.

Haridra Daruharidra Kashaya *(Sushruta Samhita)* is a decoction made from **Haridra root** (turmeric / *Curcuma longa)* and **Daruharidra bark** (barberry / *Berberis nepalensis)*, taken with honey.

Haridra Kashaya *(Sushruta Samhita)* is a decoction made from **Patha root** *(Stephania hernandifolia)*, **Agaru wood** (eaglewood / *Aquilaria agallocha)* and **Haridra root** (turmeric / *Curcuma longa).*

Haritakivarti *(Chakradatta)* is an eyesalve made from **Haritaki fruit** *(Terminalia chebula)*, **Hardira root** (turmeric / *Curcuma longa)*, **Pippali fruit** *(Piper longum)* and saindhava.

Haritala Nisha Nimbakalka is made from **Haritala Bhasma** (orpiment / purified yellow arsenic trisulphide), **Haridra root** (turmeric / *Curcuma longa)*, **Nimba leaf** (neem / *Azadirachta indica)* and **Patola fruit** *(Trichosanthes dioica).*

Kaishora Guggulu Vati *(Sharangadhara Samhita)* contains **Haritaki fruit** *(Terminalia chebula)*, **Bibhitaki fruit** *(Terminalia belerica)*, **Amalaki fruit** (Indian gooseberry / amla / *Emblica officinalis)*, **Guduchi stem** *(Tinospora cordifolia)*, and purified **Guggulu gum resin** *(Commiphora wightii).* It also contains small amounts of **Pippali fruit** (long pepper / *Piper longum)*, **Maricham seed** (black pepper / *Piper nigrum)*, **Shunthi root** (dry ginger / *Zingiber officinalis)*, **Vidanga seed** *(Embelia ribes)*, **Danti seed** *(Baliospermum montanum)* and **Trivrit root** (Indian rhubarb /*Operculina turpethum).*

Kakubha Chandana Kashaya *(Sushruta Samhita)* is a decoction made from **Arjuna bark** *(Terminalia arjuna)* and **Chandanam wood** (white sandalwood / *Santalum album)*, taken with honey.

Kalaka Yoga *(Charaka Samhita)* is made from **Yavakshara alkaline ash** (barley plant / *Hordeum vulgare*, **Patha root** *(Stephania hernandifolia)*, **Trikatu** *(Piper longum, Piper nigrum, Zingiber officinalis)*, **Daruharidra extract** (barberry / *Berberis nepalensis)*, **Chavyam fruit** *(Piper chaba)*, **Triphala** *(Phyllanthus emblica / Terminalia belerica / Terminalia chebula)*, **Lodhram bark** *(Symplocos paniculata)*, **Grihadhuma** (black soot), and **Chitraka root** (leadwort, white flower / *Plumbago zeylanica)* mixed with honey.

Kamalakilyana contains **Swarnapatri leaf** (senna / *Cassia auriculata)*, **Pippali root** (long pepper / *Piper longum)*, **Chitraka root** (leadwort, white flower / *Plumbago zeylanica)*, **Amalaki fruit** (Indian gooseberry / amla / *Phyllanthus emblica)*, and **Haritaki fruit** *(Terminalia chebula)*, **Vasaka leaf** (Malabar nut / *Adhatoda vasica)*, **Shukti Bhasma** (oyster shell ash /*Ostrea gigas)* and **Mandura Bhasma** (purified iron ore oxide), and **Yavasa** *(Alhagi maurorum).*

Kanakabindwaristam contains **Khadira extract** (catechu / *Acacia catechu*, white), **Ghrita** (Ghee), **Triphala** *(Phyllanthus emblica / Terminalia belerica / Terminalia chebula)*, **Vidanga seed** *(Embelia ribes)* and **Mustaka tuber** *(Cyperus rotundus).*

Kanchanara Guggulu Vati contains **Guggulu gum resin** *(Commiphora wightii)* and **Kanchanara bark** (mountain ebony / *Bauhinia tomentosa).* It also contains **Triphala** *(Emblica officinalis / Terminalia belerica / Terminalia chebula),* **Trikatu, Varuna bark/stem** (Three-leaved caper / *Crataeva religiosa),* **Ela fruit** (greater cardamon / *Amomum subulatum),* **Twak bark/stem** (Cinnamon / *Cinnamomum zeylanicum)* and **Patram leaf** (cassia / *Cinnamomum tamala).*

Kankayana Vati *(Chakradatta)* contains **Danti seed** *(Baliospermum montanum),* **Karchura tuber/seed** (zedoary /*Curcuma zedoaria),* **Nilotpalam flower** (blue lotus / *Iris nepalensis)* **Vidanga seed** *(Embelia ribes),* **Dadima rind** (pomegranate / *Punica granatum),* **Haritaki fruit** *(Terminalia chebula),* **Chitraka root** (Leadwort, white flower / *Plumbago zeylanica),* **Amlavetasa root** (rhubarb / *Rheum emodi),* **Shunthi root** (dry ginger / *Zingiber officinalis),* **Yavani seed** (wild omum / *Trachyspermum ammi),* **Jirakam seed** (cumin / *Cuminum cyminum),* **Dhanyakam seed** (coriander / *Coriandrum sativum),* **Aparajita seed/root** (butterfly pea / *Clitoria ternatea),* **Ajamoda seed** (wild celery / *Carum roxburghianum),* **Krishnajiraka seed** (black cumin / *Nigella sativa),* **Hingu gum** (asafoetida / *Ferula narthex),* **Yavakshara alkaline ash** (barley plant / *Hordeum vulgare),* **Yavasa alkaline ash** *(Alhagi maurorum),* **Lavanapanchakam** and **Trivrit root** (Indian rhubarb /*Operculina turpethum),* ground with the juice of **Matulunga fruit** (Citron / *Citrus medica).*

Karpurasava *Bhaishajya Ratnavali)* contains **Sukshmaila seed** (cardamom / *Elettaria cardamomum),* **Musta tuber** *(Cyperus rotundus),* **Hriverum plant** *(Pavonia odorata),* **Yavani seed** (wild omum / *Trachyspermum ammi),* **Maricham seed** (black pepper / *Piper nigrum),* **Karapura leaf exudate** (camphor / *Cinnamomum camphora).* These herbs are mixed with alcohol and tinctured.

Kasturadi Vati *(Charaka Samhita)* is made from **Kasturi** (deer musk / *Moschus moschiferus),* **Khadira extract** (catechu / *Acacia catechu,* white), **Sphutikarika** (purified alum), **Patram leaf** (Cassia cinnamon / *Cinnamomum tamala),* **Jatiphalam** (nutmeg / *Myristica fragrans),* **Lavangam seeds** (clove / *Syzigium aromaticum),* **Ela fruit** (greater cardamon / *Amomum subulatum),* **Sukshmaila seed** (cardamom / *Elettaria cardamomum),* **Nagakeshara seed** (Ironwood tree / *Mesua ferrea),* **Madhukam root** (licorice / *Glycyrrhiza glabra),* **Babbula bark** (gum arabic / *Acacia Arabica)* and **Patram leaf** (Cassia cinnamon / *Cinnamomum tamala).* In parts of the world where **deer musk** is not available or illegal because of the Musk deer's endangered status the pills can be made without it.

Krimighna Yoga *(Chakradatta)* is made from **Haritaki fruit** *(Terminalia chebula),* **Bibhitaki fruit** *(Terminalia belerica),* **Vacha rhizome** (acorus / *Acorus calamus),* **Kutaja bark** *(Holarrhena antidysenterica),* **Pippali fruit** (long pepper /

Piper longum), and **Maricham seed** (black pepper / *Piper nigrum)*, mixed with **Aja paya** (goat milk).

Krimimudgararasa Vati contains **Rasasindura** (red crystal of mercury sulphide), **Gandhaka Bhasma** (purified sulfur oxide), **Ajamoda seed** (wild celery / *Carum roxburghianum)*, **Vidanga seed** *(Embelia ribes)*, **Kuchila seed** (purified nux vomica /*Strychnos nuxvomica)* and **Hastikarnapalasa seed** (bastard teak / *Butea monosperma)*.

Krishna Vati *(Bhavaprakasha Samhita)* contains **Kumari** (aloe leaf gum extract / *Aloe barbadensis)*, **Maricham seed** (black pepper / *Piper nigrum)* and **Tankana Bhasma** (purified borax).

Kshyakesarirasa contains **Maricham seed** (black pepper / *Piper nigrum)*, **Sphutikarika** (purified alum), **Vatsanabha** (aconite tuber, purified / *Aconitum palmatum)*, and **Nrisara** (purified ammonium chloride).

Kushmandavaleha *(Bhaishajya Ratnavali)* contains a special preparation of **Kushmanda fruit** (wax gourd / *Benincasa hispida)*, **Ghrita** (clarified butter, **Madhu** (honey), and **Vetasa** (cane sugar / *Saccharum officinarum)* into which the following powders are added: **Pippali fruit** (long pepper / *Piper longum)*, **Shunthi root** (dry ginger / *Zingiber officinalis)*, **Jirakam seed** (cumin / *Cuminum cyminum)*, **Dhanyakam seed** (coriander / *Coriandrum sativum)*, **Patram leaf** (Cassia cinnamon / *Cinnamomum tamala)*, **Sukshmaila seed** (cardamom / *Elettaria cardamomum)*, **Maricham seed** (black pepper / *Piper nigrum)* and **Twak bark** (Cinnamon / *Cinnamomum zeylanicum)*.

Lauha Triphala *(Chakradatta)* is made by combining **Lauha Bhasma** (purified iron oxide) with **Triphala** *(Phyllanthus emblica / Terminalia belerica / Terminalia chebula)*.

Lauhasava *(Sharangadhara Samhita)* is a fermentation made from **Lauha Bhasma** (purified iron oxide), **Trikatu** *(Piper longum, Piper nigrum, Zingiber officinalis)*, **Triphala** *(Phyllanthus emblica / Terminalia belerica / Terminalia chebula)*, **Yavani seed** (wild omum / *Trachyspermum ammi)*, **Vidanga seed** *(Embelia ribes)*, **Mustaka tuber** *(Cyperus rotundus)*, **Chitraka root** (Leadwort, white flower / *Plumbago zeylanica)*, and **Madhu** (honey).

Lavanapanchakam contains **Samudram** (sea salt), **Saindhvam** (mineral salt), **Sauvarchalam** (black salt), **Romaka** (salt of Roma lake) and **Vidam** (salt made from Amalaki fruit - *Phyllanthus emblica)*.

Lavangadi Churna *(Chakradatta)* contains **Lavangam seeds** (clove / *Syzigium aromaticum)*, **Gajapippali fruit** *(Piper chaba)*, **Ushira root** *(Andropogon muricatum)*,

Chandanam wood (white sandalwood / *Santalum album*), Vamshalochana (Bamboo manna / *Bambusa breviflora*), Twak bark (Cinnamon / *Cinnamomum zeylanicum*), Patram leaf (Cassia cinnamon / *Cinnamomum tamala*), Sukshmaila seed (cardamom / *Elettaria cardamomum*), Nagakeshara seed (Ironwood tree / *Mesua ferrea*), Trikatu *(Piper longum, Piper nigrum, Zingiber officinalis)*, Utpala *(Nymphaea stellate)*, Jirakam seed (cumin / *Cuminum cyminum*), Krishnajiraka seed (black cumin / *Nigella sativa*), Agaru wood (eaglewood / *Aquilaria agallocha*), Padmam stamen (white lotus / *Nelumbo nucifera*), Tagara bark *(Erytania coronarea)*, Bilwa fruit (bael / *Aegle marmelos*), Hriverum plant *(Pavonia odorata)*, Karapura leaf (camphor / *Cinnamomum camphora*), Jatiphalam (nutmeg / *Myristica fragrans*), Bhringaraja plant *(Eclipta alba)*, and Vetasa (cane sugar / *Saccharum officinarum)*.

Maha Yogaraja Guggulu Vati *(Bhaishajya Ratnavali)* are made primarily from Guggulu gum resin *(Commiphora wightii)*, and Triphala *(Terminalia chebula, Terminalia belerica*, and *Emblica officinalis)*. Small amounts of the following herbs and purified minerals are also added: Nagaram rhizome (Indian cyperus / *Cyperus pertenuis)*, Pippali fruit (long pepper / *Piper longum)*, Chavyam stem *(Piper chaba)*, Pippali root (long pepper / *Piper longum)*, Chitraka root (leadwort, white flower / *Plumbago zeylanica)*, Hingu gum (asafoetida / *Ferula narthex)*, Ajamoda seed (wild celery / *Carum roxburghianum)*, Sarshapa seed (turnip / *Brassica campestris)*, Jirakam seed (cumin / *Cuminum cyminum)*, Krishnajiraka seed (black cumin / *Nigella sativa)*, Renuka fruit *(piper aurantiacum)*, Indrayava seed *(Holarrhena antidysenterica)*, Patha root *(Stephania hernandifolia)*, Vidanga seed *(Embelia ribes)*, Gajapippali fruit *(Scindapsus officinalis)*, Kutki rhizome (Indian gentian / *Picrorhiza kurroa)*, Ativisha tuber, purified (aconite / *Aconitum heterophyllum)*, Bhargi root (Turk's turban / *Clerodendron serratum)*, Vacha rhizome (acorus / *Acorus calamus)*, Murva plant *(Bauhinia vahlii)*, Vanga Bhasma (purified tin oxide), Rajata Bhasma (purified silver oxide), Naga Bhasma (purified lead oxide), Mandura Bhasma (purified iron ore oxide), Abhraka Bhasma (purified mica oxide), Lauha Bhasma (purified iron oxide), Rasasindura (red crystal of mercury sulphide).

Mahousadhayoga Anjana contains powders of Shunthi root (dry ginger / *Zingiber officinalis)*, Pippali fruit (long pepper / *Piper longum)*, and Musta tuber *(Cyperus rotundus)* mixed with juice of Matulunga fruit (Citron / *Citrus medica)*.

Mandura Vati contains Vasaka leaf (Malabar nut / *Adhatoda vasica)*, Shukti Bhasma (oyster shell ash / *Ostrea gigas)* and Mandura Bhasma (purified iron ore oxide).

Manduravataka contains **Vasaka leaf** (Malabar nut / *Adhatoda vasica*), **Shukti Bhasma** (oyster shell ash /*Ostrea gigas*), and **Mandura Bhasma** (purified iron ore oxide).

Manjishtha Chandana Kashaya *(Sushruta Samhita)* is a decoction made from **Manjishtha plant** (Indian madder / *Rubia cordifolia)* and **Chandanam wood** (white sandalwood / *Santalum album).*

Manohwa Yoga *(Sushruta Samhita)* contains **Manashila Bhasma** (purified realgar), **Kashisa** (ferrous sulfate), **Trikatu** *(Piper longum, Piper nigrum, Zingiber officinalis)*, **Rasanjana** (Daruharidra bark extract / *Berberis nepalensis)*, and **Saindhavam** (mineral salt), mixed with honey.

Mriddhika Kashaya *(Sushruta Samhita)* is a decoction made from **Triphala Churna** *(Phyllanthus emblica / Terminalia belerica / Terminalia chebula)* cooked with **Amalaki fruit** (Indian gooseberry / amla / *Phyllanthus emblica)* and **Draksha fruit** (grape / *Vitis vinifera).*

Mrigamadasava *(Arka Prakasha)* is an alcohol-based medicine made with **Pippali fruit** (long pepper / *Piper longum)*, **Maricham seed** (black pepper / *Piper nigrum)*, **Lavangam seeds** (clove / *Syzigium aromaticum)*, **Twak bark** (Cinnamon / *Cinnamomum zeylanicum)*, **Jatiphalam** (nutmeg / *Myristica fragrans)*, **Madhu** (honey), and **Kasturi** (deer musk / *Moschus moschiferus).*

Mrityunjayarasa Vati *(Bhavaprakasha Samhita)* is made from **Vatsanabha** (aconite tuber, purified / *Aconitum palmatum)*, **Gandhaka Bhasma** (purified sulfur oxide), **Pippali fruit** (long pepper / *Piper longum)*, **Maricham seed** (black pepper / *Piper nigrum)*, **Tankana Bhasma** (purified borax), and **Hingulu Bhasma** (cinnabar / purified red cinnabar sulphide), ground with the juice of **Adrakam root** (ginger / *Zingiber officinalis)* and made into pills.

Nagara Yoga *(Sushruta Samhita)* is made from **Nagaram rhizome** (Indian cyperus / *Cyperus pertenuis)*, **Sarshapi seed** (black mustard / *Sinapis juncea)*, **Triphala** *(Phyllanthus emblica / Terminalia belerica / Terminalia chebula)* and **Musta tuber** *(Cyperus rotundus)* mixed with **Daruharidra bark/extract** (barberry / *Berberis nepalensis).*

Narayana Taila *(Bhaishajya Ratnavali)* contains **Goukshira** (cow milk), **Shatavari root** (wild asparagus / *Asparagus racemosus)*, and **Tila seed oil** (sesame / *Sesamum indicum)*, along with small amounts of **Ashwagandha root** *(Convolvulus arvensis / Withania somnifera)*, **Bala root** (country mallow / *Sida cordifolia)*, **Bilwa fruit** (bael / *Aegle marmelos)*, **Patala root** *(Stereospermum personatum)*, **Brihati root** (vrihati / *Solanum indicum)*, **Kantakari herb** (Black nightshade / *Solanum* xanthocarpum), **Gokshura fruit** (*Tribulus terrestris*), **Atibala plant** *(Sida rhombifolia)*, **Nimba leaf** (neem / *Azadirachta indica*), **Shyonaka root** (Indian trumpet flower / *Oroxylon indicum*), **Punarnava root** *(Boerhavia difusa)*, **Agnimantha root** *(Premna integrifolia)*, **Kustha root** *(Saussurea lappa)*, **Ela fruit** (greater cardamon / *Amomum subulatum*), **Chandanam wood** (white sandalwood / *Santalum album*), **Jatamansi rhizome** (spikenard /*Nardostachys jatamansi*), **Saindhavam** (mineral salt), **Vacha rhizome** (acorus / *Acorus calamus*), **Rasna root/leaf** *(Vanda roxburghii)*, **Shatapushpa seed** (anise / *Pimpinella anisum*), **Devadaru wood** (Himalayan cedar / *Cedrus deodara*), **Shalaparni plant** *(Desmodium gangeticum)*, **Prishniparni plant** *(Uraria lagopoides)* and **Tagara bark** *(Erytania coronarea)*.

Narikela Lavanam *(Chakradatta)* is made by opening a hole in a **Narikela** (coconut / *Cocos nucifera)*, and putting in **Saindhavam** (mineral salt), then sealing and cooking.

Navarasa Vati *(Satmya Darpana)* contains **Abhraka Bhasma** (purified mica oxide), **Rasasindura** (red crystal of mercury sulphide), **Gandhaka Bhasma** (purified sulfur oxide), **Sukshmaila seed** (cardamom / *Elettaria cardamomum)*, **Nagakeshara seed** (ironwood tree / *Mesua ferrea)*, **Matshya bile** (fish bile), **Kumkumam stamen** (saffron / *Crocus sativum)*, **Praneshwara** (standard anti-fever compound), **Vamshalochana** (bamboo manna / *Bambusa breviflora)*, and **Kasturi** (deer musk / *Moschus moschiferus)*. Pills are made by grinding the formula with the juice of **Brahmi** (gotu kola / *Hydrocotyle asiatica /Centella asiatica)*.

Nimbadi is made from **Nimba leaf** (neem / *Azadirachta indica)*, **Vasaka leaf** (Malabar nut / *Adhatoda vasica)*, **Bibhitaki fruit** *(Terminalia belerica)*, and **Shukti Bhasma** (oyster shell ash /*Ostrea gigas)*.

Nimba Kashaya *(Sushruta Samhita)* is a decoction made from **Nimba leaf** (neem / *Azadirachta indica)* and taken with **Madhu** (honey).

Nishadi Taila *(Chakradatta)* is made from oil cooked with **Haridra root** (turmeric / *Curcuma longa)*, **Lodhram bark** *(Symplocos paniculata)*, **Priyangu seed** *(Prunus mahaleb)*, and **Madhukam root** (licorice / *Glycyrrhiza glabra)*.

Nyagrodhadi Kashaya *(Sushruta Samhita)* is a decoction made from **Pippali fruit** (long pepper / *Piper longum)*, **Arjuna bark** *(Terminalia arjuna)*, **Amrataka fruit** *(Spondias magnifera)*, **Madhukam root** (licorice / *Glycyrrhiza glabra)*, **Kutaki rhizome** (Indian gentian / *Picrorhiza kurroa)*, **Bhallataka** (marking nut tree / *Semecarpus anacardium)*, and **Palasha seed** (bastard teak / *Butea frondosa)* and any one of the herbs from the *Ficus* genus. These include **Udumbara** *(Ficus glomerata)*,

Vata bark (banyan tree / *Ficus bengalensis*) and **Ashwattha bark** (bodhi tree / *Ficus religiosa*).

Panchamulam ('five roots' compound) is comprised of equal parts **Bilwa root** (bael / *Aegle marmelos*), **Shyonaka root** (Indian trumpet flower / *Oroxylon indicum*), **Agnimantha root** *(Premna integrifolia)*, **Patala root** *(Stereospermum personatu)* and **Kashmari root** *(Gmelina arborea)*

Pippalyadi Churna is made from **Pippali fruit** (long pepper / *Piper longum*), **Haritaki fruit** *(Terminalia chebula)*, **Musta tuber** *(Cyperus rotundus)*, **Dhanyakam seeds** (coriander / *Coriandrum sativum*), **Shunthi root** (dry ginger / *Zingiber officinalis)* and **Vidam** (Salt made from **Amalaki fruit** - *Phyllanthus emblica*). This compound is more effective if given with **Nrisara** (purified ammonium chloride).

Pitaka Yoga *(Charaka Samhita)* is made from **Manashila Bhasma** (purified realgar), **Yavakshara alkaline ash** (barley plant / *Hordeum vulgare*), **Haritala Bhasma** (orpiment / purified yellow arsenic trisulphide), **Saindhavam** (mineral salt from Sindhu), and **Daruharidra bark extract** (barberry / *Berberis nepalensis*) mixed with honey and suspended in the scraped top layer of **Ghrita** (Ghee).

Pratisarana Yoga *(Sushruta Samhita)* is made from **Trikatu** *(Piper longum, Piper nigrum, Zingiber officinalis)*, **Saurvarchalam** (black salt), **Yavakshara alkaline ash** (barley plant / *Hordeum vulgare*), and **Sarjikakshara**(sodium bicarbonate). These ingredients are combined with honey and made into a paste.

Priyangu Yoga *(Sushruta Samhita)* is made from **Priyangu seed** *(Prunus mahaleb)*, **Triphala** *(Phyllanthus emblica / Terminalia belerica / Terminalia chebula)*, **Lodhram bark** *(Symplocos paniculata)* and honey.

Punarnavadi Yoga *(Chakradatta)* is made from **Punarnava plant/root** *(Boerhavia difusa)*, **Shunthi root** (dry ginger / *Zingiber officinalis*), **Trivrit root** (Indian rhubarb /*Operculina turpethum)*, **Guduchi stem** *(Tinospora cordifolia)*, **Rajavriksha** (Indian laburnum /*Cassia fistula)*, **Haritaki fruit** *(Terminalia chebula)*, and **Devadaru wood** (Himalayan cedar / *Cedrus deodara*) taken with **Guggulu gum resin** *(Commiphora wightii)* and **Goumutra** (cow urine).

Rajavriksha Kashaya *(Sushruta Samhita)* is the decoction of **Rajavriksha pod pulp** (Indian laburnum /*Cassia fistula)*.

Rasa Churna is made from 50 parts of **Twak bark** (cinnamon / *Cinnamomum zeylanicum)* and one part of **Rasakarpura** (white crystal of mercury sulphide / mineral camphore) ground in **Nimbu juice** (lemon / *Citrus limonium*). This compound is toxic and is only prescribed in small doses.

Rasanjana *(Chakradatta)* is made from a condensed extract of **Daruharidra bark** *(Berberis nepalensis)* or **Darvi root** *(Berberis asiatica)*.

Rasanjana Taila *(Sushruta Samhita)* is made from oil cooked with **Rasanjana** (condensed extract of **Daruharidra bark** - *Berberis nepalensis* or **Darvi root** - *Berberis asiatica)*, **Ativisha tuber, purified** (aconite / *Aconitum heterophyllum)*, and **Musta tuber** (nut grass / *Cyperus rotundus)*

Samudradi Churna *(Chakradatta)* is made from **Yavakshara alkaline ash** (barley plant / *Hordeum vulgare)*, **Lavanapanchakam** (the five salts), **Danti seed** *(Baliospermum montanum)*, **Lauha Bhasma** (purified iron oxide), **Mandura Bhasma** (purified iron ore oxide), **Trivrit root** (Indian rhubarb /*Operculina turpethum)*, **Shurana tuber** (telugo potato / *Amorphophallus campanulatus)*, and **Goumutra** (cow urine), mixed with **Dadhi** (yogurt) and **Goukshira** (cow milk).

Samudraphenanjanam *(Sushruta Samhita)* is made from **Samudraphenam** (sea foam / *Sepia species)*, **Saindhavam** (mineral salt from Sindhu), **Shankha Bhasma** (purified conch shell ash, *Turbinella pyrum)*, **Mudga bean** (mung bean / *Phaseolus mungo)*, and **Sobhanjan** *(Moringa oleifera)*.

Shadbindu Taila *(Bhaishajya Ratnavali)* contains **Bhringaraja juice** *(Eclipta alba)* with **Krishnatilam seed oil** (black sesame / *Sesamum indicum)* and **Aja paya** (goat milk). Small amounts of the following ingredients are added: **Eranda root** (Castor oil plant / *Ricinus communis)*, **Tagara stem** *(Erytania coronarea)*, **Shatapushpa seed** (anise / *Pimpinella anisum)*, **Jivanti root** *(Leptadenia reticulate)*, **Rasna root/leaf** *(Vanda roxburghii)*, **Saindhavam** (mineral salt from Sindhu), **Twak bark** (Cinnamon / *Cinnamon zeylanicum)*, **Vidanga seeds** *(Embelia ribes)*, **Madhukam root** (licorice / *Glycyrrhiza glabra)*, and **Shunthi root** (dry ginger / *Zingiber officinalis)*.

Shankha Vati contains **Yavani seed** (wild omum / *Trachyspermum ammi)*, **Saindhavam** (mineral salt), **Haritaki fruit** *(Terminalia chebula)*, **Shunthi root** (dry ginger / *Zingiber officinalis)*, **Shankha Bhasma** (purified conch shell ash, *Turbinella pyrum)*, **Maricham seed** (black pepper / *Piper nigrum)*, **Pippali fruit** (long pepper / *Piper longum)*, **Hingu gum** (asafoetida / *Ferula narthex)*, **Vidanga seed** *(Embelia ribes)*, **Vijaya leaf** (hemp / *Cannabis sativa)*, **Nagaram rhizome** (Indian cyperus / *Cyperus pertenuis)*, **Chitraka root** (Leadwort, white flower / *Plumbago zeylanica)*, **Dhanyakam seed** (coriander / *Coriandrum sativum)*, **Amalaki fruit** (Indian gooseberry / amla / *Phyllanthus emblica)* and **Ahiphenam seed** (poppy / *Papaver somniferum)*.

Sannipata Vairava Vati *(Sharangadhara Samhita)* contains **Rasasindura** (red crystal of mercury sulphide), **Gandhaka Bhasma** (purified sulfur oxide), **Abhraka Bhasma** (purified mica oxide), **Vanga Bhasma** (purified tin oxide), **Sobhanjan**

(Moringa oleifera), **Hemakshiri plant** (Swarnakshiri / *Argemone Mexicana)*, **Aparajita seed/root** (butterfly pea / *Clitoria ternatea)*, **Devadali herb** *(Luffa echinota)*, **Pippali fruit** (long pepper / *Piper longum)*, **Tagara bark** *(Erytania coronarea)*, **Jatamansi rhizome** (spikenard / *Valeriana jatamansi* / *Nardostachys jatamansi)* and **Tanduliyakam plant** *(Amaranthus polyganus)*.

Sariva paste *(Sushruta Samhita)* is made from **Sariva plant** *(Trachelospermum fragrans)*, **Utpala** (any type of lotus flower), **Madhukam root** (licorice / *Glycyrrhiza glabra)*, **Lodhram bark** *(Symplocos paniculata)*, **Agaru wood** (eaglewood / *Aquilaria agallocha)* and **Rakta Chandanam wood** (red sandalwood / *Pterocarpus santalinus)*.

Sarvajwaraharalauha Vati *(Bhavaprakasha Samhita)* contains **Lauha Bhasma** (purified iron oxide) with **Jatiphalam bark** (nutmeg / *Myristica fragrans)*, **Chitraka root** (Leadwort, white flower / *Plumbago zeylanica)*, **Trikatu** *(Piper longum, Piper nigrum, Zingiber officinalis)*, **Vidanga seed** *(Embelia ribes)*, **Musta tuber** *(Cyperus rotundus)*, **Gajapippali fruit** *(Scindapsus officinalis)*, **Pippalamulam** (long pepper root / *Piper longum)*, **Varuna bark** (Three-leaved caper / *Crataeva religiosa)*, **Devadaru wood** (Himalayan cedar / *Cedrus deodara)*, **Kiratatiktam plant** *(Swertia chirata)*, **Hriverum plant** *(Pavonia odorata)*, **Kutki rhizome** (Indian gentian / *Picrorhiza kurroa)*, **Kantakari herb** (Black nightshade / *Solanum xanthocarpum)*, **Sobhanjan** *(Moringa oleifera)*, **Madhukam root** (licorice / *Glycyrrhiza glabra)* **Kutaja bark** *(Holarrhena antidysenterica)* and **Indrayava seed** *(Holarrhena antidysenterica)*. Standard dosage is 2 pills twice daily.

Shambukadi Vati are made from **Shankha Bhasma** (purified conch shell ash, *Turbinella pyrum)*, **Maricham seed** (black pepper / *Piper nigrum)*, **Dhanyakam seeds** (coriander / *Coriandrum sativum)*, **Pippali fruit** (long pepper / *Piper longum)*, **Shunthi root** (dry ginger / *Zingiber officinalis)* **Jirakam seed** (cumin / *Cuminum cyminum)*, **Amalaki fruit** (Indian gooseberry / amla / *Phyllanthus emblica)*, **Hingu gum** (asafoetida / *Ferula narthex)*, **Saindhavam** (mineral salt), **Vidam** (Salt made from **Amalaki fruit**), and **Yavakshara alkaline ash** (barley plant / *Hordeum vulgare)*.

Shatavariyoga is made from **Shatavari root** (asparagus / *Asparagus racemosus)*, **Vacha rhizome** (acorus / *Acorus calamus)*, **Amalaki fruit** (Indian gooseberry / *Phyllanthus emblica)*, **Brahmi leaf/root** (gotu kola / *Centella asiatica)*, and **Ashwagandha root** *(Convolvulus arvensis / Withania somnifera)*.

Shatpala Ghrita contains **Pippali fruit** (long pepper / *Piper longum)*, **Pippalamulam** (long pepper root / *Piper longum)*, **Chavyam fruit** *(Piper chaba)*, **Kiratatiktam plant** *(Swertia chirata)*, **Shunthi root** (dry ginger / *Zingiber officinalis)*, **Yavakshara alkaline ash** (barley plant / *Hordeum vulgare)*, and

Saindhavam (mineral salt) cooked in **Goukshira** (cow milk) and **Ghrita** (Ghee / clarified butter).

Shatyadigana Churna *(Chakradatta)* contains **Karchura** (zedoary /*Curcuma zedoaria)*, **Pushkaram tuber** *(Inula racemosa)*, **Duralambha bush** *(Fragonia cretica)*, **Guduchi stem** *(Tinospora cordifolia)*, **Nagaram rhizome** (nut grass / *Cyperus pertenuis)*, **Patha root** *(Stephania hernandifolia)*, and **Kiratatiktam plant** *(Swertia chirata)*.

Shilajatu Rasayana contains **Shilajatu**, **Triphala** *(Phyllanthus emblica / Terminalia belerica / Terminalia chebula)*, **Guggulu gum resin** *(Commiphora wightii)*, and **Swarna Bhasma** (purified gold).

Shimshapa Kashaya *(Sushruta Samhita)* is the decoction of **Shimshapa bark** (rosewood / *Dalbergia sisso)*.

Shitarasa Vati *(Rasatarangini)* are made from **Shilajatu Rasayana**, **Daruharidra bark extract** (rasanjana / *Berberis nepalensis)*, **Shala resin** (sal tree /*Shorea robusta)*, and **Snigdhajeera seed** *(Plantago ovate)*.

Shrivestaka Yoga *(Sushruta Samhita)* is made from **Shala resin** (sal tree /*Shorea robusta)*, **Devadaru wood** (Himalayan cedar / *Cedrus deodara)*, **Guggulu gum resin** *(Commiphora wightii)*, and **Madhukam root** (licorice / *Glycyrrhiza glabra)*.

Siddhapraneshwar contains **Vamshalochana** (Bamboo manna / *Bambusa breviflora)*, **Abhraka Bhasma** (purified mica oxide), **Kajjali** (mercury powder ground with pure sulphur), and **Lavanapanchakam** (the five salts).

Shirashuladivajrarasa Vati contains **Guggulu gum resin** *(Commiphora wightii)*, **Rasasindura** (red crystal of mercury sulphide), **Gandhaka Bhasma** (purified sulfur oxide), **Lauha Bhasma** (purified iron oxide), **Tamra Bhasma** (purified copper oxide), **Triphala** *(Phyllanthus emblica / Terminalia belerica / Terminalia chebula)*, **Madhukam root** (licorice / *Glycyrrhiza glabra)*, **Trivrit root** (Indian rhubarb /*Operculina turpethum)*, **Pippali fruit** (long pepper / *Piper longum)*, **Shunthi root** (dry ginger / *Zingiber officinalis)*, **Gokshura fruit** *(Tribulus terrestris)*, **Vidanga seed** *(Embelia ribes)*, **Agnimantha** *(Premna integrifolia)*, **Bilwa root** (bael / *Aegle marmelos)*, **Shyonaka** (Indian trumpet flower / *Oroxylon indicum)*, **Patala root/bark** *(Stereospermum personatum)*, **Kashmari** *(Gmelina arborea)*, **Shalaparni plant** *(Desmodium gangeticum)*, **Prishniparni plant** *(Uraria lagopoides)*, **Brihati shrub** (vrihati / *Solanum indicum)*, and **Kantakari herb** (Black nightshade / *Solanum xanthocarpum)*.

Sitopaladi Churna *(Charaka Samhita)* is made from **Twak bark** (Cinnamon / *Cinnamomum zeylanicum)*, **Sukshmaila seed** (cardamom / *Elettaria cardamomum)*, **Pippali fruit** (long pepper / *Piper longum)*, **Vamshalochana** (Bamboo manna / *Bambusa breviflora)*, and **Vetasa** (cane sugar / *Saccharum officinarum)*.

Sringarabhraka Yoga contains **Mrigashringa horn ash** (deer / *Cervus Nippon)* and **Abhraka Bhasma** (purified mica oxide) as the main ingredients. It also contains **Karapura leaf** (camphor / *Cinnamomum camphora)*, **Jatiphalam seed** (nutmeg / *Myristica fragrans)*, **Jatiphalam bark** (nutmeg / *Myristica fragrans)*, **Hriverum plant** *(Pavonia odorata)*, **Gajapippali fruit** *(Scindapsus officinalis)*, **Twak bark** (Cinnamon / *Cinnamomum zeylanicum)*, **Jambu seeds** *(Syzygium jambolanum)*, **Jatamansi rhizome** (spikenard / *Nardostachys jatamansi)*, **Rohitaka stem** (rhododendron / *Rhododendron arboretum)*, **Patram leaf** (Cassia cinnamon / *Cinnamomum tamala)*, **Nagakeshara seed** (Ironwood tree / *Mesua ferrea)*, **Kustha root** *(Saussurea lappa)*, **Dhataki flower** *(Woodfordia fruticosa)*, **Triphala** *(Terminalia chebula, Terminalia belerica, Phyllanthus emblica)*, **Trikatu** *(Piper longum, Piper nigrum, Zingiber officinalis)*, **Sukshmaila seed** (cardamom / *Elettaria cardamomum)*, **Gandhaka Bhasma** (purified sulfur oxide), and **Kajjali** (mercury powder ground with pure sulphur for purification).

Sudarshana contains **Kiratatiktam plant** *(Swertia chirata)* as the major ingredient (about one third), along with **Triphala** *(Phyllanthus emblica / Terminalia belerica / Terminalia chebula)*, **Haridra root** (turmeric / *Curcuma longa)*, **Daruharidra bark/extract** (barberry / *Berberis nepalensis)*, **Brihati shrub** (vrihati / *Solanum indicum)*, **Kantakari herb** (Black nightshade / *Solanum xanthocarpum)*, **Karchura tuber/seed** (Zedoary /*Curcuma zedoaria)*, **Trikatu** *(Piper longum, Piper nigrum, Zingiber officinalis)*, **Pippalamulam** (long pepper root / *Piper longum)*, **Murva plant** *(Bauhinia vahlii)*, **Guduchi stem** *(Tinospora cordifolia)*, **Duralambha bush** *(Fragonia cretica)*, **Kutki rhizome** (Indian gentian / *Picrorhiza kurroa)*, **Parpata herb** *(Fumaria indica)*, **Musta tuber** *(Cyperus rotundus)*, **Hriverum plant** *(Pavonia odorata)*, **Nimba leaf** (neem / *Azadirachta indica)*, **Pushkaram tuber** *(Inula racemosa / Iris germanica)*, **Madhukam root** (licorice / *Glycyrrhiza glabra)*, **Indrayava seed** *(Holarrhena antidysenterica)*, **Kutaja bark** *(Holarrhena antidysenterica)*, **Bhargi root resin** (Turk's turban / *Clerodendron serratum)*, **Sobhanjan seed** *(Moringa oleifera)*, **Sphutikarika** (purified alum), **Vacha rhizome** (acorus / *Acorus calamus)*, **Twak bark** (Cinnamon / *Cinnamomum zeylanicum)*, **Padmakam heartwood** *(Betula alnoides)*, **Ushira root** *(Andropogon muricatum)*, **Chandanam wood** (white sandalwood / *Santalum album)*, **Ativisha tuber, purified** (aconite / *Aconitum heterophyllum)*, **Bala plant** (country mallow / *Sida cordifolia)*, **Shalaparni plant** *(Desmodium gangeticum)*, **Prishniparni plant** *(Uraria lagopoides)*, **Vidanga seed** *(Embelia ribes)*, **Tagara bark** *(Erytania coronarea)*, **Chitraka root** (Leadwort, white flower / *Plumbago zeylanica)*, **Devadaru wood** (Himalayan cedar / *Cedrus deodara)*, **Gajapippali fruit** *(Piper chaba)*, **Patram leaf** (Cassia cinnamon /

Cinnamomum tamala), **Patola leaf** *(Trichosanthes dioica)*, **Jivaka bulb** (wild garlic / *Allium wallichii,* small), **Lavangam seeds** (clove / *Syzigium aromaticum)*, **Vamshalochana** (Bamboo manna / *Bambusa breviflora)*, **Padmam plant** (lotus / *Nelumbo nucifera)*, **Kakoli bulb** *(Fritillaria cirrhosa)*, **Palasha seed** (bastard teak / *Butea frondosa)*, **Jatiphalam seed/bark** (nutmeg / *Myristica fragrans)* and **Rohitaka stem** (rhododendron / *Rhododendron arboretum)*. Standard dosage is 1-2 grams twice daily.

Sukhavativarti *(Chakradatta)* is made from **Kataka fruit** *(Strychnos potatorum)*, **Shankha Bhasma** (purified conch shell ash, *Turbinella pyrum)*, **Trikatu** *(Piper longum, Piper nigrum, Zingiber officinalis)*, **Saindhavam** (mineral salt), **Vetasa** (cane sugar / *Saccharum officinarum)*, **Samudraphenam** (sea foam / *Sepia species)*, **Rasanjana** (extract of *Berberis nepalensis)*, **Madhu** (honey), **Vidanga seed** *(Embelia ribes)*, **Manashila Bhasma** (purified realgar), and **Kukkuta andam** (chicken egg shell).

Shulanirmulanarasa Vati are made from **Trikatu** *(Piper longum, Piper nigrum, Zingiber officinalis)*, **Gandhaka Bhasma** (purified sulfur oxide), **Shankha Bhasma** (purified conch shell ash, *Turbinella pyrum)*, **Saindhavam** (mineral salt), **Rasasindura** (red crystal of mercury sulphide), **Jirakam seed** (cumin / *Cuminum cyminum)*, **Amlavetasa root** (rhubarb / *Rheum emodi)* and **Kuchila seed** (purified nux vomica /*Strychnos nuxvomica)* ground with **Adrakam juice** (ginger / *Zingiber officinalis)*.

Surasadigana *(Sushruta Samhita)* contains **Dronapuspi herb** *(Leucus cephalotus)*, **Kasamarda plant** *(Cassia sophera)*, **Vidanga seed** *(Embelia ribes)*, **Tulsi plant** (holy basil / *Ocimum sanctum)*, **Kuchila seed** (nux vomica /*Strychnos nuxvomica)*, **Nirgundi plant** *(Vitex negundo,* white), **Mushikaparni root/rhizome** *(Ipomoea reniformis)*, and **Bhargi root/resin** (Turk's turban / *Clerodendron serratum)*.

Talishadyam Churna *(Chakradatta)* contains **Talisham leaf** (rhododendron / *Rhododendron setosum)*, **Maricham seed** (black pepper / *Piper nigrum)*, **Shunthi root** (dry ginger / *Zingiber officinalis)*, **Pippali fruit** (long pepper / *Piper longum)*, **Twak bark** (Cinnamon / *Cinnamomum zeylanicum)* and **Ela fruit** (greater cardamon / *Amomum subulatum)* mixed with **Vetasa** (cane sugar / *Saccharum officinarum)*.

Tinduksthi Kashmarya *(Sushruta Samhita)* is made from **Tinduka bark** *(Dyospyros cordifolia)*, **Madhukam root** (licorice / *Glycyrrhiza glabra)* and **Kashmari bark** *(Gmelina arborea)*

Trikatu contains **Pippali fruit** (long pepper / *Piper longum)*, **Maricham fruit** (black pepper / *Piper nigrum)*, and **Shunthi root** (dry ginger / *Zingiber officinalis)*.

Trikaturasayana Vati are made from **Gandhaka Bhasma** (purified sulfur oxide), **Jirakam seed** (cumin / *Cuminum cyminum)*, **Saindhavam** (mineral salt), **Trikatu** *(Piper longum, Piper nigrum, Zingiber officinalis)*, **Hingu gum** (asafoetida / *Ferula narthex)* and **Lashunam bulb** (garlic / *Allium sativum)*, ground with **Nimbu juice** (lemon / *Citrus limonium)*.

Triphala is the classic formula comprised of the three rejuvenating fruits: **Amalaki** *(Phyllanthus emblica)*, **Bibhitaki** *(Terminalia belerica)*, and **Haritaki** *(Terminalia chebula)*. It can be prepared as a Churna (powder) or as an aqueous extract, and is commonly fond as an ingredient in many other formulas.

Triphala Guggulu Vati are made from **Guggulu gum resin** *(Commiphora wightii)*, **Triphala,** and **Pippali fruit** (long pepper / *Piper longum)*.

Triphaladi Ghritam *(Bhaishajya Ratnavali)* is made with **Triphala, Vasaka leaf** (Malabar nut / *Adhatoda vasica)*, **Bhringaraja plant** *(Eclipta alba)*, **Shatavari root** (asparagus / *Asparagus racemosus)*, **Guduchi stem** *(Tinospora cordifolia)*, **Amalaki fruit** (Indian gooseberry / amla / *Phyllanthus emblica)* and **Aja paya** (goat milk). Other herbs added in small measure are **Maricham seed** (black pepper / *Piper nigrum)*, **Draksha fruit** (grape / *Vitis vinifera)*, **Chandanam wood** (white sandalwood / *Santalum album)*, **Saindhavam** (mineral salt), **Bala plant** (country mallow / *Sida cordifolia)*, **Kakoli bulb** *(Fritillaria cirrhosa)*, **Pippali fruit** (long pepper / *Piper longum)*, **Shunthi root** (dry ginger / *Zingiber officinalis)*, **Vetasa** (cane sugar / *Saccharum officinarum)*, **Padmam** (white lotus / *Nelumbo nucifera)*, **Nilotpalam flower** (Blue lotus / *Iris nepalensis)*, **Punarnava plant/root** *(Boerhavia difusa)*, **Daruharidra bark extract** (barberry / *Berberis nepalensis)*, **Haridra root** (turmeric / *Curcuma longa)*, **Madhukam root** (licorice / *Glycyrrhiza glabra)* and **Ghrita** (Ghee / clarified butter). It is typically taken with milk as an anupana.

Ushakadigana contains **Shilajatu complex**, **Saindhavam** (mineral salt), **Kashisa** (ferrous sulfate), **Hingu gum** (asafoetida / *Ferula narthex)*, and **Tutthakam Bhasma** (purified copper sulphate).

Vachadiyoga Churna *(Sushruta Samhita)* is made from **Vacha rhizome** (acorus / *Acorus calamus)*, **Shatavari root** (asparagus / *Asparagus racemosus)* and **Amalaki fruit** (Indian gooseberry / amla / *Phyllanthus emblica)*.

Vakuchyadi Vati *(Chakradatta)* contains **Vakuchi seed** *(Psoralia corylifolia)*, **Khadira extract** (catechu / *Acacia catechu*, white), and **Bibhitaki fruit** *(Terminalia belerica)*.

Varunadigana *(Sushruta Samhita)* is a solidified decoction containing **Varuna bark** (Three-leaved caper / *Crataeva religiosa*), **Sobhanjan** *(Moringa oleifera)*, **Agnimantha** *(Premna integrifolia)*, **Apamarga herb** *(Achyranthes aspera)*, **Gajapippali fruit** *(Piper chaba)*, **Shatavari root** (asparagus / *Asparagus racemosus)*, and **Bilwa fruit** (bael / *Aegle marmelos).*

Vatakulantakrasa is made from **Manashila Bhasma** (purified realgar), **Rasasindura** (red crystal of mercury sulphide), **Gandhaka Bhasma** (purified sulfur oxide), **Jatiphalam** (nutmeg / *Myristica fragrans)*, **Ela fruit** (greater cardamon / *Amomum subulatum)*, **Lavangam seeds** (clove / *Syzigium aromaticum)*, **Abhraka Bhasma** (purified mica oxide), and **Bibhitaki fruit** *(Terminalia belerica)*. This compound is more powerful when taken with **Kasturi** (deer musk / *Moschus moschiferus).*

Vishamajwarahara Vati *(Rasatarangini)* contains one part **Shankha Visha Bhasma** (arsenic) with 100 parts of **Latakaranja seed /** *(Caesalpinia sepiaria)*. This medicine is poisonous, and used only for a short period of time.

Vishatinduka Taila is made from **Kuchila seed** (purified nux vomica */Strychnos nuxvomica)* and **Tila seed oil** (sesame / *Sesamum indicum).*

Yavaniyoga contains **Bibhitaki fruit** *(Terminalia belerica)*, **Gandhaka Bhasma** (purified sulfur oxide), **Shukti Bhasma** (oyster shell ash */Ostrea gigas)*, **Kiratatiktam plant** *(Swertia chirata)*, **Swarnapatri leaf** (senna / *Cassia auriculata)* and **Amalaki fruit** (Indian gooseberry / amla / *Phyllanthus emblica)*

Treatment with Rasayana

The branch of Ayurveda called Rasayana Tantra (health and longevity division) developed many restorative medicines, both individual herbs as well as formulas, all of which have wide medical applications. That is, they can be used with great benefit for many diseases, over a long period of time, and virtually without side effects. Some of these do contain purified metals, which may be considered toxic or illegal for clinical use in different jurisdictions. Examples of Rasayana herbs and minerals include:

1. **Abhraka Bhasma** (purified mica oxide).
2. **Agaru wood** (eaglewood / krishnagaru / *Aquilaria agallocha).*
3. **Amalaki fruit** (Indian gooseberry / amla / *Phyllanthus emblica).*
4. **Ashwagandha root** *(Convolvulus arvensis / Withania somnifera).*
5. **Bala plant** (country mallow / *Sida cordifolia).*
6. **Brahmi leaf/root** (gotu kola / *Hydrocotyle asiatica /Centella asiatica).*
7. **Dadima rind** (pomegranate / *Punica granatum).*

8. **Gandhaka Bhasma** (purified sulfur oxide).
9. **Gokshura fruit** *(Tribulus terrestris).*
10. **Guduchi stem** *(Tinospora cordifolia).*
11. **Guggulu gum resin** *(Commiphora wightii).*
12. **Haritaki fruit** (chebulic myrobalan / *Terminalia chebula).*
13. **Kasturi** (deer musk / *Moschus moschiferus).*
14. **Lauha Bhasma** (purified iron oxide).
15. **Madhukam root** (licorice / *Glycyrrhiza glabra).*
16. **Shatavari root** (asparagus / *Asparagus racemosus).*
17. **Shilajatu Rasayana**.
18. **Vanga Bhasma** (purified tin oxide).
19. **Bibhitaki fruit** *(Terminalia belerica).*

Commonly Used Rasayana Formulas
1. **Alarasayana.**
2. **Chandanadi Churna.**
3. **Gokshuradi Guggulu Vati**.
4. **Kaishora Guggulu Vati.**
5. **Kanchanara Guggulu Vati.**
6. **Shilajatu Triphala Vati** (**Shilajatu** with **Triphala**).
7. **Trikatu Vati** *(Piper longum, Piper nigrum, Zingiber officinalis).*
8. **Triphala Vati** *(Phyllanthus emblica / Terminalia belerica / Terminalia chebula).*
9. **Triphala Guggulu Vati.**
10. **Yogaraja Guggulu Vati.**

Rasayana Formula Differentiation
While all the above Rasayana medicines can be used for longevity and good health, many of these as well as others also have special applications, listed as follows:

Anti-cancer Rasayanas - Chandraprabha Vati, Kaishora Guggulu Vati, Guggulu gum resin, Shilajatu Triphala Vati, Shilajatu Rasayana, and Kanchanara Guggulu Vati.

Anti-toxin Rasayanas - Chandraprabha Vati, Kaishora Guggulu Vati, Guduchi stem, Madhukam root, Shilajatu Rasayana, Gandhaka Bhasma and Bibhitaki fruit.

Blood Rasayanas - Dadima rind, Shilajatu Rasayana, Abhraka Bhasma, Vanga Bhasma and Alarasayana.

Bowel Rasayanas – Haritaki fruit and Triphala Vati.

Brain Rasayanas - Shilajatu Rasayana, Vanga Bhasma, Kasturi, Brahmi, Shatavari root, and Ashwagandha root.

Complex disease (Sannipata) Rasayanas – Any of the Guggulu or Shilajatu compounds, and Chandraprabha Vati.

Digestive Rasayanas – Haritaki fruit and Trikatu Vati.

Energy Rasayanas - Shilajatu Triphala Vati, Bala plant, Ashwagandha root, and Chandanadi Churna.

Eye Rasayanas – Triphala Vati, Shatavari root, and Punarnava root

Heart Rasayanas – Amalaki fruit, Kasturi, Abhraka Bhasma, Vatakulantaka Rasa, Shatavari root, and Guduchi stem.

Kidney Rasayanas - Shilajatu Rasayana, Shilajatu Triphala Vati, Kaishora Guggulu Vati, Chandraprabha Vati, and Shitarasa Vati.

Liver Rasayanas – Kaishora Guggulu Vati, Chandraprabha Vati, Shilajatu Rasayana, Lauha Bhasma, Guggulu gum resin, and Guduchi stem.

Lung Rasayanas - Amalaki fruit and Chyavanaprasha

Nerve Rasayanas – Yogaraja Guggulu Vati, Ashwagandha root, Bala plant, Agaru wood, Shatavari root, Gokshura with Ashwaghanda.

Skin Rasayanas – Haritala Bhasma, Kaishora Guggulu Vati, Gandhaka Bhasma, Alarasayana, and Nimbadi.

Throat Rasayana - Madhukam root (chewed).

Urinary system Rasayanas - Gokshuradi Guggulu Vati, Vanga Bhasma, and Chandanadi Churna

Diagnosis and Treatment

Chapter 10: Classification and Treatment of Disease

This section gives a complete overview of the understanding of disease etiology in Ayurveda, i.e. how diseases are grouped and then differentiated according to the principles of proper treatment. There are about 700 diseases identified according to the theory of Tridosha Siddhanta, following the categories established in the *Charaka Samhita* and *Sushruta Samhita*, and expanded by later texts such as the *Madhava Nidana* (circa 700 CE).

Based upon this, and after more than 40 years of clinical medical practice, I have found a congruence between the classical diseases described in Ayurveda and various diseases described in Western medicine. The process of establishing theses correlations began in the 1950's and continued until the writing of this book. I use the term 'congruence' because an exact concordance between Ayurveda and Western medicine is not possible, although many connections between them can be made. In 1996 an American board-certified ophthalmologist reviewed my text on the treatment of eye disease, and the medical terms assigned to the set of symptoms described in Ayurveda was found to be highly accurate.

There are several issues necessary to fully understand this process of disease classification. In some cases the disease described in Ayurveda is so closely identical to a Western medical disease that there is no question as to its equivalency. Arthritis of the hand (Viswachi) is a good example. In other cases the diseases are similar enough that a congruency better describes this relationship. For example, many fevers in Ayurveda share symptoms with specific types of fever encountered in modern medicine, but there is no certainty that the viral or bacterial agents identified in modern disease are also the cause of these fevers in Ayurveda. In some cases a single Western disease is divided by Ayurveda into several groups, and vice versa. As well, there are diseases in Ayurveda that have no Western equivalent, such as Abhicharaja Jwara, defined as a fever caused by black magic. In this case the disease can only be given a descriptive term.

In addition to this system of classification, brief descriptions of each disease and standard methods of treatment are also presented. These general descriptions of the treatments methods used for specific diseases will mention specific treatments and/or the general categories of herbs to use, such as digestive herbs (page 173) or antipyretic herbs (page 154).

For many diseases, proper treatment requires the use of specific treatments or formulas combined with the standard treatments for Vata, Pitta, and Kapha. Normally, the choice of which general and specific treatments to choose from, as well as the order in which to use them, depends upon the skill and judgment of the physician. For example, if a standard herbal formula is given for bronchitis, one method is to combine some Vata-reducing herbs to the formula if it is Vataja bronchitis, Pitta-reducing herbs if it is Pittaja bronchitis, and Kapha-reducing herbs if it is a Kaphaja bronchitis. It is also possible to use standard formula(s) alone, or to use both standard and specific treatments side by side.

Chapter 11: Treatment of Fever (Jwara Roga)

According to Ayurveda, the generator of the bodily temperature is located in the forehead. In Ayurveda, a disturbance to the regulation of body temperature is called Jwara, which is correlated to the medical concept of fever. In most cases fever relates to a situation of diminished heat inside the stomach (i.e. the Amashaya), and a high peripheral temperature. According to Ayurveda, fever can either be a disease or a symptom of another disease. As a disease fever is classified into eight categories, including Vata, Pitta, Kapha, Vata-Pitta, Vata-Kapha, Pitta-Kapha, Vata-Pitta-Kapha, and Aghantuja. Fever as a symptom is found in infectious diseases or diseases classified with the character of Pitta.

General Rules for Fever Management

In general, fasting or light food is recommended at the beginning stage of all fevers except those of Vata character. Fasting stimulates the stomach to draw heat away from the periphery to the center by increasing the digestive fire (i.e. Agni).

Warm water is prescribed to drink except for fevers with the character of Pitta, and is beneficial to maintain the balance of heat inside the stomach. Useful foods in the management of fever include a warm liquid diet including barley, sago or vegetable soup. Anything that is astringent in taste is prohibited to take at the beginning stages of fever.

The prescription of antipyretic medicines (page 154) is prohibited during the beginning stages of a fever. Such cooling medicines lower the temperature inside the stomach, defeating the primary strategy to restore the digestive fire. It is permitted, however, to use other types of antipyretic remedies made from poisonous plants or minerals, or to prescribe cooling herbs along with digestive or appetizing remedies (page 173). The word 'poison' in Ayurveda means an agent that quickly penetrates into the body without needing to be digested, and poisonous antipyretic medicines thus do not weaken the digestive fire in order to be effective. The addition of digestive and appetizing agents (page 173) to an herbal formula will neutralize the weakening effect of cooling herbs on digestion.

General Therapies in the Treatment of Fever

The standard compound used to treat fever is **Sudarshana Churna**, which is found in the classic text the *Bhaishajya Ratnavali*, taken in doses of 1-2 grams twice daily. In addition to the other treatments mentioned here, this formula can be used to treat almost any type of fever. Another simple fever treatment is **Vasaka leaf** (*Adhatoda vasica*) mixed with 10% **Shukti Bhasma** (oyster shell ash /*Ostrea gigas*), taken in doses of 1-2 grams twice daily with warm water.

Vataja Jwara (Seasonal Fever of the Monsoon)

Fever with the character of Vata is concerned with the aggravated function or the loss of control of the nervous system. Symptoms include excited or throbbing pulse, shivering, fluctuating fever, dry lips and throat, a feeling of generalized dryness, body ache, an astringent taste in the mouth, and yawning. It is common in the monsoon season (after summer), during the Vata times of day in the morning and afternoon, and after digestion. Other causes for Vataja fever include the suppression of natural urges (e.g. defecation, urination, flatus, sleep), in mental agony and depression, excessive exercise, the misuse of laxatives, and the overconsumption of foods with an astringent, bitter and pungent taste. Although Vataja fever is easy to treat, this same type of fever when found in another season is more difficult to cure.

Vataja fever is treated with general treatments and diet to reduce Vata (page 56) along with antipyretic herbs (page 154). A typical formula for treating Vataja fever is **Sudarshana Churna**, 1-2 grams twice daily. Based on signs and symptoms, treatment can be modified by using specific herbs such as **Nagarmotha** *(Cyperus rotundus)* and **Pippali** *(Piper longum)* or a decoction of **Guduchi** *(Tinospora cordifolia)* and **Punarnava** *(Boerhavia difusa)*.

Pittaja Jwara (Seasonal Fever of Autumn)

Jwara with the character of Pitta is concerned with the aggravated function of the venous system. Symptoms include a high fever, burning sensations, dizziness, diarrhea, nausea or vomiting, sweating, and a bitter taste in mouth, all of which are more prominent during mid-day, or in the middle of the night. Pitta fever is caused by factors including excessive exercise, excessive exposure to heat, fire or the sun, and the excessive consumption of pungent and salty foods and beverages, including alcohol. It is common during the season following the Monsoon season called Sharat, as well as in summer, and is easy to cure. If however the same fever occurs in a different season it becomes more difficult to cure.

Pitta fever treated with general treatments and diet to reduce Pitta (page 67) along with general antipyretic herbs (page 154). Specific formulations include equal parts **Sudarshana Churna** and **Chandanadi vasa yoga**, given in doses of 1-2 grams twice daily. Another simple formulation is equal parts **Kutki rhizome** *(Picrorhiza kurroa)* and **Indrayava seed** *(Holarrhena antidysenterica)*, 1-2 grams twice daily, taken with honey.

Kaphaja Jwara (Seasonal Fever of Spring)

Jwara with the character of Kapha is concerned with the aggravated function of the arterial system. Symptoms include a feeling of heaviness, lethargy, coldness, nausea, difficult respiration, a sweet taste in the mouth, and whitish discoloration of the eyes, all of which are more prominent mid-morning and evening. Kapha fever is common in the Spring and is easy to cure, but if this same fever occurs during another season, however, it becomes difficult to cure. It is caused by the excessive consumption of cold foods and beverages, foods and beverages with a sweet, sour or salty taste, sleeping during the day, and a lack of physical exercise. Kaphaja fever is treated with general treatments and diet to reduce Kapha (page 77) along with the general antipyretic medicines (page 154). Herbal therapy for Kapha fever includes **Sudarshana Churna**, as well as specific herbs such as **Amalaki fruit** *(Phyllanthus emblica)*, **Haritaki fruit** *(Terminalia chebula)* and **Chitraka herb** *(Plumbago zeylanica)*.

Vata-Pittaja Jwara (Paratyphoid fever type A)

Jwara with the characters of Vata and Pitta is concerned with the aggravated functions of the nervous and venous systems, manifesting symptoms including headache, joint pain, burning sensation thirst, and dizziness. It is curable with effort, treated with combined Vata and Pitta treatments and diet (page 81) along with the general antipyretic medicines (page 154). Typical herbal therapy includes **Sudarshana Churna**, or a simple formula such as equal parts **Shunthi rhizome** *(Zingiber officinalis)*, **Guduchi vine** *(Tinospora cordifolia)*, **Nagarmotha rhizome** *(Cyperus rotundus)*, and **Kiratatiktam plant** *(Swertia chirata)*.

Vata-Kaphaja Jwara (Paratyphoid fever type B)

Jwara with the character of Vata and Kapha is concerned with the aggravated functions of the nervous and arterial systems, manifesting symptoms including heaviness of body, headache, cold, cough, and a slow fever. It is curable with effort. It is treated with combined Vata and Kapha methods and diet (page 81) along with the general antipyretic medicines (page 154). Useful herbal therapies include equal parts **Sudarshana Churna** and **Mrityunjayarasa Vati**, 1-2 grams, taken with honey. Other useful herbs include **Pippali fruit** *(Piper longum)*, **Pippalamula root** *(Piper longum)*, **Chavyam fruit/stem** *(Piper chaba)*, **Chitraka herb** *(Plumbago zeylanica)*, and **Nagaram rhizome** (nut grass / *Cyperus pertenuis)*.

Pitta-Kaphaja Jwara (Paratyphoid fever type C)

Jwara with the character of Pitta and Kapha is concerned with the aggravated functions of the venous and arterial systems, manifesting symptoms including coldness, sweating, loss of appetite, bitter taste, and drowsiness. It is curable with effort. It is treated with the combined Pitta and Kapha treatments and diet (page 81), along with along with the general antipyretic remedies (page 154). Useful herbs include **Guduchi vine** *(Tinospora cordifolia)*, **Neem leaf** *(Azadirachta indica)*, **Dhanyakam seed** (coriander / *Coriandrum sativum)*, **Padmakam heartwood** *(Betula alnoides)*, and **Chandanam wood** (white sandalwood / *Santalum album)*.

Vata-Pitta-Kapha (Sannipataja) Jwara (Typhoid Fever)

Jwara with the character of Sannipata is concerned with the simultaneous aggravated function of the nervous, venous, and arterial systems. Symptoms may include a high fever, with alternating feelings of heat and cold, joint pain, headache, red eyes, sore throat, dry tongue, physical exhaustion, infrequent defecation and urination, burning sensation, and a heavy feeling. If all the symptoms develop then it is difficult to cure, but if only some develop the patient will get better quickly. If there is lymphatic swelling in the armpit or parotid involvement then it is considered to be fatal, as this is the last symptom of sannipata fever. In regards to the treatment of this sort of complicated fever, Ayurveda points out that the Kapha system (arterial function and mucus) has to be controlled as soon as possible with Kapha treatments and diet along with the specific herbal formulas against typhoid fever. Once this is accomplished, it is found that the aggravated functions of the nervous and venous systems are easier to control with appropriate herbal formulas. Traditional physicians report that the specific formulas against typhoid fever have clear therapeutic value for control of the fever and its complications, although the effect is not powerful enough for a complete cure. Treatments based upon the theory of balance combined with specific medicine formulations side by side is the most effective way to treat typhoid fever.

Some specific formulas against typhoid fever:

1. **Shatyadigana Churna**, 1-2 grams twice daily.
2. **Brihatyadigana Churna**, 1-2 grams twice daily.
3. **Navarasa Vati**, 2 pills twice daily.
4. **Sudarshana Churna**, 1-2 grams twice daily.
5. **Sannipata Vairava Vati**, 2 pills twice daily.

Aghantuja Jwara (Externally Caused Fever)

Externally caused fever (Aghantuja) is classified into four groups: Abhighataja, Abhicharaja, Abhishapaja, and Abhisangaja.

Abhighataja Jwara (Traumatic fever)

Traumatic fever or fever caused by injuries is concerned with the aggravated function of the nervous system. It is treated with the methods used for monsoon seasonal fever (see page 148).

Abhicharaja Jwara (Fever caused by black magic)

Fever caused by black magic develops the same symptoms as typhoid fever. Spiritual healing is the correct remedy for it. The regular medicines of typhoid fever worsen the symptoms.

Abhishapaja Jwara (Fever caused by curse)

Fever caused by a curse develops the same symptoms of typhoid fever. Spiritual healing is the remedy for it. The regular medicines against typhoid fever worsen the symptoms.

Abhisangaja Jwara (Fever caused by emotion, poison, pollen and/or unseen biological forces)

There are several subdivisions within this group. Fevers caused by emotion are called either Kamaja, Shokaja, Bhayaja, and Krodhaja. A fever caused by poison is called Vishaja. Hay fever caused by pollen is called Osadhigandhaja. Fever caused by unseen biological forces is called Bhutaja.

Kamaja Jwara (Fever caused by romantic/sexual desire)

Kamaja fever is caused by romantic desires and/or excessive sexual arousal, causing symptoms including mental disturbance, emotional intoxication, tiredness, loss of appetite, and pain in the heart. Stimulating anger in the patient or advising sexual intercourse are the main remedies. It can also be treated the same as fever with the character of Vata (see page 148).

Shokaja Jwara (Fever caused by grief)

Fever caused by grief develops from tragedy among family and friends due to excessive emotional attachment, causing symptoms including crying, weeping, muttering along with typical Vataja symptoms. Sex and/or inducement to anger are the remedies for it. It is also treated with the methods for seasonal monsoon fever (see page 148).

Bhayaja Jwara (Fever caused by fear)

Fever caused by fear develops from situations in which the patient has experienced great fear, manifesting as typical Vataja symptoms including shivering and muttering to oneself. Sex or inducement to anger (or both) are the remedies for Bhayaja fever. It is also treated with the methods used for seasonal monsoon fever (see page 148).

Krodhaja Jwara (Fever caused by anger)

Fever caused by anger is caused by the expression of angry emotions, manifesting as typical Pitta symptoms including redness of face and excessive muscle tension. Sexual activity will cure it, or it can be treated with the methods for seasonal fever of autumn, described on page 148.

Osadhigandhaja Jwara (Hay fever)

Hay fever develops from exposure to certain pollens, which function as a kind of biological toxin causing symptoms including sneezing, continual nasal discharge (runny nose) with little or no infection, as well as headache or even fainting.

Antitoxin (Ama-reducing) remedies are the remedies used for it (page 155). Also used are:

1. **Mrityunjayarasa Vati**, 2 pills twice daily.
2. **Alarasayana,** 2 pills twice daily.
3. **Yavaniyoga**, 2 pills twice daily.

Vishaja Jwara (Fever caused by poison)

Fever caused by poison is caused from exposure to a number of different poisons, including poisonous mushrooms, heavy metals or animal toxins. Symptoms include blackening of the face, diarrhea, burning sensations, thirsty, body ache, and fainting. Typical treatment rests upon the use of antitoxin (blood purifying) remedies (page 155), vamana therapy, and other therapies specific to the symptoms manifest.

Vishama Jwara

Vishama Jwara relates to fevers that have an alternating pattern in which the signs and symptoms of fever come and go. It is often a very serious disorder, and has two basic causes. The first of these causes relates to an affliction of the Bhuta and the disturbance of the mind, whereas the second relates to the continued influence of small amounts of toxic wind, bile, or mucus found in the blood and tissues of the body. Fever caused by the Bhutas occurs in patients that express weakness, timidity, and loneliness, causing symptoms such as inexplicable laughing or weeping, with shivering and other Vataja symptoms.

Fever caused by either the Bhuta or imbalances in the blood are divided into Santata, Satataka, Anyedyuska, Tritiyaka, and Chaturthaka, and are identified on the basis of the following symptoms:

1. Santata Jwara: continuous fever for 7, 10 or 12 days;
2. Santaka Jwara: high fever twice day time and night time;
3. Anyedyusk Jwara: high fever once a day;
4. Tritiyaka Jwara: fever every alternate day;
5. Chaturthaka Jwara: fever every after two days.

Santata Jwara (Epidemic typhoid fever)

Typhoid fever found during an epidemic develops the same symptoms as Sannipata Jwara, or regular typhoid fever. Epidemic typhoid fever is not easy to cure. If the diet is poor it can be fatal. The temperature from this fever can stay for seven days, ten days, or twelve days. If the symptoms of an aggravated nervous system (Vata) are prominent, the fever will stay for seven days. If the symptoms of an aggravated arterial system (Kapha) are prominent, the fever will stay for ten days. If the symptoms of an aggravated venous system (Pitta) are prominent, the fever will stay for twelve days. This timing is a general rule, based on the observations of traditional physicians treating typhoid fever cases during epidemics. In general, the removal of pathogenic defects in the plasma (Rasa) are the basis for treatment, using the methods for typhoid fever along with the remedies for malaria fever. Spiritual healing is also a method of treatment.

Santataka Jwara (Malarial fever, A type)

A type malaria fever is concerned with pathogenic defects of the blood. In this case, the temperature will spike up twice every twenty-four hours. Spiritual healing or specific remedies such as the ones listed below are effective against malaria:

1. **Vishamajwarahara Vati,** 2 pills twice daily
2. **Sarvajwaraharalauha Vati,** 2 pills twice daily
3. **Mrityunjayarasa Vati,** 2 pills twice daily

Anyedyuska Jwara (B type malaria fever)

B type malaria fever is concerned with the pathogenic defects of the blood and the muscular tissue. In this case, the temperature goes up one time each twenty-four hours. It is treated with the same remedies of A type malaria fever with the addition of laxative remedies (page 174).

Tritiyaka Jwara (C type malaria fever)

Analysis of C Type malaria fever from the perspective of Ayurveda relates to pathogenic defects in the blood, muscular tissues, and fatty tissues. The fever alternates i.e. one day with fever, one day without fever. It is classified into three categories: alternating malarial fever with the characters of Vata-Pitta, Vata-Kapha, and Pitta-Kapha. Spiritual healing or the specific remedies against malaria fever are prescribed. In addition, the treatments based upon the theory of balance must also be prescribed side by side.

Chaturthaka Jwara (D type malaria fever)

D type malaria fever relates to pathogenic defects of blood, fatty tissues, bone, and marrow. In this case, the temperature goes up with a gap of two days (one day fever, two days no fever). There are two categories: one with the symptoms of the aggravated nervous system and another with the symptoms of the aggravated arterial system. This kind of malaria fever is very difficult to cure. However, it is treated with the spiritual healing techniques, the specific remedies against malarial fever, and treatments based upon the theory of balance. A variation on this type of fever is Chaturthaka Viparya, in which the fever stays for two days, followed by one day of no fever, and then a return of two days of fever. The remedies for this are the same as those for D type malaria fever.

Jirna Jwara (Chronic Fever)

Any fever, whatever its cause or character, can become chronic if not properly treated along with proper diet. Neglect of fever usually causes the nervous system

(Vata) to become overactive. Use of medicated Ghee preparations made with heat reducing herbs (antipyretics - page 154) is the best remedy. **Sudarshana Churna** with warm water can also be used.

Sometimes patients with chronic fevers such as pulmonary TB fever become aware of the times when the fever will recur, and induce it as a result. This is very common. Use of pleasant entertainment or other similar diversions is the method used to break this memory-induced fever.

List of Antipyretic Herbs

1. **Musta tuber** *(Cyperus rotundus).*
2. **Atirasa root/plant** (dandelion / *Taraxacum officinalis).*
3. **Vasaka leaf** (Malabar nut / *Adhatoda vasica).*
4. **Nimba leaf** (neem / *Azadirachta indica).*
5. **Parpata herb** *(Fumaria indica).*
6. **Kutki rhizome** (Indian gentian / *Picrorhiza kurroa).*
7. **Tulsi plant** (holy basil / *Ocimum sanctum).*
8. **Rakta Chandanam wood** (red sandalwood / *Pterocarpus santalinus).*
9. **Guduchi stem** *(Tinospora cordifolia).*
10. **Kantakari herb** (Black nightshade / *Solanum xanthocarpum).*
11. **Kiratatiktam plant** *(Swertia chirata).*
12. **Nirgundi plant** *(Vitex negundo,* white).
13. **Ushira root** *(Andropogon muricatum).*
14. **Sahadeva** *(Auslaea latifolia).*
15. **Dhatura herb** (downy datura /*Datura metal).*
16. **Shalaparni plant** *(Desmodium gangeticum).*
17. **Duralambha bush** *(Fragonia cretica).*
18. **Hriverum plant** *(Pavonia odorata).*
19. **Priyangu seed** *(Prunus mahaleb).*
20. **Brihati shrub** *(Solanum indicum).*
21. **Patha root** *(Stephania hernandifolia).*
22. **Patola fruit** *(Trichosanthes dioica).*
23. **Latakaranja seed/leaf** *(Caesalpinia sepiaria).*
24. **Yavasa** *(Alhagi maurorum).*
25. **Chandanam wood** (white sandalwood / *Santalum album).*
26. **Sariva plant** *(Trachelospermum fragrans).*

List of Antitoxin and Blood Purifying Herbs and Formulae

1. **Agasti bark/flower/leaf** *(Sesbania grandiflora)*.
2. **Arjuna bark** *(Terminalia arjuna)*.
3. **Asana wood** *(Terminalia tomentosa)*.
4. **Atirasa root/plant** (dandelion / *Taraxacum officinalis*).
5. **Ativisha tuber, purified** (aconite / *Aconitum heterophyllum*).
6. **Badari fruit** (jujube / *Zizyphus jujube*).
7. **Bhutakeshi herb** *(Valeriana wallichii)*.
8. **Brihati shrub** (vrihati / *Solanum indicum*).
9. **Chandanam wood** (white sandalwood / *Santalum album*).
10. **Guduchi stem** *(Tinospora cordifolia)*.
11. **Guggulu gum resin** *(Commiphora wightii)*.
12. **Haridra root** (turmeric / *Curcuma longa*).
13. **Jatamansi rhizome** (spikenard / *Valeriana jatamansi* / *Nardostachys jatamansi*).
14. **Kanchanara bark** (mountain ebony / *Bauhinia tomentosa*).
15. **Kapittha fruit** (wood apple / *Feronia limonia*).
16. **Kumari** (aloe leaf gum extract / *Aloe barbadensis*).
17. **Kustha root** *(Saussurea lappa)*.
18. **Lodhram bark** *(Symplocos paniculata)*.
19. **Madhukam root** (licorice / *Glycyrrhiza glabra*).
20. **Manashila Bhasma** (purified realgar).
21. **Manjishtha plant** (Indian madder / *Rubia cordifolia*).
22. **Nakuli herb** (mugwort / *Artemisia vulgaris*).
23. **Nilika herb** *(Indigofera tinctoria)*.
24. **Nirgundi plant** *(Vitex negundo*, white).
25. **Priyangu seed** *(Prunus mahaleb)*.
26. **Rakta Chandanam wood** (red sandalwood / *Pterocarpus santalinus*).
27. **Sanapushpi seed** (rattle-box / *Crotolaria juncea*).
28. **Shirisha flower/seed/bark** *(Albizzia lebbeck)*.
29. **Suvarma Bhasma** (purified gold oxide).
30. **Tanduliyakam plant** *(Amaranthus polyganus)*.
31. **Triphala** (standard formula).
32. **Varuna bark** (Three-leaved caper / *Crataeva religiosa*).

Chapter 12: Diseases of the Digestive System (Annavahasrota Roga)

The Digestive Fire

There are many medical terms for digestive problems, but the fundamental cause of all of them is directly related to abnormal functioning of Agni. Agni is defined as the digestive fire, the heat producing physical element present in the alimentary system that is responsible for cooking the foods we eat. For digestion to function properly, the digestive fire should be regular in both amount and activity. Problems with the digestive fire are the root cause for most alimentary system diseases. In addition, the toxins (Ama) produced by digestive problems can be causative factors in many other diseases. For example, the acid toxins produced from undigested greasy foods can be a cause of rheumatoid arthritis. A list of digestion-enhancing herbs is found on page 173.

Some basic standard compounds used for digestive fire problems are:

1. For irregular digestive fire (Vishamagni): **Trikaturasayana Vati**, 2 pills twice daily.
2. For overactive digestive fire (Tikshnagni): **Avipattikara Churna**, 1-2 grams twice daily.
3. For sluggish digestive fire (Mandagni): **Pippalyadi Churna,** 1-2 grams twice daily.

Aruchi (Loss of appetite / Anorexia)

Aruchi is loss of appetite, and is divided into five categories by Ayurveda: Aruchi with the character of Vata, Pitta, Kapha, Sannipata, and Aghantuja.

Vataja Aruchi

Loss of appetite with the character of Vata is detected by the presence of an astringent taste in the mouth. It is treated with digestive, appetizing remedies that are sweet, sour, and salty in taste. Bitter taste should be avoided. Choose sweet and sour remedies from the list of digestive remedies on page 173. Salts can be added for added benefit. Enema therapy (Vasti Karma) can also be helpful.

Pittaja Aruchi

Loss of appetite with Pitta character causes a bitter taste in the mouth. It is treated with appetizing remedies that are sweet, bitter, and astringent in taste.

Choose from the list on page 173. Purgation therapy (Virechana Karma) can also be helpful.

Kaphaja Aruchi

Loss of appetite with the character of Kapha causes a sweet taste in the mouth. It is treated with appetizing remedies that are bitter, pungent, and astringent in taste. Sweet tastes should be avoided. Choose from the list on page 173. Emetic therapy (Vamana Karma) can also be helpful.

Sannipataja Aruchi

Loss of appetite with Sannipata character causes miscellaneous abnormal tastes in the mouth. It is treated with compounds of various appetizing herbs. In this case putting the patients into a situation with pleasant surroundings is very important.

Aghantuja loss of appetite

Aghantuja loss of appetite is caused by fear, shock, anger, bad smells, bad tastes, and unpleasant atmosphere. It is treated by presentation of tempting and delicious food, appetizing fermented beverages, and living in pleasant, clean surroundings.

Ajirnam (Indigestion)

Ajirnam is correlated with indigestion, and is classified into four categories: Ama, Vidagdha, Vistambha, and Rasashesa. There are many general medicines used to strengthen digestion (see list on page 173). A specific medicine to improve digestion is the standard compound **Dhanyapanchakam**, 1-2 grams given with warm water twice daily.

Amaja Ajirnam

Indigestion caused by Amajirna (undigested greasy foods) is related to Kapha. Symptoms include a heavy feeling in the stomach, nausea, puffiness under the eye and cheeks, belching with sweet taste and/or the same taste as the previous meal. It is treated with Kapha treatments along with digestive remedies. Fasting from food and taking lime juice with salt is helpful. **Hingwastak Churna** taken in doses of 1-2 grams twice daily can also help to resolve Amaja indigestion.

Vidagdha Ajirnam

Indigestion in the form of Vidagdha is concerned with a Pitta imbalance. Symptoms include burning sensation in the stomach, sour-tasting reflux, dizziness, and thirst. When neglected this condition gives rise to Amlapittam ('gastritis'). It is treated with Pitta treatments along with digestive remedies. One useful remedy is **Pippalyadi Churna**, taken in doses of 1-2 grams twice daily with food.

Vistambha Ajirnam

Indigestion in the form of Vistambha is caused by Vata. Symptoms include colicky pain, bloating, constipation, and discomfort. Vata treatments are used along with digestive remedies. Salty-tasting medicines are useful. Heavy, greasy, and cold foods should be avoided.

Rasashesa Ajirnam

Indigestion in the form of Rasashesa is concerned with inactive stomach function. Symptoms include weakness and fatigue, loose stool, nausea, body ache, and a cold feeling. It is treated with laxative and digestive remedies. Cold, watery foods such as melon, cucumber, and banana should be strictly avoided.

Vilambika (Achlorhydria)

Achlorhydria is concerned with the aggravated functions of the nervous system (Vata) and arterial system (Kapha) that results in a lack of digestion of food in the stomach. It is treated with digestive remedies that are sour, salty, and pungent in tastes to stimulate the digestive juice (Pachaka Pitta) of the stomach. Choose from the list on page 173. It is difficult to cure.

Chardi (Vomiting)

Chardi refers to vomiting as a disease, and is classified into five categories with the characters of Vata, Pitta, Kapha, Sannipata, and Dwistarth. Whatever may be the cause and condition of vomiting, at the beginning fasting is a very important step to stop the upset, followed by the antiemetic remedies listed on page 174.

One useful remedy is 125 mg of **Tamra Bhasma** (purified copper oxide) combined with one gram of the freshly ground powder of **Ela fruit** (greater cardamom / *Amomum subulatum)*, or with one of the laxative medicines (see page 174), taken twice daily.

Examples of other possible remedies include:

1. **Dashamula** decoction, 60-90 mL twice daily.
2. Equal parts decoction of **Kutaki rhizome** (Indian gentian / *Picrorhiza kurroa)* and **Chitraka root** (leadwort, white flower / *Plumbago zeylanica)*, 30-60 mL twice daily.
3. One part decoction of **Nagaram rhizome** (nut grass / *Cyperus pertenuis)* taken with one part either **Dhanyakam seed** (coriander / *Coriandrum sativum)* or **Guduchi stem** *(Tinospora cordifolia)*, 60-90 mL twice daily.
4. Powder of **Pippali fruit** (long pepper / *Piper longum)*, 500-1000 mg, taken with **Madhu** (honey) twice daily.
5. Powder of **Murva plant** *(Bauhinia vahlii)* with **Madhu** (honey), 500-1000 mg, taken with **Madhu** (honey) twice daily.

6. Decoction of equal parts **Madhukam root** (licorice / *Glycyrrhiza glabra*), **Arjaka leaf/extract** (white mint plant / *Mentha spp.)*, and **Dhanyakam seed** (coriander / *Coriandrum sativum)*, 60-90 mL twice daily.

Vataja Chardi

Vomiting with the character of Vata is concerned with the aggravated function of the nervous system. It is treated with the regular Vata treatments and diet (page 56) along with mild laxatives and emetics (to rid the body of toxins), followed by the antiemetic remedies (see page 174). A specific medicine to use is the fresh juice of **Amalaki fruit** (Indian gooseberry / amla / *Phyllanthus emblica)*, 10-15 mL taken with **Ghrita** (Ghee / clarified butter) and **Saindhavam** (mineral salt).

Pittaja Chardi

Vomiting with the character of Pitta is concerned with the aggravated function of the venous system (inflammation). It is treated using Pitta treatments and diet along with sweet purgative remedies (to rid the body of toxins - page 174) and the antiemetic remedies. One specific remedy is a decoction of **Panchamula** (the 'five roots' compound), 30-60 mL, mixed with **Madhu** (honey) when cool, two to three times daily depending on the severity of symptoms.

Kaphaja Chardi

Vomiting with the character of Kapha is concerned with the aggravated function of the arterial system (excess exudation) or mucous membranes (edema). It is treated with the regular Kapha treatments and diet (page 77) along with the emetic remedies (to aid in quickly removing excess mucus) and antiemetic remedies (see page 174). Remedies can be chosen from the **Aragwadhadigana group** (page 271.)

Sannipataja Chardi

Vomiting with the character of Sannipata is concerned with the simultaneous aggravated functions of the nervous, venous, and arterial systems. It is difficult to cure if blood is vomited. Otherwise it can be treated with combined remedies along with the antiemetic remedies.

Dwistartha Chardi

Vomiting with the character of Dwistartha is caused by unpleasant food and/or atmosphere, car fumes, or any similar disgusting condition (rancid smells etc). Avoiding the condition which caused the upset is the best remedy for it.

Amlapittam (Gastritis and Gastric ulcer)

Amlapittam can be correlated with gastritis, with or without ulcer. Amlapittam without ulcer is called Adhoga Amlapitta whereas with ulcer it is called Urdhwaga Amlapitta. Adhoga Amlapitta manifests as nausea with a sour taste, acid reflux, and a burning sensation in the esophagus. Urdhwaga Amlapitta manifests as a burning sensation in the stomach region, pain, bloating, and a burning sensation upon defecation. Both are treated with the regular Pitta treatments and diet (page 67) along with antacid remedies, symptomatic treatments, and specific medicines. Useful antacid remedies to treat Amlapittam include **Churnahh Bhasma** (purified limestone ash), **Pravala Bhasma** (purified coral oxide), **Shankha Bhasma** (purified conch shell ash, *Turbinella pyrum*), and **Shukti Bhasma** (oyster shell ash /*Ostrea gigas*).

One specific remedy for either type of Amlapittam is as follows, taken in doses of 1-2 grams, with milk or water as an Anupana:

1. **Avipattikara Churna** 10 parts;
2. **Shankha Bhasma** 4 parts;
3. **Pravala Bhasma** 2 parts;
4. **Shukti Bhasma** 2 parts;
5. **Churnahh Bhasma** 1 part.

Gastric ulcer is very difficult to cure, especially in the advanced stage. Curing it requires regeneration of the mucous membrane or the development of a new membrane to replace the inflamed and eroded area. The same medicines as for gastritis are used, but in the example of the above formula, ½ part **Tamra Bhasma** (purified copper oxide) is added.

Parinamashulam (Duodenal ulcer)

Parinamashulam is correlated with duodenal ulcer, characterized by similar symptoms as Amlapittam along with a gnawing hunger pain. It is treated with the same remedies for gastric ulcer (see page 160), along with specific remedies against Parinamashulam. Some simple medicines against duodenal ulcer are:

1. Cereal made from **Yava flour** (barley / *Hordeum vulgare)* is taken in **Kalaya soup** (fresh pea / *Pisum sativum).*
2. **Aparajita Churna** (butterfly pea / *Clitoria ternatea)* taken with water.

Specific formulas to treat Parinamashulam include:

1. **Aparajita Churna**, 1000 mg twice daily.
2. **Samudradi Churna,** 250 mg twice daily.
3. **Narikela Lavanam,** 250 mg twice daily.
4. **Lauha Bhasma (1 part)** and **Triphala** (10 parts), 1-2 grams twice daily.
5. **Shulanirmulanarasa Vati**, 3 pills twice daily.

Annadravashulam (Peptic ulcer)

Peptic ulcer characterized with constant pain is treated with the same remedies used for gastric ulcer along with the remedies for Shulam (page 162).

Vibandha (Constipation)

Vibandha is constipation, and is usually caused by Ajirnam (indigestion). Digestive remedies with laxatives are the normal remedies for it - refer to the lists of digestive and laxative remedies on page 173. The formula Triphala is commonly prescribed but is only really effective in mild cases. In chronic constipation Triphala can be combined with more powerful laxatives such as Trivrit *(Operculina turpethum)*. Other approaches include:

1. **Chandraprabha** Vati, 2 pills twice daily, taken with Pippalydai Churnam, **Swarnapatri leaf** (senna / *Cassia auriculata)* and Saindhava.
2. Equal parts **Amalakyadi Churna** and **Arkalavanam**, 1-2 grams daily.

In its acute form Vibandha is called Alasaka. The treatments are the same, but also include the use of enemas and/or herbal suppositories.

Anaha (Tympanites)

Anaha refers to tympanities, and refers to the swelling of the abdomen with gas. The general treatment is similar to that of Vibandha, utilizing a combination of carminative remedies (page 175), along with laxative and digestive remedies (page 173). One helpful formula to alleviate gas and flatulence is Dhanyapanchakam.

Udavarta (Reversed function of the digestive tract)

Although constipation and gas is usually caused by Ajirnam (indigestion), it can also be caused by the reversed function of the digestive tract, called Udavarta. Caused by a vitiation of Vata, Udavarta manifests as a witholding of or inability to express the urges to defecate or to expel gas, causing constipation and tympanites. It is treated with hot abdominal compress, enema, and laxative and carminative remedies (page 175).

Shulam (Abdominal colic)

The term Shulam corresponds with abdominal colic, and generally is the result of blockage in the function of the nervous system. It is classified into seven categories: Vata, Pitta, Kapha, Sannipata, Kukshishula, Vitshula, and Amashula.

Treatment of Shulam

When treating colic pain, whatever the cause, it is important to first of all control the pain caused by the aggravated function of the nervous system. Some specific remedies used against Shulam include:

1. **Pippalyadi Churna**, 2 grams with warm water twice daily.
2. **Shulanirmulanarasa Vati**, 3 pills with warm water twice daily.
3. **Samudradi Churna**, 250 mg with warm water twice daily.
4. **Karpurasava**, 10 drops with water 2-3 times daily.
5. **Ahiphenasava**, 5 drops twice daily.
6. **Vachadiyoga Churna**, 1000 mg with water twice daily.

Vataja Shulam

Colic with the character of Vata is caused by the blockage of gas in either the stomach or the intestine. It is treated with hot compress, carminative remedies (page 175) and the remedies described for Shulam.

Pittaja Shulam

Colic with the character of Pitta is concerned with inflammation. It is treated with cold compress, laxatives, and the remedies described for the treatment of Shulam. In Pittaja Shulam the medicines used should only be given after inducing vomiting, typically by drinking ice cold water. This is an important consideration.

Kaphaja Shulam

Colic with the character of Kapha is concerned with local edema of any part of the alimentary system. It is treated with hot compress, emetic remedies (page 175), and the remedies under Shulam.

Sannipataja Colic

Colic with the character of Sannipata is concerned with deadly symptoms. It is not curable.

Kukshishulaja Colic

Colic with the character of Kuksishula is caused by indigestion. It is treated with digestive, carminative, laxative, and emetic remedies (page 173), hot compress, and the remedies under Shulam.

Vitshulaja Colic

Colic with the character of Vitshula is caused by obstruction of the stool. It is treated with hot compress, purgative remedies (page 174), enema, and the remedies under Shulam. In severe cases this has to be treated as soon as possible to break the blockage, otherwise it can be the cause of death.

Amashulaja or Annadoshaja

Colic with the character of Amashula or Annadoshaja is concerned with overeating. It is treated with hot compress, fasting, emetic remedies (page 175), digestive remedies (page 173), and the remedies under Shulam.

Tuni and Pratuni (Spasmodic colic of the colon / Irritable bowel syndrome)

Tuni and Pratuni refer to spasm of the colon, radiating either downward (Tuni) or upward (Pratuni), and concern the aggravated function of the nervous system. Both are treated with hot compress, intake of warm salty water with oils, carminative remedies (page 175), and greasy enema.

Atisara (Diarrhea)

Atisara is correlated with diarrhea, and in general is the result of indigestion. It is divided into six categories: Vata, Pitta, Kapha, Sannipata, Bhayaja, and Shokaja. Diarrhea in the beginning stages should not be stopped with astringent remedies or antidiarrhea remedies, during which time the body is eliminating unwanted substances. Immediate stoppage of diarrhea can be the cause of many problems including anemia, sprue, hemorrhoid, fever, and an enlarged spleen and/or liver (see Grahani, page 167). An electrolyte rich, liquid diet is prescribed for all types of Atisara, such as a watery rice soup prepared with salt.

Some simple treatments for diarrhea include:

1. **Bilwa fruit** (bael / *Aegle marmelos*) with 10% **Shankha Bhasma** (purified conch shell ash, *Turbinella pyrum*), taken with water. Dosage is 500 mg twice daily.
2. One **Amram seed** (mango / *Magnifera indica*) is roasted in a fire, and is taken over a day in divided doses, 2-3 times per day.
3. **Karpurasava**, 10 drops taken with warm water, twice daily.

Vataja Atisara (Diarrhea with gas)

Diarrhea with gas is related to aggravated function of the nervous system. Symptoms include small amounts of stool with undigested food and gas, with a pale, light color. It is treated with antidiarrhea remedies, along with carminatives (page 175), and digestives (page 173).

Pittaja Atisara (Dysentery)

Pittaja Atisara is correlated with dysentery, and is concerned with intestinal inflammation (aggravated function of the venous system). Symptoms include a yellow or multi-colored stool with burning sensations. It is treated with the antidiarrhea remedies (above), along with digestives (page 173) and antipyretics (page 154). Some specific medicines against dysentery include:

1. The powders of **Musta tuber** (*Cyperus rotundus*), **Hriverum plant** (*Pavonia odorata*), **Kiratatiktam plant** *Swertia chirata*), **Kutaja bark** (*Holarrhena antidysenterica*), **Shatapushpa seed** (anise / *Pimpinella anisum*), and **Bilwa fruit** (bael / *Aegle marmelos*) can be given with warm

water. Standard dosage is 1-2 grams twice daily. This compound is especially good for bacillary dysentery. For amoebic dysentery, use the methods for Kaphaja Atisara below.

2. **Anandabhairavarasa Vati**, 2 pills twice daily.
3. **Karpurasava,** 10 drops taken with warm water, twice daily.

Kaphaja Atisara (Colitis)

Kaphaja Atisara can be correlated with colitis, and is concerned with the aggravated function of the arterial system and the mucous membranes of the colon. Symptoms include an offensive smelling, white-colored stool. It is treated with digestive (page 173) and antidiarrhea remedies along with specific medicines such as **Dhanyapanchakam** given with **Shatapushpa tea** (anise / *Pimpinella anisum*). **Dhanyapanchakam** is more effective if given with the standard compounds **Rasa Churna** and **Shambukadi Vati**.

Sannipataja Atisara (Bacillary dysentery)

Sannipataja can be correlated with bacillary dysentery, and is concerned with aggravated of all three Doshas (Sannipataja). Symptoms include a pale or flesh colored stool with white particles, along with severe exhaustion. Is difficult to cure, however, it is treated with digestive, carminative, and antipyretic remedies (See lists on pages 154, 173, and 175), and the remedies mentioned under Atisara above.

Bhayaja Atisara (Diarrhea caused by fear)

Bhayaja Atisara is diarrhea caused by fear, and is treated with carminatives (page 175), digestives (page 173) and the remedies mentioned under Atisara. In this case, encouragement, and showing of consideration and love to the patient is very important.

Shokaja Diarrhea (Diarrhea caused by shock)

Shokaja Atisara is diarrhea caused by shock is treated just like the diarrhea of fear. It is difficult to cure quickly.

Jwaratisara (Gastroenteritis)

Jwaratisara can be correlated with gastroenteritis, manifesting as diarrhea (Atisara) with fever (Jwara). It is treated with the methods used for Pitta Atisara (see page 165).

Pravahika (Amebic dysentery)

Pravahika can be correlated with amebic dysentery, and is concerned with aggravated function of the mucous membranes and nervous system of the colon. It is treated with the medicines for Kaphaja Atisara (page 165) along with carminative spices (page 175). If there is presence of blood and mucus in stool, it has to be treated with the principles and medicines used for Pitta Atisara (page 164).

Raktatisara (Proctitis)

Raktatisara is a form of proctitis, manifesting as inflammation of the rectum secondary to Atisara (diarrhea). It is treated with the medicines used for Pitta Atisara along with antihemorrhagic remedies (see page 258). One useful remedy is equal parts **Bilwa fruit** (bael / *Aegle marmelos)* and **Vasaka leaf** (Malabar nut / *Adhatoda vasica)*, given as tea in doses of 60-90 mL 2-3 times daily.

Visuchika (Cholera)

The treatment of cholera does not respond well to typical interventions, although in general is related to indigestion. Fasting and the use of liquid preparations (tinctures or decoctions) made from digestive remedies (page 173) with salt can be used as general remedies. Emetic (page 174) and laxative remedies (page 174) are found beneficial to prescribe, and it is very important to keep the patient near a heat source (in ancient times the patient was kept near a fire). **Bilwa fruit** (bael / *Aegle marmelos)* can be used as a tea along with **Kathini Bhasma** (purified white chalk / calcium carbonate) and **Shankha Bhasma** (purified conch shell ash, *Turbinella pyrum)*. In the advanced stage with severe symptoms of dehydration, these general medicines have no effect. Spiritual healing has been reported be helpful in some cases, especially during epidemic conditions. Surgeons have found that keeping the heel (and foot) hot by placing close to a very strong heat source is an effective strategy.

Krimi (Parasites)

Ayurveda has identified twelve types of parasites (Krimi) that can be found in the stool. These parasites are divided into two groups: parasites that active in the mucous membrane and parasites that are active in the stool. The parasites that are active in the mucous membrane are called:

1. Antrada (Hookworm).
2. Udarada (Roundworm).
3. Hridayachara (Larva of roundworm or hookworm which can be found in the heart).
4. Churna (Threadworm, large).
5. Darbhapushpa (Threadworm, small).
6. Saugandhika (Whipworm).
7. Mahaguda (Tapeworm).

The parasites that are active in stool are called:

1. Kakeruka.
2. Lehika.
3. Sashulaka.

4.   Sausurada.

These last four parasites are the larvae and ova of the same parasites that are active in the mucous membrane. All these parasites, whatever may be their names and forms, are all treated with anthelmintic remedies (see page 175) and bitter, pungent remedies. Symptomatic treatments are also given combined with digestive remedies (page 173). One simple formula is **Vidanga seed** *(Embelia ribes)* given with 10% **Shringaputa** (deer horn ash / *Cervus nippon)* given in doses of 1-2 grams 2-3 times daily. A stronger medicine is the standard combination **Krimimudgararasa Vati**, 2 pills given with warm water twice daily.

Grahani (Chronic diarrhea / Sprue)

Grahani corresponds to chronic diarrhea, sprue and malabsorptive syndromes. Ayurveda states that when diarrhea is treated too soon, or if after treatment the patient is careless in diet, the result can be Grahani. In this case the stomach acid secretion is elevated and the alkaline reaction in the small intestine becomes weak. Grahani is divided into four categories: Vata, Pitta, Kapha and Sannipata.

The compound **Shankha Vati** can be taken with warm water for simple sprue, 2-3 pills twice daily. It is sometimes necessary to control the commonly found symptom of an excessively strong appetite. In this case warm water is not used. Instead, the drinking of Ghee with cold water is prescribed. Another simple medicine contains powder of **Bilwa fruit** (bael / *Aegle marmelos)* and 10% **Shankha Bhasma** (purified conch shell ash, *Turbinella pyrum)*, 1-2 grams twice daily given with **Kanjika** (whey). These treatments used can be modified according to signs and symptoms.

Vataja Grahani

Grahani with the character of Vata is treated with carminative (page 175), digestive (page 173), antidiarrhea (page 164) and antacid remedies (page 160). One useful medicine is **Siddhapraneshwar**, given in doses of 2 pills twice daily.

Pittaja Grahani

Grahani with the character of Pitta is treated with the methods used for Pitta Atisara (page 164) along with antacid remedies (page 160). One useful remedy is **Kathini Bhasma** (purified white chalk / calcium carbonate) and **Shankha Bhasma** (purified conch shell ash, *Turbinella pyrum)*, given with an infusion of **Vasaka leaf** (Malabar nut / *Adhatoda vasica).*

Kaphaja Grahani

Grahani with the character of Kapha is treated with the methods and medicines for Kapha Atisara (page 165) along with antacid remedies (page 160).

Sannipataja Sprue

Complex Grahani (Sannipataja) is difficult to cure. However, it is treated with the methods used for bacillary dysentery (see page 165) along with antacid remedies (page 160).

Arsha (Hemorrhoid)

Arsha refers to hemorrhoids, which are varicosity of the extremity of the portal vein around the anus. Ayurveda divides hemorrhoids into six categories: Vata, Pitta, Kapha, Sannipata, Raktaja, and Sahaja.

Hemorrhoid Treatment

At the beginning, hemorrhoidal bleeding should not be suddenly stopped with astringent remedies. This can be the cause of complications including liver problems and anemia. During treatment of hemorrhoids, whatever the cause, digestive and appetizing remedies (page 173) are very important to prescribe to prevent blood congestion in the extremity of the portal vein. To prevent blood accumulation in the distal portal vein the liver must function properly. The digestive and appetizing remedies support complete digestion and ease the work of the liver, and so play a major role in the treatment of hemorrhoids.

Some individual remedies against hemorrhoids include:

1. **Shurana tuber** (*Amorphophallus campanulatus*) (never given alone).
2. **Kutaja bark/seed** (*Holarrhena antidysenterica*).
3. **Bilwa fruit** (bael / *Aegle marmelos*).
4. **Ativisha tuber, purified** (aconite / *Aconitum heterophyllum*).
5. **Daruharidra bark/extract** (barberry / *Berberis nepalensis*).

Formulas include:

1. **Chandraprabha Vati**, 2 pills twice daily.
2. **Dhanwayasa compound**, 1-2 grams twice daily.
3. **Avipattikara Churna**, 1-2 grams twice daily.
4. Equal parts **Vasaka leaf** (Malabar nut / *Adhatoda vasica*) and **Shatavari root** (asparagus / *Asparagus racemosus*) can be used to stop bleeding, 1-2 grams twice daily.

For external application to the anus, the following can be used:

1. A paste made from **Haridra root** (turmeric / *Curcuma longa*) with the milk of **Arka** (milkweed / *Calotropis gigantea*).
2. The standard oil preparation **Narayana Taila** mixed with a pinch of **Sphutikarika** (purified alum).

3. To relieve pain, apply ice cold fresh **Dadhi** (yogurt) with cotton, along with the use of a mild laxative internally (see page 174).

In the advanced stage, it is necessary to remove hemorrhoids by surgical operation or corrosive alkaline (lime) thread binding.

Vataja Hemorrhoid

Hemorrhoids with the character of Vata is concerned with the aggravated function of the nervous system, and manifests with a dull, aching pain with small bluish colored hemorrhoids. It is treated with digestive (page 173) and carminative herbs (page 175) along with the specific remedies against hemorrhoids. Other methods include hot compress, corrosive plasters and burning with strong corrosive alkali or heated plate.

Pittaja Hemorrhoid

Hemorrhoid with the character of Pitta character involves more severe inflammation of the anus, with a sharp burning pain and reddish-colored hemorrhoids. It is treated with general Pitta treatments and diet (page 67) along with venesection (see page 92), sedative plasters, digestive remedies (page 173), antihemorrhagic remedies, surgery and specific remedies against hemorrhoid.

Kaphaja Hemorrhoid

Hemorrhoid with the character of Kapha develops with aggravated function of the arterial system. The influence of Kapha promotes edema and pronounced swelling, a whitish discoloration, and itchiness rather than pain. It is treated with the regular Kapha treatments and diet (page 77) along with hot compress, corrosive plaster, burning with strong alkali or heated instrument, digestive remedies (page 173), surgery and specific remedies against hemorrhoid.

Sannipataja Hemorrhoid

Hemorrhoid with Sannipataja character (complex symptoms) develops due to aggravated function of the nervous system along with inflammation and edema. It is not curable. However it can be maintained with the specific remedies again hemorrhoid and various symptomatic treatments.

Raktaja Hemorrhoid

Raktaja hemorrhoid involves pathogenic defects of blood, causing passive hemorrhaging of the affected tissues. It is treated with the same principle of hemorrhoid with the character of Pitta.

Sahaja Hemorrhoid

Sahaja hemorrhoid refers to a hemorrhoid caused by 'congenital' (Sahaja) factors. It is not curable. However it can be maintained with digestive remedies (page 173) and the specific remedies against hemorrhoid.

Gudabhramsha (Prolapse of the anus)

Gudabhramsha refers to the prolapse of the anus, and is usually the result of neglected chronic diarrhea or dysentery. It is treated with internal digestive remedies (page 173) along with external washing with astringent remedies such as **Khadira extract** (catechu, white / *Acacia catechu*) and **Sphutikarika** (purified alum). Plastering the affected area with the fat of cow or Ghee is also helpful.

Sanniruddhaguda (Stricture of the anus)

Sanniruddhaguda refers to stricture of the anus, and is concerned with the aggravated function of the nervous system. It is treated by insertion of a pipe into the anus through which oily medications that reduce Vata are applied, such as **Narayana Taila**. If the case is severe, surgical operation is advised.

Vidradhi (Abscess)

Vidradhi corresponds to an abscess, either internal or external, and is concerned with pathogenic defects of the blood. In the beginning stage Vidradhi can be treated with the same remedies used for Dukshijavidradhi (appendicitis). An abscess of the colon, especially of the appendix, is called Kukshijavidradhi, whereas an abscess of the alimentary system affecting the small intestine around the navel is called Navijavidradhi. The latter of these is not curable if it bursts. Useful formulas include **Varunadigana** and **Ushakadigana**, given in doses of 1-2 grams 2-3 times daily. **Sobhanjan root** *(Moringa oleifera)* and **Varuna bark** (Three-leaved caper / *Crataeva religiosa)* can also be used externally as an antiseptic.

Dukshijavidradhi (Appendicitis)

Dukshijavidradhi refers to inflammation of the appendix, or appendicitis, and is considered curable. It is treated as soon as possible with strong purgative remedies (page 174) along with venesection practices, greasy enema, hot compress and specific remedies against internal abscess. Also, in more advanced conditions it is treated with the methods for abdominal tumor with the character of Pitta (see page 172) and surgery. In addition to the remedies against Vidradhi (see above) **Samudradi Churna** is also prescribed, five one gram doses given over a 12 hour period.

Baddhagudodara (Intestinal obstruction)

Either a twisted intestine or a physical blockage causes intestinal obstruction. It is curable only by operation. In some cases, if the intestine is not severely twisted, it can be treated with urine therapy (see below), strong purgative remedies (page 174), enema and hot compress.

Chhidrodara (Perforation of the intestine)

Perforation of the intestine is curable only with operation. In some condition, it can be treated with the regular Kapha treatments (page 77) along with drainage of the accumulated water from the peritoneum.

Udararoga (Peritonitis)

Peritonitis, in general, is concerned with the blockage of the lymphatic duct system attached with the alimentary system. It is classified in to four categories: Vataja, Pittaja, Kaphaja and Sannipataja.

All the forms of peritonitis are treated with urine therapy, enema, laxative, digestive and antiedema remedies. To balance the Doshas, symptomatic treatments should also be carried out side-by-side to restore balance to the nervous (Vata), vein (Pitta) or artery (Kapha) system. Peritonitis with the character of Sannipata is not curable.

Peritonitis of all types is very difficult to cure. Urine therapy combined with use of digestive and appetizing remedies (page 173) is very important. A specific digestive medicine against peritonitis is **Pippalyadi** given with **Soraka** (Potassium chloride).

Urine therapy is the drinking of the urine of a cow, buffalo, camel, horse, Each type of urine has different medical properties. In the advanced stages of peritonitis, these regular medicines have no effect, and only snake poison is beneficial to prescribe. However, use of snake poison is very dangerous.

Jalodara (Ascites)

Ascites is related to peritonitis. It is treated with the same remedies for peritonitis, but along with the addition of alkali remedies and the Kapha treatments and diet. The fluid accumulation should be taken out repeatedly.

Some common alkali remedies:

1. **Yavakshara alkaline ash** (barley plant / *Hordeum vulgare*).
2. **Shukti Bhasma** (oyster shell ash / *Ostrea gigas*).
3. **Sarjikakshara** (sodium bicarbonate).
4. **Churnahh** (Limestone Bhasma).

A specific treatment for ascites is **Amalakyadi Churna**, given in doses of 1-2 grams twice daily.

Antravriddhi (Hernia)

Antravriddhi refers to herniation of the intestine through the inguinal canal, and is caused by several factors including traumatic injury, as well as excessive sexual activity, bowel problems such as constipation and chronic coughing. More common in men, the protrusion can extend down into the scrotum and interfere with testicular function. It is treated with specific remedies against hernia along with venesection (see page 92) from the temple area, right above the ear. Some specific remedies against hernia are **Airanda Taila**, taken internally and applied topically, as well as **Balasiddha payonwitan**. For external treatment, the root of **Arka** (milkweed / *Calotropis gigantea)* ground with vinegar can be plastered onto the affected area. Another plaster is made from **Vacha rhizome** (acorus / *Acorus calamus)* and **Sarshapi seed** (black mustard / *Sinapis juncea)*. If the condition is unresponsive to treatment surgical measures are typically applied.

Gulma (Abdominal tumor)

Gulma refers to an abdominal tumor, and is classified into four categories: tumor with the character of Vata, Pitta, Kapha and Sannipata. No matter what the cause and condition when treating abdominal tumors, the aggravated function of the nervous system has to be controlled as soon as possible with digestive (page 173) and carminative remedies (page 175). It is an empirical observation in Ayurveda that if the digestive power is maintained and strengthened, tumor growth will be greatly inhibited. Some specific remedies against abdominal tumors are:

1. **Kankayana Vati**, 2 pills twice daily.
2. **Samudradi Churna**, 1-2 grams twice daily.
3. **Amalakyadi Churna**, 2 grams twice daily.

For pain the remedies for colic are prescribed (page 162).

Vataja Gulma (Gastrointestinal adenomatous polyp)

Vataja gulma can be compared to a gastrointestinal adenomatous polyp, and is defined by Ayurveda as being an unrooted tumor. It is concerned with the aggravated function of the nervous system. It is treated with the regular Vata treatments and diet (page 56) along with hot compress, enema, digestive (page 173) and carminative remedies (page 175) and symptomatic treatments. In advanced stage, venesection (page 92) is beneficial to stop the abnormal growths. The specific remedies against tumor are also prescribed.

Pittaja Gulma (Ulcerative gastric tumor)

Pittaja gulma can be compared with ulcerative gastric tumor, and is related to the aggravated function of the venous system (i.e. a tumor with gastric inflammation). It is treated with the regular Pitta treatments and diet (page 67) along with enema, venesection (see page 92) and the remedies for gastritis (160). It can also be treated with the treatments used for internal abscess (see page 170). In the advanced stage, if there is hemorrhage, it is curable only with surgical treatments. The specific remedies against tumors are always prescribed side by side with all the general treatments.

Kaphaja Gulma (Gastroadenoma)

Kapha gulma can be compared with gastroadenoma, and is concerned with the aggravated function of the arterial system (tumor with gastric edema). It is treated with the regular Kapha treatments and diet (page 77) along with fasting, hot compress, emetic remedies (see page 175), alkaline remedies (page 171), enema and pressure massage to dissolve the abnormal growth. It the advanced stage, venesection (see page 92) and cauterization of the elevated area of the tumor is beneficial. The specific remedies against tumor are always prescribed side by side with all the general treatments.

Sannipataja Gulma (Malignant gastric tumor)

Sannipataja corresponds with malignant gastric tumor and is concerned with aggravated function of the nervous system, inflammation and edema of the stomach. It is not curable. However, fatality can be delayed with venesection (see page 92) and symptomatic treatments.

Asthila (Tumor of the colon or intestine)

A tumor of the colon is called Pratyasthila, and a tumor of the intestine is called Vatashthila. Both are concerned with the aggravated function of the nervous system (Vata), and the remedies for them are the same as for abdominal tumor. With these diseases the digestive power has to be maintained by all means possible.

List of Digestive Herbs
1. **Ela fruit** (greater cardamon / *Amomum subulatum).*
2. **Yavani seed** (wild omum / *Trachyspermum ammi).*
3. **Ajamoda seed** (wild celery / *Carum roxburghianum).*
4. **Adrakam root** (ginger / *Zingiber officinalis).*
5. **Chavyam fruit/stem** *(Piper chaba).*
6. **Chitraka root** (leadwort / *Plumbago zeylanica).*
7. **Dhanyakam seeds** (coriander / *Coriandrum sativum).*
8. **Jirakam seed** (cumin / *Cuminum cyminum).*
9. **Krishnajiraka seed** (black cumin / *Nigella sativa).*
10. **Lavangam seeds** (cloves / *Syzigium aromaticum).*
11. **Maricham seed** (black pepper / *Piper nigrum).*
12. **Musta tuber** *(Cyperus rotundus).*
13. **Pippali fruit** (long pepper / *Piper longum).*
14. **Pippalimulam** (long pepper root / *Piper longum).*
15. **Shatapushpa seed** (anise / *Pimpinella anisum).*

16. **Sukshmaila seed** (cardamom / *Elettaria cardamomum*).
17. **Trikatu** (three pepper formula).
18. **Twak bark** (Cinnamon / *Cinnamon zeylanicum*).

List of Laxative and Purgative Herbs

Laxative and purgative remedies are used to help remove toxins. Patients are usually given greasy foods or oils such as **Ghrita** (Ghee) or **Tila oil** (sesame seed / *Sesamum indicum*) to lubricate the system prior to administration of laxatives. Small amounts of these remedies can also be added to formulas to help with removal of Pitta Dosha during treatment. Both methods can be used according to signs and symptoms. Use of strong purgatives should not be used with weak or elderly patients without proper knowledge. For a mild effect, use **Haritaki fruit** (*Terminalia chebula*) because it has a restorative effect, or use low doses of the moderate laxatives.

Strong Purgatives
1. **Amlavetasa root** (rhubarb / *Rheum emodi*).
2. **Arka milk** (milkweed / *Calotropis gigantea*).
3. **Danti seed** (*Baliospermum montanum*).
4. **Eranda oil/root/seed** (Castor / *Ricinus communis*).
5. **Snuhi cactus milk** (*Euphorbia nerifolia*).
6. **Swarnapatri leaf** (senna / *Cassia auriculata*).
7. **Trivrit root** (Indian rhubarb /*Operculina turpethum*).

Moderate Laxatives
1. **Indravaruni fruit** (bitter apple / *Citrullus colocynthis*).
2. **Kampillaka pollen** (kamala / *Mallotus philippinensis*).
3. **Kumari** (aloe leaf gum extract / *Aloe barbadensis*).
4. **Kutki rhizome** (Indian gentian / *Picrorhiza kurroa*).
5. **Nilika herb** (*Indigofera tinctoria*).
6. **Rajavriksha pod pulp** (Indian laburnum /*Cassia fistula*).
7. **Tanduliyakam plant** (*Amaranthus polyganus*).
8. **Triphala** (*Phyllanthus emblica* / *Terminalia belerica* / *Terminalia chebula*).
9. **Varuna bark** (Three-leaved caper / *Crataeva religiosa*).
10. **Bibhitaki fruit** (*Terminalia belerica*).
11. **Haritaki fruit** (*Terminalia chebula*).

List of Antiemetic Herbs
1. **Ela fruit** (greater cardamon / *Amomum subulatum*).
2. **Adrakam root** (ginger / *Zingiber officinalis*).
3. **Ashwattha bark alkali** (bodhi tree / *Ficus religiosa*).
4. **Atirasa root/plant** (dandelion /*Taraxacum officinalis*).
5. **Jambu seeds** (*Syzygium jambolanum*).

6. **Kasturi** (deer musk / *Moschus moschiferus).*
7. **Lavangam seeds** (clove / *Syzigium aromaticum).*
8. **Matulunga fruit/root** (Citron / *Citrus medica).*
9. **Priyangu seed** *(Prunus mahaleb).*
10. **Sukshmaila seed** (cardamom / *Elettaria cardamomum).*

List of Antihelmintic Herbs
1. **Apamarga herb** *(Achyranthes aspera).*
2. **Chitraka root** (leadwort, white flower / *Plumbago zeylanica).*
3. **Hastikarnapalasa seed** (bastard teak / *Butea monosperma)* with sugar.
4. **Kampillaka pollen** (kamala / *Mallotus philippinensis).*
5. **Karanja bark/seed oil** (Indian beech / *Pongamia pinnata).*
6. **Lashunam bulb** (garlic / *Allium sativum).*
7. **Mahanimba leaf** (Perisan lilac / *Melia azadirachta).*
8. **Maricham seed** (black pepper / *Piper nigrum).*
9. **Methika seed** (fenugreek / *Trigonella foenum-graecum).*
10. **Palasha seed** (bastard teak / *Butea frondosa).*
11. **Sobhanjan bark/root/flower/seed oil/gum** *(Moringa oleifera).*
12. **Vasaka leaf** (Malabar nut / *Adhatoda vasica).*
13. **Vidanga seeds** *(Embelia ribes).*

List of Emetic Herbs
1. **Vacha rhizome** (acorus / *Acorus calamus).*
2. **Kovidara flower** *(Bauhinia variegata).*
3. **Sanapushpi herb** (rattle-box / *Crotolaria juncea).*
4. **Madanam fruit** *(Randia dumetorum).*
5. **Katukalabu fruit** (bitter bottle gourd / *Lagenaria siceria).*
6. **Nimba leaf** (neem / *Azadirachta indica).*

List of Carminative Herbs
1. **Ela fruit** (greater cardamon / *Amomum subulatum).*
2. **Yavani seed** (wild omum / *Trachyspermum ammi).*
3. **Ajamoda seed** (wild celery / *Carum roxburghianum).*
4. **Dhanyakam seeds** (coriander / *Coriandrum sativum).*
5. **Fennel seed** (madhurika / *Foeniculum vulgare).*
6. **Hingu gum** (asafoetida/ *Ferula narthex).*
7. **Jirakam seed** (cumin / *Cuminum cyminum).*
8. **Jatiphalam seed** (nutmeg / *Myristica fragrans).*
9. **Karchura tuber/seed** (Zedoary /*Curcuma zedoaria).*
10. **Krishnajiraka seed** (black cumin / *Nigella sativa).*
11. **Lavangam seeds** (cloves / *Syzigium aromaticum).*
12. **Nagaram rhizome** (Indian cyperus / *Cyperus pertenuis).*
13. **Shatapushpa seed** (anise / *Pimpinella anisum).*

14. **Sukshmaila seed** (cardamom / *Elettaria cardamomum*).
15. **Trikatu** *(Piper longum, Piper nigrum, Zingiber officinalis)*.
16. **Tumburu seed** *(Zanthozylum armatum)*.
17. **Twak bark** (Cinnamon / *Cinnamon zeylanicum)*.

Chapter 13: Diseases of the Liver and Spleen (Yakrita Pliha Roga)

According to the theory of Ayurveda, liver and spleen disorders are often due to neglect of Pandu, a metabolic disorder correlated with the various types of anemia (page 256). Persons who over-exert themselves, eat excessive amounts of sour and salty foods, drink alcohol or do other things that vitiate the blood are subject to this group of diseases.

Yakridvriddhi (Enlarged liver)

Yakridvriddhi refers to an enlargement of the liver, caused by its hyperactivity, and is most often the result of other serious diseases. It is treated with combinations of purgative (page 174, diuretics (page 195), digestive (page 173) and alkali remedies (page 171), depending on signs and symptoms. These are taken with the specific medicines.

Some specific medicines include:

1. **Shatpala Ghrita**, 1-2 grams twice daily.
2. **Shukti Bhasma** (oyster shell ash /*Ostrea gigas)*, 500 mg given with warm water, twice daily.
3. An infusion is made from one part **Rohitaka stem** (rhododendron / *Rhododendron arboreum)* and two parts **Triphala** *(Phyllanthus emblica / Terminalia belerica / Terminalia chebula)* soaked in water or **Goumutra** (cow urine). Dose is 60-90 mL twice daily.
4. **Arkalavanam**, 1 gram given with warm water, twice daily.

Kamala (Jaundice / Hepatitis)

The disease of Kamala refers to both jaundice, which is related to an aggravation of hepatic venous system that causes inflammation, and hepatitis, in which there is an aggravation of both the hepatic vein and arterial systems, causing inflammation and swelling. Jaundice is treated with the regular Pitta treatments and diet (page 67) along with purgative remedies (page 174), diuretics (page 195), anti-inflammatories such as **Vasaka leaf** (Malabar nut / *Adhatoda vasica)*, and the remedies against Pandu (anemia) (page 256). These treatments help open the bile duct and remove the jaundice.

Hepatitis is treated with the principles and diet used for Pitta and Kapha treatment (page 81) along with purgative (page 174), diuretics (page 195), alkaline remedies (page 171) and specific remedies against hepatitis. Treatments for hepatitis involve initially treating hepatic edema or swelling of the liver to open the blockage of the bile duct system, followed by use of anti-inflammatories and liver restoratives.

Some specific compounds against hepatitis are:

1. **Mandura Vati**, 2-3 pills twice daily.
2. **Kamalakilyana**, 1000 mg twice daily.

After initial treatment of hepatitis (removing jaundice and liver blockage), liver restoratives are added, such as the standard compound **Shilajatu Rasayana**, given in doses of 2 pills twice daily.

Kumbhakamala (Chronic Hepatitis)

If Kamala or hepatitis is not properly treated, it can become chronic with symptoms including fatigue and bleeding problems. Chronic hepatitis is very difficult to cure. However, it can be treated with the same remedies for hepatitis along with anti hemorrhagic remedies (page 258) and liver restoratives including:

1. **Chandraprabha Vati**, 2-3 pills twice daily.
2. **Shilajatu Rasayana**, 2 pills twice daily.

Halimaka (Biliary Cirrhosis)

Biliary cirrhosis is concerned with the aggravated hepatic venous and nervous systems. It is treated with the principles used for Pitta and Vata treatment (page 81) along with the remedies for hepatitis. It is difficult to cure. Two useful remedies include:

1. **Chandraprabha Vati,** 2-3 pills twice daily.
2. **Kaishora Guggulu Vati,** 2 pills twice daily.

These two formulas can be given together, and taken with grape juice as an anupana.

Parshwashula (Liver pain with swelling)

Parshwashula refers to flank pain. If this pain occurs primarily on the right side of the abdomen and shoulder it is correlated with the liver. Colic pain of the liver can be caused by cholecystitis, gallstones, or cirrhosis of the liver. These diseases are characterized by aggravated functions of the nervous and arterial systems that cause swelling and blockage in the liver. They are treated with the medicines for Vata and Kapha colic (see page 162) along with alkali remedies (page 171), laxative remedies (see page 174) and the remedies for gastritis (page 160). Colic pain of the liver caused by liver cirrhosis is often related to alcoholism. This condition can be treated with the methods used for the medicines for cirrhosis (above) along with those used for alcoholism (below).

Madatyaya (Alcoholism)

Although generally celebrated for its digestive-enhancing and rejuvenating properties, Ayurveda has long warned about the dangers of alcoholic intoxication (madatyaya). For treatment of alcoholism the following remedies are useful:

1. Powder of **Amlavetasa root** (rhubarb / *Rheum emodi)* is given in doses of 1000 mg with water several times per day.
2. Also used is a paste made from equal parts dried **Draksha fruit** (raisin / *Vitis vinifera)*, **Kharjura fruit** (date / *Phoenix dactylifera)*, **Tintidika fruit** (tamarind / *Tamarandus indica)*, **Dadima rind** (sour pomegranate / *Punica granatum)*, and **Amalaki fruit** (Indian gooseberry / amla / *Phyllanthus emblica)* mixed with a little water. This is given in doses of 1-2 grams.

Pittashmari (Gallstone / Gallbladder stone)

Pittashmari refers to gallstones, which is considered to be a Pitta disorder. Some remedies include:

1. For pain relief, use **Shatavari root Churna** (wild asparagus / *Asparagus racemosus)*, 1-2 grams with water, twice daily.
2. To remove the stones, use the standard compound **Narikela Lavanam**, 500 mg twice daily.
3. Another remedy is one part of the standard compound **Samudradi Churna** taken with five parts of the standard compound **Amalakyadi Churna**, given in doses of 1-2 grams twice daily. For added benefit one part each **Shukti Bhasma** (oyster shell ash /*Ostrea gigas)* and **Nrisara** (purified ammonium chloride) can be added to this formula.

Yakridvidradhi (Abscess of the liver)

Yakridvidradhi refers to an abscess of the liver, and is very difficult to cure. It is treated with the same remedies used for internal abscess of the alimentary system (Vidradhi) (page 170).

Yakritodara (Neoplasm of the liver)

Yakritodara refers to cancer of the liver, and is primarily caused by the exudation of the tainted blood into the liver or by peritonitis. The term however can also refer to advanced pre-cancerous swelling and inflammation as well. Yakritodara is treated with alkali remedies (page 171), purgative remedies (page 174), enema, hot compress, venesection (page 92) and the remedies for peritonitis (page 171). Specific remedies against cancer of the liver should also be prescribed. In the advanced stage, it is treated with snake venom but this is an extremely dangerous method. Liver cancer with ascites, bleeding and coma is not curable.

Cancer of the liver is very difficult to cure. Use of venesection from the vein of the right wrist (page 92) is considered important. The blockage of the lymphatic duct system has to be opened as soon as possible with alkali remedies (page 171), purgative remedies (page 174) and urine therapy.

Some specific remedies against the cancer of the liver are:

1. **Sharapunkha** (*Tephrosia purpurea*), 500 mg twice daily.
2. **Rohitaka stem** (rhododendron / *Rhododendron arboreum*), 1-2 grams twice daily.
3. **Pippali fruit** (long pepper / *Piper longum*), 500 mg twice daily.
4. **Rohitakasava**, 20-30 mL after food, twice daily.
5. **Rohitaka Ghritam**, 3-5 grams twice daily.

Plihavriddhi (Enlargement of the spleen)

Plihavriddhi refers to the enlargement of the spleen, and is treated with the same remedies used for enlargement of the liver above (Yakridvriddhi) (page 177).

Plihavidradhi (Abscess of the spleen)

Plihavidradhi refers to an abscess of the spleen, and is very difficult to cure. It is treated with same remedies used for the internal abscess of the alimentary system (Vidradhi) (page 170).

Plihodar (Cancer of the spleen)

Plihodar refers to cancer of the spleen, with the causes being essentially the same as of those for cancer of the liver. It is treated with the same remedies, including the treatments of peritonitis. The only difference is that the venesection (page 92) has to be carried out from the left hand.

Raktaja Plihavriddhi (Splenitis)

Raktaja Plihavriddhi can be correlated with splenitis (spleen inflammation), and is a Raktaja disease. Some useful medicines are:

1. **Shukti Bhasma** (oyster shell ash /*Ostrea gigas*), 250 mg taken with warm water, twice daily.
2. An infusion is made by soaking **Rohitaka stem** (rhododendron / *Rhododendron arboreum*) and **Triphala** (*Phyllanthus emblica* / *Terminalia belerica* / *Terminalia chebula*) into water or **Goumutra** (cow urine) for seven days. Dose is 60-90 mL twice daily.
3. The standard compound **Arkalavanam**, made from fresh leaf of **Arka** (milkweed / *Calotropis gigantea*) cooked with **Saindhavam** (mineral salt), is given in doses of 500 mg, twice daily with warm water.

Chapter 14: Diseases of the Respiratory System (Uro Roga)

Inhalation of smoke, dust or polluted air, excess exercise, suppression of natural urges, and overuse of dry foods can produce cough or respiratory irritation. Neglect of cough can lead to more serious lung conditions.

Kasa (Cough / Bronchitis)

Kasa refers to coughs, and are caused by irritation of the respiratory system. Cough can be a symptom of any number of diseases, but in the form of bronchitis it is classified into five categories: Vata, Pitta, Kapha, Kshayaja and Kshataja. If not treated properly, bronchitis can become a chronic disease that is very difficult to cure, regardless of the cause. Chronic bronchitis has to be treated with both Rasayanas (restoratives) and the specific medicines for bronchitis, including:

1. **Duralambha bush** *(Fragonia cretica).*
2. **Karkatashringi fruit gall** (Insect gall / *Pistacia intergerrima).*
3. **Kantakari herb** (Black nightshade / *Solanum xanthocarpum).*
4. **Punarnava plant/root** *(Boerhavia difusa).*
5. **Tamalaki herb** *(Phyllanthus niruni).*
6. **Pippali fruit** (long pepper / *Piper longum).*
7. **Haritaki fruit** *(Terminalia chebula).*
8. **Amalaki fruit** (Indian gooseberry / *Phyllanthus emblica).*

Some useful formula against cough/bronchitis include are:

1. **Chaturdasanga Churna,** 2 grams taken with honey if the cough is with mucus or salty water if the cough is dry. In serious cases this remedy is combined with the **Rasasindura** (red crystal of mercury sulphide).
2. **Sringarabhraka compound,** 500 mg taken with honey or meat soup.
3. To stop irritation in the throat, the patient is given **Shambukadi Vati** as a lozenge.

Vataja Bronchitis

Bronchitis with the character of Vata is concerned with the aggravated function of the bronchial nervous system, manifesting as a dry cough. It is treated with the standard Vata treatments and diet along with the specific remedies against bronchitis.

Pittaja Bronchitis

Bronchitis with the character of Pitta is concerned with the aggravated function of the bronchial venous system, with symptoms of cough with heat and inflammation. It is treated with the standard Pitta treatments and diet along with the specific remedies against bronchitis.

Kaphaja Bronchitis

Bronchitis with the character of Kapha is concerned with the aggravated bronchial arterial system, with cough, swelling and mucus. It is treated with the standard Kapha treatments and diet along with specific remedies against bronchitis.

Kshayaja Bronchitis

Bronchitis with the character of Kshayaja is related to tuberculosis. It is treated with the same the remedies of pulmonary TB (page 184) along with the specific remedies against bronchitis.

Kshataja Bronchitis

Bronchitis with the character of Kshataja involves lesions in the lungs. It is difficult to cure. It is treated with the remedies for TB (see page 184), Rasayanas, anti-hemorrhagic remedies (page 258) and the remedies for hemoptysis (page 185).

Shwasa (Asthma)

Shwasa can be correlated with asthma, and in general, is the condition of rapid or poor respiration. It is divided into five categories: Kshudrashwasa, Tamakashwasa, Chhinnashwasa, Urdhwashwasa and Mahashwasa.

While treating cases of asthma, regardless of the cause, the aggravated functions of the nervous system (Vata) and arterial system (Kapha) have to be maintained with appropriate remedies, along with remedies that have heat-producing, vaso-dilatory effect. In the case of allergic asthma, the antipyretic remedies should be made from poisonous plants, based on the notion that small doses of toxic plants neutralize the toxic response to otherwise benign allergens.

Some specific remedies against asthma are:

1.   **Karkatashringi fruit gall** (insect gall on *Pistacia intergerrima).*
2.   **Karchura tuber/seed** (zedoary / *Curcuma zedoaria).*
3.   **Pushkaram tuber** *(Inula racemosa).*
4.   **Amlavetasa root** (rhubarb / *Rheum emodi).*
5.   **Ela fruit** (greater cardamon / *Amomum subulatum).*
6.   **Agaru wood** (eaglewood / *Aquilaria agallocha).*
7.   **Tulsi plant** (holy basil / *Ocimum sanctum).*
8.   **Tamalaki herb** *(Phyllanthus niruni).*

Some useful compounds in asthma include:

1. **Bibhitaki fruit** *(Terminalia belerica)*, 1-2 g with honey.
2. **Apamarga alkali** *(Achyranthes aspera)*, 500 mg with honey.
3. Two parts of the standard compound **Chaturdasanga Churna** with one part **Vasaka leaf** (Malabar nut / *Adhatoda vasica)*, 1000 mg with honey.

Kshudrashwasa (Dyspnea)

Kshudrashwasa or dyspnea is in general caused by aggravation of the functions of the bronchial nervous system (Vata) and arterial system (Kapha), causing breathing difficulty. It is treated with the standard Vata and Kapha treatments and diet (page 81) along with inhalation of steam, smoking of medicated remedies and the specific remedies against asthma.

Tamakashwasa (Bronchial Asthma)

Tamakashwasa or bronchial asthma is related to aggravated functioning of the bronchial arterial system (Kapha), with symptoms of swelling and blockage with mucus discharge. It is treated with the standard Kapha treatments and diet along with the remedies for bronchitis (above), laxatives (page 174), emetics (page 175) and the specific remedies against asthma. It is difficult to cure.

Pratamakashwasa (Allergic asthma)

Pratamakashwasa or allergic asthma is mostly related to winter or cold climate. This kind of asthma by nature gets better in the summer or in a hot climate. It is treated with the same remedies used for bronchial asthma, along with antipyretic remedies (page 154) and antitoxin remedies. It is difficult to cure.

Incurable Asthmas

There are three additional forms of asthma called Chhinnashwasa (asthma with asphyxia), Urdhwashwasa (asthma with the contraction of the spinal cord), and Mahashwasa (deep asthma). These forms of asthma lead to death and are not curable.

Hikka (Hiccup)

Hikka or hiccup, refers to the spasm of the diaphragm, and is caused by a blockage in the stomach or trachea, by food or the Doshas. It is divided into five categories: Annaja, Yamala, Kshudra, Gambhira and Maha Hikka. While treating hiccup, whatever the cause, it is very important to control the aggravated function of the nervous system (Vata) and arterial system (Kapha) as soon as possible with appropriate remedies.

Some anti-hiccup remedies are:

1. **Karchura tuber/seed** (zedoary / *Curcuma zedoaria).*
2. **Kantakari herb** (black nightshade / *Solanum xanthocarpum).*

3. **Duralambha bush** *(Fragonia cretica)*.
4. **Karkatashringi fruit gall** (Insect gall / *Pistacia intergerrima*).
5. **Brihati shrub** (vrihati / *Solanum indicum*).
6. **Haritaki fruit** *(Terminalia chebula)*.
7. **Pippali fruit** (long pepper / *Piper longum*).
8. **Pushkaram tuber** *(Inula racemosa)*.
9. **Sauvira Bhasma** (purified antimony sulfide).
10. **Bodhibrikshya Bhasma** *(Ficus religiosa* ash).
11. **Muyurapuccha Bhasma** (peacock feather ash).

One compound that can be used is equal parts **Haritaki fruit** *(Terminalia chebula)* and **Nagaram rhizome** (Indian cyperus / *Cyperus pertenuis*), 1-2 grams given with warm water. This compound is more powerful if given with 5% **Sauvira Bhasma** (purified antimony sulfide).

Annaja (Hiccup caused by food)
Hiccup caused by food blockage or coldness is stopped by drinking water. It is not serious.

Yamala (Double hiccup)
Double hiccup is considered to be a real disease. It is difficult to cure and sometimes can be a cause of death. It is treated with the same remedies used for asthma along with the antihiccup remedies.

Kshudra (Common hiccup)
Common hiccup is treated with the remedies of asthma along with the antihiccup remedies.

Gambhira (Deep hiccup)/Maha Hikka (Severe hiccup)
These two kinds of hiccups cause death and have no cure.

Rajayakshma (Pulmonary Tuberculosis)
Rajayakshma is correlated with pulmonary tuberculosis (TB), and is concerned with the aggravated functions of the nervous system (coughing and weakness), venous system (infection) and arterial system (swelling) of the lungs. Basic symptoms may include emaciation, cough with fever, chest pain, difficult breathing and blood in the sputum. Pulmonary TB develops with a blockage in the entry of the essence of food supply into the vascular system causing emaciation. It is divided into two categories:

- Rajayakshma with eleven symptoms, including hemoptysis; and
- Rajayakshma with six symptoms, without hemoptysis.

The first of these two categories is highly progressive and difficult to cure. In general, these forms of Rajayakshma are treated with digestive and appetizing remedies (page 173) and Rasayanas (see Chapter 27), along with symptomatic treatments, i.e. the specific remedies for fever, cough, hemoptysis, common cold and general debility, all depending upon circumstances.

While treating Rajayakshma the most important initial thing to do is maintain the function of the nervous system with the general treatments and diet for Vata (page 56), along with digestive (page 173) and antipyretic remedies (page 154). Once the more difficult symptoms are under control it becomes possible to treat the venous system (Pitta) and the arterial system (Kapha) with the indicated remedies. The specific remedies against Rajayakshma are not powerful unless prescribed in combinations according to symptoms.

Some specific remedies against Rajayakshma include:

1. **Chyavanaprasha paste**, 2 grams with milk as a lung restorative.
2. **Drakshyasava**, 30 mL after meals for energy, vitality & good blood circulation.
3. **Kshyakesarirasa**, 200 mg with warm water for fever.
4. **Kushmandavaleha**, 2 grams as a lung and brain restorative.
5. **Lavangadi Churna**, 2 grams as a specific remedy to reduce cough.
6. **Madhutapyadi Churna**, 1000 mg to reduce lung exudation.
7. **Nagabala plant, wild** (country mallow / *Sida cordifolia*) 1000 mg as a general nerve restorative.
8. **Sitopaladi Churna,** 1-2 grams with honey and Ghee for relief of chest pain, cough, asthma, dyspepsia and hemoptysis.
9. **Sudarshana Churna**, 500 mg with warm water for fever.
10. **Talishadyam Churna**, 1000 mg to reduce chest infection, cough and asthma.
11. **Vayasajangha** (bird meat soup) as a lung restorative and to improve circulation.

Vranashosa (Pulmonary Tuberculosis with cancerous tubercles)

Pulmonary TB with cancerous tubercles is a very serious complicated lung lesion. Although it is not curable the patient can be maintained with the same methods used for pulmonary TB along with anti hemorrhagic remedies (page 258) and the remedies used for healing complicated wounds (page 89).

Urakshata (Hemoptysis)

Urakshata refers to hemoptysis, and indicative of some kind of injury to the lungs. It is treated with the same methods for pulmonary TB along with specific remedies including:

1. **Laksha insect secretion** *(Coccus lacca)*, 500 mg twice daily
2. **Vasa leha** *(Adhatoda vasica)*, prepared by cooking the fresh juice or fine powder of Vasa in a base of Ghee and adding honey when cool. Dose is 1-2 grams twice daily.

Uroghata (Pneumonia)

Uroghata or pneumonia is inflammation of the lungs caused by the common cold or influenza. It is divided into four categories: Vata, Pitta, Kapha and Sannipata. The general approach to the treatment of pneumonia emphasizes the proper control of the arterial system with remedies that create heat and dryness. Some specific remedies against pneumonia are:

1. **Mrigamadasava**, 10 drops twice daily.
2. **Mritunjayarasa**, 3 pills twice daily.
3. **Chaturdasanga Churna**, 1-2 grams twice daily.

Vataja Pneumonia

Pneumonia with the character of Vata involves aggravation of the nervous system. It is treated with the specific remedies against pneumonia and pleurisy, along with addition of carminative remedies (page 175), mild laxatives (page 174), and/or the remedies for the common cold (page 294). Choices among these depend upon signs and symptoms.

Pittaja Pneumonia

Pneumonia with the character of Pitta is concerned especially the aggravated function of the venous system (inflammation). It is treated with the specific remedies against pneumonia, to which laxative remedies (page 174) and antipyretic remedies (page 154) are added.

Kaphaja Pneumonia

Pneumonia with the character of Kapha is concerned especially with the aggravation of arterial system, which causing swelling and edema. It is treated with the specific remedies against pneumonia to which medicines for edema (page 257) are added.

Sannipataja Pneumonia

Pneumonia with the character of Sannipata is congruent with double pneumonia. It is difficult to cure. It is treated with the specific remedies against pneumonia with addition of other herbs dependent upon signs and symptoms.

Parshwashula (Pleurisy)

Parshwashula refers to flank pain. If this pain occurs primarily over the lungs it is correlated with pleurisy, and is concerned with the aggravated functions of the nervous and arterial systems (exudation of water into the pleura). It is treated generally with the basic Vata and Kapha treatments (page 81) along with the remedies for pneumonia (above), steam, plaster, and venesection practices (page 92). Specific remedies against pleurisy include:

1. **Chaturdasanga Churna**, 2 grams twice daily.
2. **Mrityunjayarasa Vati**, 2-3 pills twice daily.
3. Decoction of **Punarnava** *(Boerhavia difusa)*, 60-90 mL, given with 500 mg **Yavakshara alkaline ash** (barley plant / *Hordeum vulgare*).
4. **Shringaputa** (deer horn ash / *Cervus nippon*).
5. **Sitopaladi Churna,** 1-3 grams twice daily.
6. **Rasna Ghritam** (Ghee preparation made from **Rasna shrub** -*Vanda roxburghii).*
7. **Bala Ghritam** (Ghee preparation made from **Bala plant** - *Sida cordifolia*).

Urovidradhi (Abscess of the lungs)

Urovidradhi refers to abscess of the lungs, and is treated with the same methods for internal abscess of the alimentary system (Vidradhi) (page 170).

Vakshauddharsa (Pulmonary emphysema)

Vakshauddharsa is correlated with pulmonary emphysema, and is concerned with the aggravated function of the nervous system that causes distention of the chest. It is treated with the general Vata treatments and diet (page 56) along with the remedies for asthma (page 182).

Chapter 15: Diseases of the Heart (Hrida Roga)

Disease of the heart and the cardiovascular system are divided into five categories, with the characters of Vata, Pitta, Kapha, Sannipata and Krimija. A general rule is that heart disease is often caused by pathogenic defects of the plasma (see page 254). These defects must be corrected, typically, by using measures such as restricting the intake of heavy and greasy foods, and by prescribing regular exercise as well as digestive (page 173) or heart-specific Rasayanas. Additional factors in disease of the heart include the regular intake of foods that are difficult to digest, anxiousness and worrying, and the suppression of natural urges. As a general rule, heart diseases are very difficult to cure. When treating heart disease of all types, pure clean air is essential to have the best results.

General Treatment of Heart Disease

Ayurveda describes several individual heart restoratives that can be used to protect the heart, or to strengthen a weak heart. These include **Shatavari root** (wild asparagus / *Asparagus racemosus)*, **Kasturi** (deer musk / *Moschus moschiferus*), **Arjuna bark** *(Terminalia arjuna)*, **Hiraka Bhasma** (purified diamond oxide) and **Badari fruit** (jujube, sour variety / *Ziziphus jujuba).* Many sour fruits have cardio-restorative properties, including pomegranate, half-ripe mango, rhubarb, citron, jujube, and orange.

The standard compound **Dadimadi Churna** given with **Ghrita** (Ghee / clarified butter) can be used to strengthen the heart, given in doses of 1-2 grams. This compound is stronger if prescribed with 200 mg of **Shringaputa** (deer horn ash / *Cervus nippon)* and 100 mg of **Rasasindura** (red crystal of mercury sulfide). If there is complete heart failure, then it is necessary to use medicines that create heat, energy and dryness, such as **Mrigamadasava**, 10 drops given with warm water. To relieve heart attack with strong palpitations herbs such as **Nagaram rhizome** (Indian cyperus / *Cyperus pertenuis)* can be used, 1-2 grams boiled in milk.

Vataja Heart Disease (Angina Pectoris)

Vataja heart disease is generally correlated with angina pectoris, manifesting as a shooting pain radiating to the arms, shoulders and neck, accompanied by sweating. Such symptoms occur as the result of the aggravated function of the cardiac nervous system, and are treated with regular Vata treatments and diet (page 56), along with general heart remedies, and specific remedies against angina pectoris. In addition to the use of the regular Vata treatments, a decoction made of digestive remedies (page 173) or **Shunthi root** (dry ginger / *Zingiber officinalis)* is prescribed to relieve sharp pain sensations in the heart. Some specific remedies against angina pectoris are:

1. **Shringaputa** (deer horn ash / *Cervus nippon*), 200 mg with **Ghrita** (Ghee/ clarified butter).
2. **Baladyam Ghritam**, 1-2 grams.
3. **Arjuna bark** *(Terminalia arjuna)*, 500 mg with honey or milk.
4. **Bala plant** (country mallow / *Sida cordifolia*), 500 mg with honey or milk.
5. **Arjuna Ghritam**, 1-2 grams.

Hricchulam (Pseudoangina / Angina pectoris vasomotoria)

Hricchulam is a kind of pseudoangina that is concerned with the presence of air bubbles in the plasma of the heart that cause aggravation of the cardiac nervous system. It is treated with the same remedies used for angina pectoris.

Hriddrava (Tachycardia)

Hriddrava corresponds with tachycardia, and is concerned with a deficiency of the blood (either plasma or the blood sugar) that causes the aggravation of the cardiac nervous system. It is treated with the normal Vata treatments and diet, along with the same remedies used for angina pectoris (above) and the herbal remedies against anemia (see page 256). If the tachycardia is caused by toxicity, infection, or other cause, the cause must be treated. One particularly useful remedy for Hriddrava is Vatakulantaka Rasa, in doses of 125-250 mg.

Pittaja Heart Disease (Myocarditis / Pericarditis)

Pittaja disease of the heart can be correlated with myocarditis and pericarditis, manifesting as a sharp burning pain that radiates to the chest and throat, mimicking the pain of gastritis. Pittaja heart disease concerns the aggravated function of the cardiac venous system, and is treated with the regular Pitta treatments and diet (page 67), along with laxative remedies (page 174) and specific remedies, including:

1. **Arjuna bark** *(Terminalia arjuna)*, 500 mg with honey or milk.
2. **Panchamulam** (five roots compound), 1000 mg with water.
3. **Bala plant** (country mallow / *Sida cordifolia*), 500 mg with honey or milk.
4. **Madhukam root** (licorice / *Glycyrrhiza glabra*), 500 mg boiled in milk.
5. **Baladyam Ghritam**, 1-2 grams.
6. **Arjuna Ghritam**, 1-2 grams.

Kaphaja Heart Disease (Cardiac hypertrophy)

Kaphaja disease of the heart concerns the aggravated function of the cardiac arterial system that causes heaviness or an increased in the size (hypertrophy) of the heart. Common symptoms include a heavy, dull pain, an increase in chest pressure, difficult respiration and sweating. It is treated with the basic Kapha treatment and diet along with emetic remedies (see page 175) and specific remedies against hypertrophy, including:

1. **Shilajatu** is a specific medicine against hypertrophy of the heart. Dose is 2 pills twice daily.
2. **Vatakulantaka Rasa**, 2-3 pills twice daily.

Hritshulam (Heart attack / Myocardial infarction)

Hritshulam refers to a myocardial infarction, and is a Rasa-Vataja disease caused by sudden constriction or blockage causing loss of blood supply and nutrition. This is a serious condition that can lead to death. For both prevention and treatment, use a restorative made from five parts **Amalaki fruit** (Indian gooseberry / amla / *Phyllanthus emblica)* and one part **Shringaputa** (deer horn ash / *Cervus nippon),* taken in doses of 1000 mg twice daily, with **Madhu** (honey). This formula can be taken with **Vatakulantaka Rasa**, 2-3 pills twice daily.

Hridayopalepa (Thrombosis)

Hridayopalepa corresponds to thrombosis, or abnormal clotting within a blood vessel, and is a Kaphaja disease. Swelling in the arteries and excess mucus exudation are the underlying causes, caused by eating an overly heavy diet with lots of fried greasy foods, poor digestion, and lack of exercise. The first step in treatment is use of emetic medicines such as **Vacha rhizome** (acorus / *Acorus calamus)* or **Nimba leaf** (neem / *Azadirachta indica).* Emesis is followed by use of digestive remedies (page 173) taken along with the restorative herbs mentioned under general treatment of heart disease (see above).

Shiragata Roga (Varicose Veins)

Shiragata roga refers to a disease of enlarged tortuous veins, particularly of the legs, and is a Vataja disease. It is treated with application of medicated steam, warm fomentation made from salt water, oil massage and nerve restoratives. These are all chosen from the general Vata medicines (page 56). Useful nerve restoratives include **Yogaraja Guggulu Vati** and **Narayana Taila**. A decoction can be prepared with **Bilwa fruit** (bael / *Aegle marmelos)* and other herbs, to be used as a herbal steam directed onto the affected areas.

Sannipataja Heart Disease (Acute endocarditis)

Sannipataja heart disease corresponds to acute endocarditis, and is caused by the simultaneous aggravation of the cardiac nervous, vein and arterial systems. It is very difficult to cure, and is treated with symptomatic treatments for heart disease based upon signs and symptoms, along with laxative or purgative remedies (page 174). Following the symptomatic treatments, certain rules of treatment should be followed:

1. If the pain of the heart is worse during digestion of food, laxative remedies prepared with oils or fats are prescribed, to clear Pitta and congestion in the bile duct and intestines.
2. If the pain of the heart is worse right after meals, **Mrigamadasava** is prescribed in doses of 10 drops 2-3 time daily, with water.
3. If the pain of the heart is worse after complete digestion, laxative remedies prepared with Triphala or Amalaki is prescribed, to reduce Vata and ease cramping.
4. If the pain of the heart is constant, use strong purgative remedies made from powerful roots such as **Danti** *(Baliospermum montanum)*, 500-1000 mg per dose.

Beside these symptomatic treatments, the other heart disease medicaments, especially heart restoratives, have to be prescribed side by side along with proper diet.

Krimija Heart Disease (Parasitic infection of the heart)

Krimija heart disease refers to a parasitic infection of the heart and is very difficult to cure. In this case, maggots can be seen developing in the affected area of the heart, a very dangerous condition. It is treated with the same remedies as Sannipataja heart disease along with anthelmintic remedies (page 175).

Pittavrita (Hypertension)

Pittavrita corresponds with hypertension, and is caused by abnormal blood vessel dilation related to aggravated nervous system (Vata) function. There are five different types of hypertension in Ayurveda related to the five types of Vital Air (Prana, see page 47), i.e. hypertension with the characters of Prana, Udana, Samana, Vyana and Apana.

Bitter plants with a dilatory effect on blood vessels and sweet plants that calm the nervous system are the general medicines for hypertension. These are given along with remedies that counteract the individual characters and issues associated with the different types of hypertension.

To quickly lower blood pressure over the short term (but not to cure), use **Sarpagandha root** *(Rauwolfia serpentina)*, starting at doses of 250 mg and gradually increasing the dose until the desired result is achieved. Strong laxative medicines (page 174) can also lower high blood pressure quickly in emergency situations.

To treat hypertension gradually, general medicines include:

1. **Shatavari root** (asparagus / *Asparagus racemosus)*, 500 mg twice daily.
2. **Shilajatu Rasayana**, 2 pills twice daily.
3. **Guduchi stem** *(Tinospora cordifolia)*, 1000 mg twice daily.
4. **Vatakulantaka Rasa**, 2-3 pills twice daily.

Pittavrita Prana (Hypertension related to inhalation)

Hypertension related to inhalation occurs when the inhalation function (Prana Vayu) becomes weak or disturbed, reducing available blood oxygen. This subsequently leads to a toxic state in the blood, which when it becomes excessive causes the blood pressure to rise, as well as causing symptoms of gastritis. The general medicines for hypertension are used, along with the remedies for gastritis (see page160).

Pittavrita Udana (Hypertension related to exhalation)

Hypertension related to exhalation function occurs when the exhalation function (Udana Vayu) becomes weak, and the buildup of carbon dioxide and inflammation in the blood causes the blood pressure to elevate. The general medicines for hypertension are used, along with the remedies for Shwasa (Asthma).

Pittavrita Samana (Hypertension related to digestion)

Hypertension related to digestive function occurs when digestive neurological function (Samana Vayu) becomes weak, affecting the portal vein. Subsequently digestive power wanes, inflammation develops and the blood pressure elevates. The general medicines for hypertension are used, along with digestive agents (see page 173).

Pittavrita Vyana (Hypertension related to excessive blood volume)

Hypertension related to excessive blood volume occurs when irritated neurological function affects the general blood circulation (Vyana Vayu), and the increased blood volume causes blood pressure to elevate. The general medicines for hypertension are used, along with nerve restoratives such as **Yogaraja Guggulu Vati.**

Pittavrita Apana (Hypertension related to excretory function)

Hypertension related to excretory function occurs when irritated neurological function affects the excretory function of the kidneys and bowels (Apana Vayu), and this blockage causes blood pressure to rise. If the problem is bowel blockage, use the regular hypertension medicines along with laxatives (page 174). If the problem is kidney blockage, use the regular hypertension remedies along with the remedies for kidney infections (page 204).

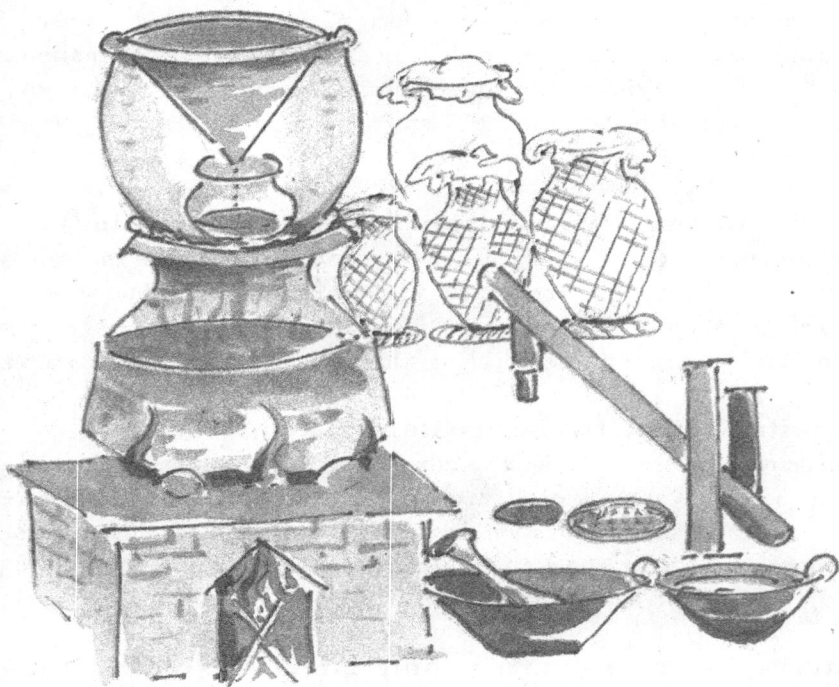

Pharmacy methods in Ayurveda, drawing by Dr. Mana

Chapter 16: Diseases of the Urinary Bladder (Mutravahasrota Roga)

Diseases of the urinary tract and kidneys are broadly classified under the heading of Mutravahasrota Roga. In general, diseases of the bladder and urethra are called Mutraghata whereas metabolic diseases marked by polyuria (excessive urination) are typically classified under the heading of Prameha. Urinary diseases under the heading Mutraghata can also be classified into thirteen categories: Vatakundalika, Vatashthila, Vatavasti, Mutratita, Mutrajathara, Mutrasanga, Mutrakshaya, Mutragranthi, Ushnavata, Vastikundalam, Vidvidhata, Mutrasada, and Ashmari. Prameha and other kidneys disorders are discussed in the next chapter.

The general remedies for disorders of the urinary tract are diuretics (mutravirechana), which promote the flow of urine and correct the downward flow of Vata Dosha. This chapter will make frequent reference to diuretics, some of which can be chosen from this list of useful remedies:

1. **Gokshura fruit** *(Tribulus terrestris).*
2. **Pashanabheda root** (rockfoil / *Bergenia ligulata).*
3. **Pueraria tuber** (vidari / *Pueraria lobata).*
4. **Punarnava plant/root** *(Boerhavia difusa).*
5. **Shilajatu Rasayana.**
6. **Shukti Bhasma** (oyster shell ash / *Ostrea gigas).*
7. **Soraka** (Potassium chloride).
8. **Yava seed** (barley / *Hordeum vulgare).*
9. **Yavakshara alkaline ash** (barley plant / *Hordeum vulgare).*

The last item on this list is **Yavakshara alkaline ash**, which is a very strong diuretic that is used only in minute quantities. For example, to make the mildly diuretic **Guduchi stem** *(Tinospora cordifolia)* into a strong diuretic, one gram of **Yavakshara** is added to 400 grams of **Guduchi**.

Besides diuretic remedies, a 'urinary pipe enema' (Uttaravasti) is also commonly used in disease of the urinary bladder. In this procedure, the enema is made with remedies that stimulate the urinary system to completely eliminate. This is given after the pre-operative procedures of Pancha Karma have been implemented, including 'oil massage' (Abhyanga) and 'steam bath' (Swedana), as well as laxatives to promote the passage of urine, feces and gas. One useful formula for urinary enema is a decoction made from two parts **Devadaru wood** (Himalayan cedar / *Cedrus deodara)* and one part **Mustaka tuber** *(Cyperus rotundus)*, mixed with one part **Madhu** (honey), one part **Saindhavam** (mineral salt) and four parts **Tila seed oil** (sesame / *Sesamum indicum*).

Medicated rectal suppositories are also used often for the same purpose of stimulating elimination. For example, a medicated suppository can be made from two parts **Sarshapi seed** (black mustard / *Sinapis juncea)*, one-half part **Trikatu** *(Piper longum, Piper nigrum, Zingiber officinalis)*, and one part **Yavakshara alkaline ash** (barley plant / *Hordeum vulgare)*, mixed with two parts **Goumutra** (cow urine) and one part **Matsyandika** (molasses).

Mutraghata

As a non-specific diagnosis, mutraghata is essentially synonymous with urethritis, as a disease of the urinary pipe. It can be divided into eight categories, with the characters of Vataja, Pittaja, Kaphaja, Sannipataja, Aghantuja, Purisaja, Shukraja, and Asmarija.

General Treatment

Whatever may be the cause and condition of urethritis, dysuria is always a symptom. Plenty of water must be drunk by the patient. Drinking water stimulates mucous membrane secretion for protection of the urethra and also causes a natural diuretic action.

There are some specific remedies against urethritis that can be prescribed in any condition, including:

1. **Gokshuradi Guggulu**, 2 pills twice daily.
2. **Shitarasa Vati**, 2 pills twice daily.
3. **Chandraprabha Vati**, 2 pills twice daily.

Vataja Urethritis

Dysuria or dysuria with the character of Vata has symptoms of dryness of the urethra. It is treated with the regular Vata treatments (page 56) along with diuretic remedies and urinary pipe enema made with greasy remedies. One useful remedy is a medicated oil prepared with equal parts **Punarnava** *(Boerhavia difusa)*, **Eranda root** (Castor / *Ricinus communis)* and **Shatavari** *(Asparagus racemosa)* in a base of Ghee or sesame oil that can be massaged over the lower pubic region.

Pittaja Urethritis

Urethritis with the character of Pitta is related to an inflamed urethra. It is treated with the regular Pitta treatments (page 67) along with diuretic remedies, enema through the urinary pipe and laxative remedies (page 174). One useful intervention is a cold fomentation applied topically to pubic region, prepared with one part **Devadaru wood** (Himalayan cedar / *Cedrus deodara)* and two parts **Amalaki fruit** (Indian gooseberry / amla / *Phyllanthus emblica)* with honey, or four parts Cucumber seed, two parts **Madhukam root** (licorice / *Glycyrrhiza glabra)* and one part **Devadaru wood** (Himalayan cedar / *Cedrus deodara)*, prepared with rice water or cold water.

Kaphaja Urethritis
Kapha urethritis is concerned with swelling of the urethra. It is treated with the regular Kapha treatments (page 77) along with diuretics and enema through the urinary pipe. Useful therapies include **Pravala Bhasma** (purified coral oxide), taken with cold water, or a cooled decoction of **Guduchi stem** *(Tinospora cordifolia)* taken with honey.

Sannipataja Urethritis
Urethritis with the character of Sannipata presents with complicated urinary symptoms. It is very difficult to cure, however is can be treated with symptomatic treatments based on the treatments for Vataja, Pittaja and Kaphaja urethritis.

Aghantuja Urethritis
Urethritis with the character of Aghantuja is concerned with a traumatic injury causing urethritis. It is treated with the same remedies of urethritis with the character of Vata, along with remedies such as **Chandraprabha Vati** (2 pills twice daily) and **Gokshuradi Guggulu Vati** (2 pills twice daily).

Purisaja Urethritis
Urethritis with the character of Purisaja is related to constipation. It is treated with the regular Vata treatments (page 56) and laxative remedies (page 174).

Shukraja Urethritis
Urethritis with the character of Shukraja is related to prostatitis. It is treated with the same remedies used for prostatitis (page 198).

Asmarija Urethritis
Urethritis with the character of Asmarija is caused by urinary lithiasis. It is treated with the same remedies used for urinary lithiasis (page 200)

Vatakundalika (Spasmodic Stricture of the Bladder)
Vatakundalika refers to a spasmodic stricture of the bladder, and is concerned with the aggravated function of the cystic nervous system. It is caused by the consumption of dry foods and the suppression of natural urges. It is treated with enema through the urinary pipe, application of steam, diuretics, carminative remedies (page 175), and the remedies that are prescribed for bladder stones (page 200).

Vatashthila (Prostatitis / Neoplasm of the prostate gland)

The Sanskrit word Vatashthila refers to both prostatitis and tumor of the prostate gland. It is concerned with the aggravated function of the cystic nervous system (Vata). It is treated with the regular Vata treatments and diet (page 56) along with enema through the urinary pipe, diuretics, application of steam, venesection (see page 92) around the affected area, and surgery. Specific medicines against prostatitis include **Gokshuradi Guggulu Vati** (2 pills twice daily), and **Shitarasa Vati** (2 pills twice daily). If the disease progresses to neoplasm (a Sannipataja disease), the general medicines for cancer (page 248) are added.

Vatavasti (Outlet obstruction of the bladder)

Vatavasti, or outlet obstruction of the bladder, is concerned with blockage in the cystic nervous system. It is treated with the regular Vata treatments (page 56) along with the use of catheter, strong diuretics, urinary pipe enema, and the application of steam or hot compress.

Mutratita (Decrease in force of urinary stream)

Mutratita, or a decrease in the force of the urinary stream is concerned with the aggravated function of the cystic nervous system. It is treated with the regular Vata treatments (page 56) along with diuretics and the application of stream or hot compress.

Mutrajathara (Distended bladder with urine and gas)

Mutrajathara refers to the distension of the urinary bladder due to the accumulation of urine and gas, and is concerned with the aggravated function of the cystic nervous system. It is treated with the regular Vata treatments (page 56) along with the use of the catheter, application of steam or hot compress, enema through urinary pipe, diuretics and medicated suppository.

Mutrasanga (Anuria)

Mutrasangha refers to the inability to urinate, or anuria, and is concerned with the aggravated function of the cystic nervous system that causes a diminution of urinary secretions. It is treated with the regular Vata treatments (page 56) along with the diuretics outlined in the beginning of this chapter. Also used are application of steam or hot compress, medicated suppository, and urinary pipe enema.

Mutrakshaya (Anuria caused by dehydration)

Anuria caused by dehydration is treated with the regular Vata and Pitta treatments (page 81) and plenty of water to drink.

Mutragranthi (Malignant neoplasm of the bladder)

Mutragranthi refers to cancer of the bladder, and is concerned with aggravation in the cystic nervous and arterial systems along with pathogenic defects of the blood. It is treated with the basic Vata and Kapha treatments and diet (page 81) together with blood cleaning remedies (page 155), venesection practices (see page 92), urinary pipe enema and the specific remedies against cancer (page 248). It is very difficult to cure. Two useful remedies include **Chandraprabha Vati** (2 pills twice daily), combined with **Gokshuradi Guggulu Vati** (2 pills twice daily).

Ushnavata (Cystitis)

Ushnavata refers to cystitis, and is concerned with the aggravated functions of the cystic venous and nervous systems. It is treated with the principles used for Pitta and Vata treatment (page 81) along with diuretics, urinary pipe enema, and specific remedies against cystitis including **Gokshuradi Guggulu Vati**, **Shitarasa Vati** (2 pills twice daily) and **Chandraprabha Vati** (2 pills twice daily).

Vastikundalam (Dislocation of the bladder)

Vastikundalam refers to the dislocation or prolapse of the bladder, and is generally concerned with the aggravated function of the cystic nervous system. It manifests with symptoms of severe pain, burning sensation, and spasm. The lower pubic region swollen resembles early pregnancy, the patient voiding urine when pressure is applied. It is very difficult to cure. However it is treated with the regular Vata treatments (page 56. With inflammation or general edema symptomatic treatments are given.

Vidvidhata (Pneumaturia)

Vidvidhata can be correlated with pneumaturia, or 'bubbles' in the urine, and is concerned with the aggravated function of the cystic nervous system that causes putrefactive gas in the urine. It is treated with the regular Vata treatments (page 56) along with hot compress, carminative remedies (page 175), and digestive remedies (page 173).

Mutrasada (Crystalluria)

Mutrasada can be correlated with crystalluria, and is divided into two categories, one with white crystals and another with yellow crystals in the urine. White crystals are related to Kapha and yellow crystals are related to 'bile' (Pitta). They are treated respectively with the regular Kapha and Pitta treatments along with the remedies for Ashmari (urinary lithiasis).

Ashmari (Urinary lithiasis)

Ashmari refers to bladder stone or urinary lithiasis, and in general develops from a bladder condition that allows sedimentation to accumulate. It is treated with specific stone breaking remedies, diuretics and symptomatic treatments. According to the color of the stone, it is classified as a Vata stone (pink), a Pitta stone (yellow) or a Kapha stone (white). If the stone is large, it must be taken out with surgery. Some useful 'stone-breaking' specific remedies are **Pashanabheda root** (rockfoil / *Bergenia ligulata)* and **Gokshura fruit** *(Tribulus terrestris)*, in doses of 1-2 grams each. Useful combinations include:

1. **500 mg of Yavakshara alkaline ash** (barley plant / *Hordeum vulgare)* combined with **Kanjika** (whey) or decoction of **Gokshura fruit** *(Tribulus terrestris)*.

2. A decoction of two parts **Gokshura fruit** *(Tribulus terrestris)* and **Punarnava** *(Boerhavia difusa)*, one part each **Pashanabheda root**, **Brihati shrub** (vrihati / *Solanum indicum)* and **Kantakari herb** (Black nightshade / *Solanum xanthocarpum)*, and one-half part **Eranda root** (Castor / *Ricinus communis)*.

Chapter 17: Diseases of the Kidneys (Mutravahasrota roga)

Diseases of the kidney as well as metabolic conditions marked by polyuria, or excess urine excretion, largely come under the heading of Prameha in Ayurveda. Prameha is a term that refers to the kidneys and their failure to properly preserve vital nutrients in the blood, allowing their excretion into the urine. It is diagnosed on the qualities of these substances found in the urine, and are broadly classified into three basic categories: Kaphaja, Pittaja and Vataja. The primary causes of Prameha are foods that are too sweet, heavy and oily in nature (which aggravate Kapha), poor digestion, lack of exercise and excessive sleep. Various toxins can also be causative.

Kaphaja Prameha

Urinary diseases related to the aggravated function of the renal arterial system are identified as Kaphaja in origin, promoting renal edema, catarrhal states, and by-products in the urine that excess the imbalanced qualities of Kapha. Ayurveda divides kidney diseases with the character of Kapha into ten subcategories: Udakameha, Ikshumeha, Sandrameha, Surameha, Pistameha, Sukrameha, Sikatameha, Shitameha, Shanairmeha, and Lalameha. They can all be treated with the basic treatments and diet for Kapha along with specific remedies.

Udakameha (Polyuria)

Udakameha or simple polyuria is concerned with the aggravated function of the renal arterial system with symptoms of excess watery urine, without a typical urine odor. It is treated with the regular Kapha treatments and diet (page 77) along with specific remedies against polyuria. It is easy to cure.

Some specific remedies against polyuria are:

1. **Parijata bark decoction** (*Erythrinia variegata*), 1-2 cups of a weak decoction.
2. **Haridra Amalirasena**, 3 pills twice daily (Vati), 2 grams twice daily (Churna).
3. **Lauhasava**, 30 mL twice daily.
4. **Shilajatu**, 2-3 pills twice daily.

Ikshumeha (Diabetes insipidus)

Ikshumeha can be correlated with diabetes insipidus, and is defined as an aggravation of the function of the renal arterial system that causes an increase of blood sugar in the urine, resembling cane sugar juice (Ikshu) in sweetness. It is treated with the general Kapha treatments and diet (page 77) along with specific remedies against diabetes insipidus. It is easy to cure. Some useful medicines for ikshumeha include:

1. **Shilajatu**, 2-3 pills several times daily.
2. Decoction of equal parts **Khadira extract** (catechu / *Acacia catechu*, white) and **Puga nut** (betel / *Areca catechu*), 60-90 mL twice daily.
3. Decoction of two parts **Triphala** *(Phyllanthus emblica / Terminalia belerica / Terminalia chebula)* and one part **Gokshura fruit** *(Tribulus terrestris)*, 60-90 mL twice daily.
4. **Vaijayanti Kashaya**, 60-90 mL twice daily.
5. **Haridra Amalirasena**, 3 pills twice daily (Vati), 2 grams twice daily (Churna).
6. **Lauhasava**, 30 mL twice daily.
7. **Chaturdasanga Churna**, 2 grams twice daily.

Surameha (Phosphaturia)

Surameha refers to urine that is frothy like beer (Sura), and can be correlated with phosphaturia. It is treated with the regular Kapha treatments and diet (page 77) along with specific remedies. It is easy to cure. Some specific remedies against surameha include:

1. **Nimba Kashaya** 30-90 mL twice daily, depending on strength of patient.
2. **Haridra Amalirasena**, 3 pills twice daily (Vati), 2 grams twice daily (Churna).
3. **Lauhasava**, 30 mL twice daily.
4. **Shilajatu**, 2-3 pills twice daily.

Pistameha (Chyluria)

Pistameha is correlated with chyluria, caused by an aggravation of renal arterial system that allows chyle in the urine, giving it a dirty-white colored urine. It is treated with the regular Kapha treatments and diet (page 77) along with specific remedies. It is easy to cure. Some specific remedies include:

1. **Haridra Daruharidra Kashaya**, 30-60 mL twice daily.
2. **Haridra Amalirasena,** 3 pills twice daily (Vati), 2 grams twice daily (Churna).
3. **Lauhasava**, 30 mL twice daily.
4. **Shilajatu**, 2-3 pills twice daily.

Shukrameha (Spermatorrhea)

Shukrameha refers to the presence of sperm (Shukra) in the urine. It is treated with the regular Kapha treatments and diet (page 77) along with specific remedies against spermatorrhea. It is easy to cure. Some specific remedies include:

1. **Kakubha Chandana Kashaya,** 60-90 mL twice daily.
2. **Haridra Amalirasena,** 3 pills twice daily (Vati), 2 grams twice daily (Churna).
3. **Lauhasava,** 30 mL twice daily.
4. **Shilajatu,** 2-3 pills twice daily.

Sikatameha (Urate, Calcium oxalate etc in the urine)

Sikatameha refers to the presence of urates or other solids in the urine caused by the aggravation of the renal arterial system. It is treated with the regular Kapha treatments and diet (page 77) along with specific remedies against solids in the urine. It is easy to cure. Some specific remedies against sikatameha include:

1. **Chitraka root** (leadwort, white flower / *Plumbago zeylanica)* decoction, 30-60 mL twice daily taken with honey.
2. **Haridra Amalirasena,** 3 pills twice daily (Vati), 2 grams twice daily (Churna).
3. **Lauhasava,** 30 mL twice daily.
4. **Shilajatu,** 2-3 pills twice daily.

Shitameha (Glycosuria)

Shitameha refers to the frequent voiding of cold (Shita) urine, and is commonly correlated with glycosuria. It is treated with the regular Kapha treatments and diet (page 77) along with specific remedies against glycosuria. It is easy to cure. Some specific remedies include:

1. **Triphala Churna,** 2 grams twice daily.
2. **Ashwagandha root** *(Convolvulus arvensis / Withania somnifera),* 2 grams twice daily.
3. **Mriddhika Kashaya,** 30-60 mL twice daily.
4. **Haridra Amalirasena,** 3 pills twice daily (Vati), 2 grams twice daily (Churna).
5. **Lauhasava,** 30 mL twice daily.
6. **Shilajatu,** 2-3 pills twice daily.

Shanairmeha (Anuresis)

Shanairmeha corresponds to anuresis, and is concerned with the aggravated function of the renal arterial system that causes suppression of urinary secretion, often with burning sensations. It is treated with the regular Kapha treatments and diet (page 77) along with specific remedies against anuresis. It is easy to cure. Some specific remedies include:

1. **Khadira** (catechu / *Acacia catechu*, white) decoction, 30-60 mL twice daily. Although it is very astringent, Khadira has been found effective for this condition.
2. **Haridra Amalirasena**, 3 pills twice daily (Vati), 2 grams twice daily (Churna).
3. **Lauhasava**, 30 mL twice daily.
4. **Shilajatu**, 2-3 pills twice daily.

Lalameha (Albuminuria)

Lalameha refers to urine that is thick and greasy resembling saliva, caused by the aggravated function of the renal arterial system that causes albumin in the urine. It is treated with the regular Kapha treatments and diet (page 77) along with specific remedies against albuminuria. It is easy to cure. Some specific remedies include:

1. **Patha root** (*Stephania hernandifolia*), 500 mg twice daily.
2. **Agaru wood** (eaglewood / *Aquilaria agallocha*), 500 mg twice daily.
3. **Haridra Kashaya**, 30-60 mL twice daily.
4. **Haridra Amalirasena**, 3 pills twice daily (Vati), 2 grams twice daily (Churna).
5. **Lauhasava**, 30 mL twice daily.
6. **Shilajatu**, 2-3 pills twice daily.

Pittaja Prameha

As the byproduct of blood decomposition, Pitta contains six physical properties that each gives rise to a specific subcategory of prameha, called Ksharameha, Kalameha, Nilameha, Raktameha, Manjishthameha and Haridrameha. All are treated with the general Pitta treatments (page 67) along with specific medicines, including:

1. **Sudarshana Churna/Vati**, 1-2 grams twice daily (Churna), 3-4 pills twice daily, with warm water.
2. **Guduchi stem** (*Tinospora cordifolia*), 1000 mg twice daily.
3. **Avipattikara Churna**, 2 grams twice daily.
4. One part **Shilajatu** and three parts **Triphala,** 1-2 grams twice daily.

Ksharameha (Alkalinuria)

Ksharameha is concerned with the aggravated function of the renal venous system that causes increased alkalinity of the urine. It is treated with the regular Pitta treatments and diet (page 67) along with specific remedies. It is difficult to cure. Some specific remedies against Ksharameha include:

1. **Triphala decoction**, 60-90 mL twice daily.
2. **Chandraprabha Vati**, 2 pills twice daily.
3. **Haridra Amalirasena**, 3 pills twice daily (Vati), 2 grams twice daily (Churna).
4. **Lauhasava**, 30 mL twice daily.
5. **Shilajatu**, 2-3 pills twice daily.

Kalameha (Porphyrinuria)

Kalameha refers to the aggravation of the function of the renal venous system that causes 'blackish' (Kala) pigments to appear in the urine, and can be correlated with porphyrinuria (porphyrins – a component of heme, bile, and cytochrome). It is treated with the regular Pitta treatments and diet (page 67) along with specific remedies. It is difficult to cure. Some specific remedies against Kalameha include:

1. **Nyagrodhadi Kashaya**, 30-60 mL twice daily.
2. **Chandraprabha Vati**, 2 pills twice daily.
3. **Haridra Amalirasena**, 3 pills twice daily (Vati), 2 grams twice daily (Churna).
4. **Lauhasava**, 30 mL twice daily.
5. **Shilajatu**, 2-3 pills twice daily.

Nilameha (Myoglobinuria)

Nilameha refers to a bluish-colored (nila) urine, caused by the aggravated function of the renal venous system that causes the excretion of myoglobin into the urine. It is treated with the regular Pitta treatments and diet (page 67) along with specific remedies. It is difficult to cure. Some specific remedies against Nilameha include:

1. **Ashwattha Kashaya**, 30-60 mL daily.
2. **Chandraprabha Vati**, 2 pills twice daily.
3. **Haridra Amalirasena**, 3 pills twice daily (Vati), 2 grams twice daily (Churna).
4. **Lauhasava**, 30 mL twice daily.
5. **Shilajatu**, 2-3 pills twice daily.

Raktameha (Hematuria)

Raktameha refers to the presence of blood in the urine, along with the general symptoms of prameha, and is concerned with the aggravated function of the renal venous system. It is treated with the regular Pitta treatments and diet (page 67) along with specific remedies. It is difficult to cure. Some specific remedies against Raktameha include:

1. **Guduchi stem** (*Tinospora cordifolia*), 1-2 grams twice daily.

2. **Chandraprabha Vati**, 2 pills twice daily.
3. **Haridra Amalirasena**, 3 pills twice daily (Vati), 2 grams twice daily (Churna).
4. **Lauhasava**, 30 mL twice daily.
5. **Shilajatu**, 2-3 pills twice daily.

The *Sushruta Samhita* recommends a decoction made from **Guduchi stem** *(Tinospora cordifolia)*, **Tinduka bark** *(Dyospyros cordifolia)*, **Kharjura fruit** (date / *Phoenix dactylifera*), and **Kashmari** *(Gmelina arborea)*, taken in doses of 30-60 mL twice daily.

Manjishthameha (Hemoglobinuria)

Manjishthameha refers to a reddish-yellow discoloration of the urine that resembles **Manjishtha root** *(Rubia cordifolia)* and is concerned with the aggravated function of the renal arterial system that causes the accumulation of hemoglobin and pus in the urine. It is treated with the regular Pitta treatments and diet (page 67) along with specific remedies. It is difficult to cure. Some specific remedies against Manjishthameha include:

1. **Manjishtha Chandana Kashaya**, 30-60 mL daily.
2. **Chandraprabha Vati**, 2 pills twice daily.
3. **Haridra Amalirasena**, 3 pills twice daily (Vati), 2 grams twice daily (Churna).
4. **Lauhasava**, 30 mL twice daily.
5. **Shilajatu**, 2-3 pills twice daily.

Haridrameha (Bilirubinuria)

Haridrameha refers to a yellowish orange discoloration of the urine that resembles **Haridra root** *(Curcuma longa),* and is concerned with the aggravated function of the renal venous system that causes the accumulation of bilirubin and pus in the urine. It is treated with the regular Pitta treatments and diet (page 67) along with specific remedies. It is difficult to cure. Some specific remedies against Haridrameha include:

1. **Rajavriksha Kashaya**, 30-90 mL twice daily, to bowel tolerance.
2. **Chandraprabha Vati**, 2 pills twice daily.
3. **Haridra Amalirasena**, 3 pills twice daily (Vati), 2 grams twice daily (Churna).
4. **Lauhasava**, 30 mL twice daily.
5. **Shilajatu**, 2-3 pills twice daily.

Vataja Prameha

Kidney diseases with the character of Vata are divided into four sub-categories: Vasameha, Majjameha, Hastimeha and Madhumeha.

Vasameha (Fatty casts in the urine)

Vasameha refers to the accumulation of fatty casts in the urine caused by the aggravated function of the renal nervous system. This problem has to be treated with the regular Vata treatments and diet (page 56) along with specific remedies. It is very difficult to cure, however, because the regular Vata treatments (which include greasy substances) are contradictory to neutralizing the fatty nature of the casts. Some specific remedies against Vasameha include:

1. **Agnimantha bark/root** *(Premna integrifolia)* decoction, 30-60 mL 1-2 times daily, less with cachexia and wasting.
2. **Shimshapa Kashaya**, 30-60 mL 1-2 times daily, less with cachexia and wasting.
3. **Haridra Amalirasena**, 3 pills twice daily (Vati), 2 grams twice daily (Churna).
4. **Shilajatu**, 2-3 pills twice daily.

Note that while **Lauhasava** is prescribed in Kaphaja and Pittaja prameha, it is avoided in Vataja prameha as it can promote a toxic state in the body.

Majjameha (Waxy casts in the urine)

Majjameha refers to marrow-like waxy casts in the urine caused by the aggravation of the renal nervous system. Like Vasameha, the regular treatments undertaken to reduce Vata acts in a contradictory fashion in Majjameha, making it very difficult to cure. Treatment is primarily the use of specific remedies made from kalkas (powder prepared from paste of green plants), including:

1. **Kustha root** *(Saussurea lappa).*
2. **Kutaja bark** *(Holarrhena antidysenterica).*
3. **Patha root** *(Stephania hernandifolia).*
4. **Hingu gum** (asafoetida/ *Ferula narthex).*
5. **Katuki rhizome** (Indian gentian / *Picrorhiza kurroa).*

The above kalkas can be used individually or in combination, equal part ingredients except for ¼ part **Hingu gum** (asafoetida/ *Ferula narthex).*
Other medicines include:

1. **Guduchi Chitraka Rasena,** 3 pills twice daily (Vati), 2 grams twice daily (Churna).

2. **Haridra Amalaki Rasena,** 3 pills twice daily (Vati), 2 grams twice daily (Churna).
3. **Shilajatu**, 2-3 pills twice daily

Hastimeha (Plasma in the urine)

Hastimeha refers to urine that is thick with Rasa (plasma) and is thus voided very slowly, moving like an elephant (hasti). It is concerned with the aggravated function of the renal nervous system that causes urinary tenesmus (sphincter spasm) in conjunction with the failure of the kidneys to prevent the loss of plasma during filtration. Theoretically Hastimeha would be treated with the regular Vata treatments and diet, but the remedies to reduce Vata are sweet and greasy, which increase the volume of plasma in the blood, thereby placing more stress on the kidneys. There are specific remedies against Hastimeh but due to the fact that they are not very powerful, this disease is considered very difficult to cure.

One medicine to treat Hastimeha is a decoction of two parts **Murva plant** *(Bauhinia vahlii)*, one part each **Tinduka bark** *(Dyospyros cordifolia)*, **Kapittha fruit** (wood apple / *Feronia limonia)*, and **Patha root** *(Stephania hernandifolia)*, and one half part each **Shirisha tree** *(Albizzia lebbeck)* and **Palasha seed** (bastard teak / *Butea frondosa)*. To this add one part either **Kantakari herb** (Black nightshade / *Solanum xanthocarpum)* or **Duralambha bush** *(Fragonia cretica)*. Dose is 30-60 mL twice daily.

Other useful remedies include:

1. Equal parts **Madhuma dhuram** and **Hastyashwa shukara sweet honey**, taken in doses of 10-15 g twice daily.
2. **Dahyama Modaka Kanda decoction** is sweet rice gruel ball made with lotus root, and is taken in doses of 30 mL.
3. **Shilajatu**, 2-3 pills twice daily.

Hastyashwa shukara sweet honey is honey and water to which is added the alkaline ashes made from the bones of elephant, horse, boar, donkey, and camel.

Madhumeha (Diabetes mellitus)

Madhumeha refers to the excretion of a very sweet urine, and hence the name Madhu (honey) meha (urine). Madhumeha is commonly linked with diabetes mellitus, and is signified by sugar in the urine with increased urinary frequency. In health the blood sugar should be primarily sweet in taste, but in the case of diabetes the blood is found to become more sweet and astringent in taste. According to Ayurveda theory the presence of astringency in the blood sugar is considered to be an effect of the aggravated function of the nervous system, and Madhumeha is thus classified as a Vataja disease.

Madhumeha is divided into two categories by Ayurveda, which closely resemble the divisions found in Western medicine:

1.	Diabetes that occurs in persons who are skinny and have a nervous disposition (Vata prakriti), called Dhatukshayaja Madhumeha, or type 1 diabetes;
2.	Diabetes caused by the excessive consumption of rich, sweet foods, causing obesity, called Avrita Madhumeha, or type 2 diabetes.

Both types of diabetes are resistant to cure because the principles of treatment are contradictory. In general, the aggravated function of the nervous system (Vata) has to be controlled with sweet remedies and rich foods. In the case of diabetes, however, such remedies are contradictory because they increase the sugar in the blood. In the same way, the remedies against Kapha contain astringent remedies that can aggravate the function of the nervous system. Nonetheless, there are certain remedies in Ayurveda that have medicinal value to maintain and prolong the lives of diabetics, except that beyond the very early stages, their effect is not powerful enough to cure. The ancient texts reveal however that Madhumeha cases can sometimes be cured or maintained with the simple practice of regular walking or hiking each day, while avoiding sweet food. This practice should continue for many, many years.

Dhatukshayaja Madhumeha (type 1 diabetes) is not curable, but it can be maintained with the specific remedies against diabetes. Avrita Madhumeha (type 2 diabetes) is curable, but it needs much effort. It is treated with the general Kapha treatments and diet (page 77) along with the specific remedies. During treatment it is important to ensure that the regular Kapha treatments and diet (page 77) do not aggravate the function of the nervous system. That is, while heavy oily foods are restricted, it is important that there is enough to maintain and balance the nervous system. Some specific remedies against Madhumeha include:

1.	**Khadirakramuka decoction**, 30 mL twice daily.
2.	**Shilajatu**, 2-3 pills twice daily.
3.	**Trikaturasayana**, 3 pills twice daily.
4.	One part **Chaturdasanga Churna,** taken with two parts **Triphala,** 1/20th part **Naga Bhasma** (purified lead oxide), and 1/10th each **Vanga Bhasma** (purified tin oxide) and **Yashada Bhasma** (purified zinc oxide). Dose is 1000 mg twice daily.

Vastija Udavarta (Kidney Failure related to Vata)

Failure of the kidneys is concerned with the aggravated function of the renal nervous system that causes the reversed function (Udavarta) of the kidney. Anuria is the main symptom. It is treated with the regular Vata treatments (page 56) along with medicated suppository, enema, greasy laxative remedies (page 174), 'steam bath' (Swedana), and diuretics (page 195).

The use of a medicated suppository is the best remedy for this problem. One example is a medicated suppository made of one part each white **Nishotha**

(Marsdenia tenacissima) and black **Nishota** *(Operculina turpethum)*, **Pippali fruit** *(Piper longum)*, **Danti seed** *(Baliospermum montanum)* and **Nila**, with ten parts of **Goumutra** (cow urine) and 2 parts molasses.

In some conditions, Vastija Udavarta has to be treated with the specific remedies mentioned in the cases of kidney diseases with the character of Vata (Vataja prameha).

Kshinakshaya (Renal tuberculosis)

Kshinakshaya is a form of nephritis that presents with a lung pathology, and most closely resembles renal tuberculosis (TB). It is treated with the remedies of pulmonary TB (page 184) along with the remedies used for kidneys diseases classified with the character of Pitta (Pittaja prameha, above).

Sharkara (Renal calculus)

Sharkara corresponds with renal calculus. It has the same etiology as Ashmari (bladder stone) and is treated with the same remedies (page 200).

Vrikkavidradhi (Renal abscess)

Vrikkavidradhi is an abscess of the kidneys. It relates to the same pathogenic defects in blood that causes Vidradhi (abscess of the alimentary system), and is treated with the same medicines (page 170).

Chapter 18: Diseases of Male Sexual Function (Purushajanendriya Roga)

Shukradosha (Defects of Semen)

Ayurveda defines eight semen defects: foamy semen, deficiency of semen, rough semen, colorful semen, putrefactive semen, viscous semen, semen mixed with blood and acids, and coagulated semen. Foamy semen, deficiency of semen or little semen, and rough or dry semen are Vata disorders, concerned with the aggravated function of the nervous system. Semen with abnormal colors (such as yellow or blue), and putrefactive semen are Pitta disorders, the result of the aggravated function of the venous system. Viscous semen is a Kapha disorder, the result of an aggravated function of the arterial system. Coagulated semen is Sannipataja, related to the aggravated function of all systems. Blood, mixed with semen is related to injury.

Defects of semen are almost always treated with the Vajikarana and Rasayana remedies for long life and good health. Combined with these remedies, after proper diagnosis, are treatments to maintain the balance of the bodily systems, i.e. the nervous system (Vata), the venous system (Pitta), and the arterial system (Kapha).

Vajikarana Remedies

1. **Ashwagandha root** (*Convolvulus arvensis, Withania somnifera*).
2. **Vijaya leaf** (hemp / *Cannabis sativa*).
3. **Guduchi stem** (*Tinospora cordifolia*).
4. **Gunja seed** (crab's eye / *Abrus precatorius*).
5. **Jivaka bulb** (wild garlic / *Allium wallichii*, small).
6. **Kakoli bulb** (*Fritillaria cirrhosa*).
7. **Kapikacchu seeds** (cowhage / *Mucuna pruriens*).
8. **Kasturi** (deer musk / *Moschus moschiferus*).
9. **Lashunam bulb** (garlic / *Allium sativum*).
10. **Musali tuber** (*Curculigo orchioides*).
11. **Pueraria tuber** (vidari / *Pueraria lobata*).
12. **Risabhaka bulb** (*Allium wallichii*, large).
13. **Shalaparni plant** (*Desmodium gangeticum*).
14. **Shilajatu Rasayana**.

Klaivyam (Impotence)

Klaivyam or Impotence is related to defects of semen, old age and general debility. It is also caused by lesions caused by sexual misconduct such as rape or excess masturbation. Abnormal sex or sexual excesses lead to impotency for mental reasons (such as guilt) as well as by injury to the nerves related to the genital organs.

It is treated according to the signs and symptoms, taking into consideration the cause of the impotence, along with aphrodisiac remedies (vajikarana) and general restoratives (rasayana, page 140). When treating cases of impotence, a peaceful atmosphere in the home is very important. Impotence caused by congenital atrophy or trauma is not curable.

Upadamsha (Syphilis)

Upadamsha or syphilis causes the eruption of lesions on the penis, and is classified into five categories, with the characters of Vataja, Pittaja, Kaphaja, Sannipataja and Raktaja. Vata Upadamsha manifests with blackish colored lesions with severe pain. Pittaja Upadamsha manifests with yellowish colored lesions and burning sensation, later developing into an oozing lesion. Syphilitic lesions with the quality of Kapha are skin coloured with swelling and itchiness. Sannipataja Upadamsha manifests with lesions that have mixed symptoms, and Raktaja Upadamsha is similar to Vataja but involves bleeding.

Syphilis of all types is treated with venesection (see page 92), specific healing plasters and laxative remedies (page 174). Blood purifying remedies (page 155) are particularly important to maintain the bodily systems, as well as Rasayanas (page 140) made with purified minerals. Syphilis with the character of Raktaja (congenital) or Sannipataja (complicated) is not curable. However, both can be treated with venesection practices and specific healing remedies to reduce symptoms and prevent worsening. Syphilis in the advanced stage has to be treated with surgery and with remedies based upon signs and symptoms in the affected organ(s).

Some specific remedies against syphilis are:

1. **Triphala** (3 fruits compound), 2 grams twice daily.
2. **Patola fruit** *(Trichosanthes dioica)*, 2 grams twice daily.
3. **Nimba leaf** (neem / *Azadirachta indica*), 2 grams twice daily.
4. **Guduchi stem decoction** (*Tinospora cordifolia*), 2 grams twice daily.
5. **Asana wood** *(Terminalia tomentosa)* made into an infusion for internal use, 2 grams twice daily.
6. **Khadira Sanabhyam** is **Khadira extract** (catechu / *Acacia catechu*, white) made into a paste form, and applied topically.
7. An external ointment can be made by burning **Triphala fruits** *(Phyllanthus emblica / Terminalia belerica / Terminalia chebula)*, then grinding with honey.

Lingavarti (Chancre)

The term Lingavarti refers to chancre, or wart-like growth(s) around the external urethral orifice. It is caused by is caused by Upadamsha or syphilis with the character of Sannipata, and is very difficult to cure.

Sarshapika (Herpes simplex genitalia)

Sarshapika refers to herpes simplex genitalia, and is concerned with the aggravated function of the genital arterial system along with pathogenic defects of blood. It is treated with the regular Kapha treatments (page 77) along with blood cleansing remedies (page 155). The standard compound **Guduchiyoga** is an effective blood purifier, and is taken in doses of 2 grams twice daily. Another important formula is **Kaishora Guggulu Vati**, 2 pills twice daily.

The blisters have to be cracked open and sprinkled with the powder of astringent remedies for proper healing. Two commonly used astringents are **Khadira extract** (catechu, white / *Acacia catechu*) and **Sphutikarika** (purified alum). A compound used for this purpose is **Khadiradi Churna** which contains bitter **Nimba leaf** (neem / *Azadirachta indica*) with some other astringents agents. Other external plasters include:

1. **Puga nut** (betel / *Areca catechu*) made into a paste.
2. **Karavira root** (sweet-scented oleander / *Nerium indicum*) made into a paste.
3. Sprinkle on powder of **Dadima rind** (pomegranate / *Punica granatum*).
4. **Rasanjana** (condensed extract of *Berberis nepalensis* or *Berberis asiatica*) made into a paste with honey.

Grathitam (Venereal granuloma)

Grathitam is correlated with Venereal granuloma, and is concerned with the aggravated function of the genital arterial system. It is treated with the application of steam, or hot compress and poultice based on remedies used against Kapha (page 77).

Kumbhika (Melanoma genitalia)

Kumbhika is correlated with Melanoma genitalia, and is concerned with the aggravated function of the genital venous system (inflammation) along with pathogenic defects of blood. It is treated with surgery. Anti-cancer (page 248) and blood cleansing remedies (page 155) may be used after surgery to prevent recurrence.

Alagi (Erysipeloid)

Alagi is correlated with erysipeloid, an acute bacterial infection of the penis, and is concerned with the aggravated function of the genital venous system (inflammation). It is treated with venesection practices and healing remedies based on the principles of Pitta treatment (inflammation - page 67).

Mriditam (Balanitis)

Mriditam is correlated with the inflammation of the glans penis, or balanitis, and is concerned with the aggravated function of the genital nervous system. It is treated with medicated oil massage and Vata-based poultices (page 56).

Sammudhapidaka (Traumatic boils of the penis)

Sammudhapidaka is correlated with traumatic boils of the penis, and is concerned with internal injury. It is treated with surgery along with venesection practices.

Avamantha (Chancroid)

Avamantha is correlated with chancroid and is concerned with the aggravated function of the genital arterial system along with blood defects. It is treated with surgery.

Pushkarika (Syphilis-like boil)

Pushkarika is a boil on the penis resembling syphilis, and is concerned with the aggravated function of the genital venous system and the pathogenic defects of blood. It is treated with venesection practices and refrigerant remedies (page 154) for both internal and external use.

Sparshahani (Numbness of the penis)

Sparshahani refers to numbness of the penis, and is concerned with the pathogenic defects of blood. It is treated with venesection practices to remove toxins along with medical plasters made of sweet remedies to nourish and heal, including sweet tasting and nourishing herbs such as **Bala plant** (country mallow / *Sida cordifolia)* and **Musali tuber** *(Curculigo orchioides)*.

Uttama (Red pimples of the penis)

Uttama refers to the appearance of red pimples of the penis, and is concerned with the aggravated function of the genital venous system along with blood defects. Cancerous in nature, it is treated with surgery. Herbal medicines are not effective.

Shataponaka (Fistula of the penis)

Shataponaka refers to a urinary fistula of the penis, and is concerned with the aggravated function of the genital nervous system along with blood defects. It is treated with surgery. Herbal medicines are not effective.

Twakpaka (Penitis)

Penitis is concerned with the aggravated function of the nervous system and venous system of the penis. It is treated with the remedies of erysipelas (page 241).

Shonitarbuda (Angioma of the penis)

Angioma of the penis is concerned with the pathogenic defects of blood. It is treated with the remedies for abscess caused by blood defects (page 246) along with venesection practices, laxative remedies (page 174) and surgery. It is very difficult to cure.

Mansarbuda (Myoma of the penis)

Myoma of the penis is concerned with the pathogenic defects of muscular tissues. It is treated with the remedies used for myoma of the skin (page 249). It is very difficult to cure.

Mansapaka (Acute penitis)

Acute penitis has complicated symptoms (Sannipataja) and is not curable.

Vidradhi (Abscess of the penis)

Abscess of the penis has complicated symptoms (Sannipataja) and is not curable. However, it can be treated with the remedies used for abscess (page 170).

Tilakalaka (Gangrene)

Tilakalaka or gangrene of the penis has complicated symptoms (Sannipataja) and is not curable.

Parivartika (Paraphimosis)

Parivartika refers to paraphimosis, in which the foreskin becomes trapped behind the glans penis and cannot be pulled back to its normal position. Parivartika is divided into two forms: one with the character of Vata and another with the character of Kapha. In general, they are treated with the application of steam, medicated oil massage, enema through the urinary pipe and poultices prepared with the regular Vata (page 56) or Kapha (page 77) remedies.

Avapatika (Tear in the prepuce)

Avapatika refers to a tear in the prepuce or foreskin is concerned with the aggravated function of the nervous system. It is treated with the same remedies used for Vataja Parivartika (paraphimosis).

Niruddhaprakasha (Phimosis)

Niruddhaprakasha or phimosis, is when the foreskin cannot be fully retracted over the glans penis. It is concerned with the aggravated function of the nervous system (Vata) that causes thickness of the foreskin and blockage of urination. It is treated by inserting a pipe through the urethra for administering a medicated oil. **Narayana Taila** or other oils beneficial for Vata can be used. In some conditions surgery is advised to remove the foreskin.

Shukrashmari (Seminal calculus)

Shukrashmari or seminal calculus is concerned with the aggravated function of the genital nervous system that causes dry semen and blockage in the passage. It is treated with the same remedies used for bladderstone (page 200).

Andavriddhi (Orchitis)

Andavriddhi refers to inflammation of the testicles, or orchitis. It is classified into five categories, with the characters of Vata, Pitta, Kapha, Meda and Rakta. Orchitis of all types is treated with specific remedies, along with general medicines based upon signs and symptoms. Laxative remedies are also essential to prescribe (page 174). **Eranda oil** (Castor / *Ricinus communis*) with milk can be used for this purpose.

Some specific internal medicines against orchitis are:

1. **Aindramula Churna Rubutailena,** made from **Aindra root** (bitter apple / *Citrullus colocynthis)* mixed with **Eranda oil** (Castor / *Ricinus communis)* and **Goukshira** (cow milk).
2. **Sudarshana Churna/Vati.**
3. **Airenda Taila,** made from **Bibhitaki fruit** *(Terminalia belerica)*, **Pippali fruit** (long pepper / *Piper longum)*, **Saindhavam** (mineral salt) and **Eranda oil** (castor / *Ricinus communis).*

For external treatment medicated poultices are used, including:

1. **Narayana Taila.**
2. **Vachasarshapa Kalka Lepa** *(Chakradatta)*, made from **Vacha rhizome** (acorus / *Acorus calamus)* and **Sarshapi seed oil** (black mustard / *Sinapis juncea)*
3. **Lajjagriddha Malabhyam Lepa** *(Chakradatta)*, made from **Lajjalu plant** (sensitive plant / *Mimosa pudica)* mixed with vulture excretion.
4. **Rupika Mulabalkam Aranalenapistam Lepa** *(Chakradatta)*, made from **Eranda root** (castor / *Ricinus communis)* mixed with **Kanjika** (whey).

Vataja Orchitis

Orchitis with the character of Vata is concerned with bladder-like (air filled) swelling of the testicles. It is treated with oil massage, application of steam, foot warming (to stimulate circulation), laxative remedies (page 174) and medicated poultice. It has to be treated with surgery if it is infected.

Pittaja Orchitis

Orchitis with the character of Pitta is concerned with inflammation of the testicles. It is treated with anti-inflammatory remedies for internal and external uses (page 155), along with laxative remedies (page 174) and venesection practices. It has to be treated with surgery if it is infected.

Kaphaja Orchitis

Orchitis with the character of Kapha is concerned with edema of the testicle. It is treated with the regular Kapha treatments (page 77) along with poultice, urine therapy and foot warming (to increase circulation). It has to be treated with surgery if it is infected (filariasis).

Medoja Orchitis

Orchitis with the character of Meda is concerned with fatty growth. It is curable only with surgery.

Raktaja Orchitis

Orchitis with the character of Rakta is concerned with the pathogenic defects of blood. It is treated with the same remedies of orchitis with the character of Pitta.

Mutravriddhi (Hydrocele)

Mutravriddhi or hydrocele is concerned with water accumulation in the testicle. It is treated with surgery to take out the fluid. Additionally, it can be treated with specific remedies against orchitis (above) along with foot warming (to stimulate circulation), and massage with **Narayana Taila**.

Vrishanakacchu (Tinea crusis)

Vrishanakacchu can be correlated with Tinea crusis, a fungal infection that is concerned with the aggravated function of the scrotal arterial system along with blood defects (see page 255). It is treated with the remedies used for Pama (eczema) (page 238).

Chapter 19: Diseases of Female Sexual Function (Stri Roga)

Note: Diseases of the female genital organ such as herpes and syphilis that are common to both sexes are discussed in the previous chapter, Chapter 18: Diseases of Male Sexual Function (Purushajanendriya Roga).

Udavartayoni (Dysmenorrhea)

Udavartayoni or dysmenorrhea is concerned with the reversed function of the uterine nervous system that causes menstrual cramps. It is treated with the regular Vata treatments (page 56) along with warming medicated pessary and specific remedies against dysmenorrhea. One specific formulation is two parts **Dadima rind** (pomegranate / *Punica granatum)* mixed with one part **Shatapushpa seed** (anise / *Pimpinella anisum)* and 1/5th part **Lauha Bhasma** (purified iron oxide), mixed with **Ghrita** (Ghee) to make pills, taken in doses of 2 pills twice daily. This medicine is taken along with **Chandraprabha Vati**, 2 pills twice daily.

Raktapradara (Menorrhagia)

Raktapradara or menorrhagia is typically related to blood defects that cause irregular menses. It is classified into four categories: menorrhagia with the character of Vata, Pitta, Kapha and Sannipata. All types of menorrhagia can be treated with specific remedies that maintain the function of the nervous system (Vata) along with remedies for hemorrhage (page 258). Some specific remedies against menorrhagia include:

1. **Ashoka bark** *(Saraca indica)*, taken as Churna (powder), 2 grams twice daily, or as a decoction, 60-90 mL twice daily.
2. **Ashokarista**, 30 mL after food, twice daily.
3. **Bala root**, 1000 mg, twice daily.
4. **Chandraprabha Vati**, 2 pills twice daily.
5. Combination of **Sauvira Bhasma** (purified antimony sulfide) 25 mg and **Vasaka leaf** (Malabar nut / *Adhatoda vasica)* 2 grams, taken twice daily.

One useful topical remedy is a medicated pessary made from **Sphutikarika** (purified alum powder) and **Pippal bark** *(Ficus religiosa)*.

Vataja Menorrhagia

Menorrhagia with the character of Vata is concerned with the aggravated function of the uterine nervous system. It is treated with the regular Vata treatments (page 56) along with medicated pessary and the remedies for hemorrhage (page 258), or proctitis (page 166), or hemorrhoid with bleeding (page 169).

Pittaja Menorrhagia
Menorrhagia with the character of Pitta is concerned with the aggravated function of the uterine venous system that causes inflammation of the uterus. It is treated with the regular Pitta treatments (page 67) along with medicated pessary and the remedies for hemorrhage (page 258).

Kaphaja Menorrhagia
Menorrhagia with the character of Kapha is concerned with the aggravated function of the uterine arterial system that causes swelling of the uterus. It is treated with the regular Kapha treatments (page 77) along with medicated pessary and the remedies for hemorrhage (page 258).

Sannipataja Menorrhagia
Menorrhagia with the character of Sannipata is concerned with complicated acute symptoms. It is difficult to cure and is treated with symptomatically.

Lohitakshaya / Atiraja (Hypermenorrhea)
Lohitakshaya or hypermenorrhea is concerned with the aggravated function of the uterine venous system that causes inflammation and excessive bleeding. It is treated with the regular Pitta treatments (page 67) along with cooling medicated pessary and the remedies against hemorrhage (page 258). Topically, Narayana Taila can be applied as a pessary.

Vandhya (Amenorrhea / Female sterility)
Vandhya refers to absent menstruation, or amenorrhea, which is usually an indication of Arajaska, or infertility. Both conditions are concerned with the impaired condition of the uterine nervous system that causes absence of menstruation. Both are treated with regular Vata treatments (page 56) along with warming medicated pessary (using herbs for Vata) and specific remedies against amenorrhea.

To enhance fertility and strengthen the body, the powders of one part **Shatavari root** (asparagus / *Asparagus racemosus)* and two parts **Ashwagandha root** *(Convolvulus arvensis / Withania somnifera)*, 2-3 grams total, taken with milk can be used to nourish the system. **Dadimadi Churna** can also be used, in doses of 2 grams, twice daily. Specific remedies against amenorrhea include:

1. **Krishna Vati**, 2 pills twice daily.
2. **Durvayah Pistakam,** comprised of **Durva** (Burmuda grass / *Cynodon dactylon)* and **Dhanyam flour** (rice / *Oryza sativa)*, given in doses of 2-3 grams twice daily.

3. **Japapushpam Sakanjikam** *(Chakradatta)*, made from **Japa flower** (Chinese hibiscus / *Hibiscus rosa-sinensis*) and **Kanjika** (whey). Dosage is two fresh flowers twice daily. A similar recipe can be used with vinegar instead of whey.

Sandi (Congenital sterility)

Sandi refers to congenital sterility, and is defined as a woman who reaches adulthood without ever having menstruated. It is not curable.

Shwetapradara (Leucorrhea)

According to Ayurveda, Shwetapradara or leucorrhea is related to menorrhagia. The main symptom is discharge of yellowish or white mucus from the vagina. It is treated with the regular Kapha treatments (page 77) along with specific remedies. If the leucorrhea is a symptom of another uterine disease it has to be treated symptomatically while the original cause is treated. Some specific remedies against leucorrhea include:

1. **Ashoka Arista** (fermented decoction of Ashoka flower / *Saraca indica*), 30 mL twice daily.
2. **Rohitaka Kalka** (rhododendron root / *Rhododendron arboreum*) with water, 30 mL twice daily.
3. **Amalakivija Kalka** (paste of **Amalaki seed** / *Phyllanthus emblica*)
4. **Bala root** (country mallow / *Sida cordifolia*), 1000 mg twice daily.

One useful formulation can be made from combining two parts **Amalaki fruit** (Indian gooseberry / amla / *Phyllanthus emblica*) and **Ashwagandha root** (*Convolvulus arvensis* / *Withania somnifera*) with 1/10th part **Vatsanabha** (aconite tuber, purified / *Aconitum palmatum*). This can be taken in doses of 2 grams twice daily, taken with twice the volume of a decoction of **Ashoka bark** (Ashoka tree / *Saraca indica*).

Acharana (Genital candidiasis)

Acharana or genital candidiasis (including other fungal infections) is concerned with aggravation of the vaginal arterial system that causes swelling and itching. It is treated with the regular Kapha treatments (page 77) along with astringent and warming medicated pessary and **Sphutikarika** (purified alum) to wash the affected tissue.

Upapluta (Trichomoniasis)

Upapluta can be correlated with trichomoniasis, and is concerned with the aggravated function of the uterine arterial and nervous systems that causes a copious, painful white discharge. It is treated with the combined principles used for

Vata and Kapha treatment (page 81) along with warming medicated pessary and specific remedies. For example **Sphutikarika** (purified alum) can be used as an external application to dry up the discharge, and **Rohitaka root** (rhododendron / *Rhododendron arboreum)* and **Dadimadi Churna** can be used as internal medicine.

Atyananda (Excessive sexual desire caused by irritation)

Excessive sexual desire as a disease is concerned with the aggravated function of the vaginal arterial system that causes itching, vaginal stimulation and a white sticky discharge. It is treated with the regular Kapha treatments (page 77) along with astringent and warming pessary as well as **Sphutikarika** (purified alum) to wash the affected tissue.

Acharana (Premature orgasm) and Aticharana (Polyorgasm)

Acharana and Aticharana also refer to both premature orgasm and polyorgasm respectively, and are concerned with the aggravated function of the clitoris arterial system. Both are treated with the regular Kapha treatments (page 77) along with astringent and warming medicated pessary.

Vamini (Early-onset miscarriage)

Vamini refers to the miscarriage of a week old embryo, expelled as a gel-like mass. It is caused by an aggravated function of the uterine venous system or general inflammation. It is treated with the regular Pitta treatments (page 67) along with cooling medicated pessary. Following this the patient is treated using a strengthening process called Santaparna, giving restorative medicines to gain weight such as **Ashwagandha root** *(Convolvulus arvensis / Withania somnifera)*, **Kapikacchu seeds** (cowhage / *Mucuna pruriens)* and **Bala plant** (country mallow / *Sida cordifolia)*.

Putraghni (Habitual miscarriage)

Putraghni refers to habitual miscarriage, and is concerned with the aggravated function of the uterine venous system (inflammation) along with blood defects (see page 255). It is treated with the regular Pitta treatments (page 67) along with cooling medicated pessary and specific remedies. A specific medicine against habitual miscarriage is five parts **Dadima rind** (pomegranate / *Punica granatum)* taken with one part **Lauha Bhasma** (purified iron oxide) and **Ghrita** (Ghee), used in doses of 2-3 grams for 3 to 6 months.

Paripluta (Dyspareunia)

Paripluta is correlated with dyspareunia or painful coitus, and is concerned with the aggravated function of the uterine nervous system. It is treated with the general Vata treatments (page 56) along with warming medicated pessary and specific remedies. A specific medicine against dyspareunia is **Dadimadi Ghrita**, 3-6 grams twice daily, taken along with **Yogaraja Guggulu Vati**, 2 pills twice daily.

Paripluta (Vaginitis)

Paripluta or vaginitis is concerned with the aggravated function of vaginal venous and nervous systems that cause painful inflammation. It is treated with the principles used for Pitta and Vata treatment (page 81) along with anti inflammatory remedies and pessary.

Bipluta (Uterine neuralgic pain / Vaginismus)

Bipluta is correlated with neuralgic pain of the uterus, or vaginismus, and is concerned of with the aggravated function of the uterine nervous system. It is treated with the general Vata treatments (page 56) along with warming medicated pessary and specific remedies. A specific medicine against neuralgic pain of the uterus or vaginismus is **Dadimadi Ghrita** (standard Ghee compound), made from **Dadima rind** (pomegranate / *Punica granatum)* with **Shatapushpa seed** (anise / *Pimpinella anisum)*, **Lauha Bhasma** (purified iron oxide) and Ghee. This is given in doses of 3-6 grams, twice daily, taken along with **Chandraprabha Vati**, 2 pills twice daily.

Aticharana (Traumatic swelling of the uterus)

Aticharana refers to the traumatic swelling of the uterus or vagina, and is concerned with the aggravated function of the uterine nervous system. It is treated with the general Vata treatments (page 56) along with warming medicated pessary and specific remedies. This condition has several causes including as allergy, inflammation, and kidney infection. Treatment is based on the specific causative factors.

Suchimukhi (Narrow uterine passageway)

Suchimukhi refers to a narrowing of the passage of the uterus, and is concerned with the aggravated function of the uterine nervous system. It is treated with the regular Vata treatments (page 56). Congenital problems causing a narrowing of the passage of the uterus is not curable.

Yonimukhashosa (Cervix atrophy)

Yonimukhashosa is correlated with atrophy of the cervix, and is concerned with the aggravated function of the uterine nervous system. It is treated with the regular Vata treatments (page 56) along with warming medicated pessary and specific remedies. A specific medicine against atrophy of the cervix is one part **Dadima rind** (pomegranate / *Punica granatum)* mixed with 1/5 part **Lauha Bhasma** (purified iron oxide), taken in doses of 2-3 grams twice daily with **Ghrita**

(Ghee). Topically, a cloth soaked in a solution of **Sphutikarika** (purified alum) can be applied topically. Treatment is ineffective for congenital causes of cervical atrophy.

Antarmukhi (Malposition of the cervix)

Antarmukhi refers to the malposition of the cervix, and is concerned with the aggravated function of the uterine nervous system. It is treated with the regular Vata treatments (page 56) along with warming medicated pessary and specific remedies. Treatment is best given in the early stages of the condition. Some specific remedies against Antarmukhi include:

1. **Ashoka bark** *(Saraca indica)*, taken as Churna (powder), 2 grams twice daily, or as a decoction, 60-90 mL twice daily.
2. **Ashokarista**, 30 mL after food, twice daily.
3. **Bala root**, 1000 mg, twice daily.
4. One part **Dadima rind** (pomegranate / *Punica granatum*) with 1/5th part **Lauha Bhasma** (purified iron oxide), in doses of 2-3 gram twice daily, taken with Ghee.

Prasramsini (Dislocation of the uterus)

Prasramsini or prolapse of the uterine is caused by aggravated function of the uterine venous system (inflammation). It is treated with the general Pitta treatments (page 67) along with cooling and astringent medicated pessary. While treating prolapse, the descending uterus has to be placed back into positions and then bandaged in the proper way. Prasramsini is a first or second degree prolapse.

Prakcharana (Uterine prolapse)

Prakcharana or uterine prolapse is caused by aggravation of the uterine nervous system. It can be caused by premature sexual intercourse, pregnancy at too early of an age, repeated abortion, and also occurs in older women as an effect of aging. It is treated with the regular Vata treatments (page 56) along with warming medicated pessary and specific remedies. Treatment is best given in the early stages of the condition. Some specific remedies against uterine prolapse include:

1. **Ashoka bark** *(Saraca indica)*, taken as Churna (powder), 2 grams twice daily, or as a decoction, 60-90 mL twice daily.
2. **Ashokarista**, 30 mL after food, twice daily.
3. **Bala root**, 1000 mg, twice daily.
4. One part **Dadima rind** (pomegranate / *Punica granatum*) with 1/5th part **Lauha Bhasma** (purified iron oxide), in doses of 2-3 gram twice daily, taken with Ghee.

Andali (Frank prolapse of the Uterus)

Andali refers to the frank prolapse of the uterus (third degree prolapse), and is concerned with the complicated symptoms caused by the aggravated functions of nervous, venous, and arterial systems. It is very difficult to cure, however can be treated with symptomatic treatments based upon the principles used for tridoshaja treatments (page 82), along with cooling and astringent medicated pessary and specific remedies based upon signs and symptoms. While treating prolapse, the descending uterus has to be placed back into positions and then bandaged in the proper way.

Raktagulma (Endometrial polyps)

Raktagulma refers to endometrial polyps, and are concerned with pathogenic defects of the blood. The disease is treated with specific alkaline remedies that have power to break the polyps, along with symptomatic treatments for hemorrhage (page 258) and blood defects (page 255), and the use of healing or balancing medicines. It has been observed by traditional physicians that endometrial polyps should not be treated immediately. This is because the polyps develop like an embryo, and it is much easier to remove them after nine months, just like childbirth. A specific medicine against endometrial polyps is **Palasha kshara**, the alkali of **Palasha seed** (bastard teak / *Butea frondosa).*

Karnini (Neoplasm of the cervix)

Karnini refers to cervical polyps, and are concerned with the aggravated function of the uterine arterial system along with pathogenic defects of the blood. It is treated with the regular Kapha treatments (page 77) and blood cleaning remedies along with astringent medicated pessary and the specific remedies against neoplasm (page 248).

Pratyasthila (Neoplasm of the ovary)

Pratyasthila refers to a neoplasm of the ovary, and is concerned with the aggravated function of the abdominal nervous system. It is treated with the regular Vata treatments (page 56) along with the remedies for abdominal tumor.

Mahayoni (Neoplasm of the uterus / Endometrial cancer)

Mahayoni can be correlated with endometrial cancer, and is caused by the aggravated function of the uterine nervous, venous, and arterial systems, resulting in neoplasm formation. It is very difficult to cure. It has been observed by traditional physicians that following the treatment of endometrial cancer, the aggravated function of the nervous system first must be controlled as soon as possible with the regular Vata treatments (page 56) and a warming medicated pessary. Following this, the aggravated functions of the venous and arterial systems will be easier to control with appropriate symptomatic and specific remedies. Some specific remedies against Mahayoni include:

1. **Dadima rind** (pomegranate / *Punica granatum)* mixed with 1/5th part **Lauha Bhasma** (purified iron oxide) and Ghee. Dosage is 3-6 grams twice daily.
2. **Chandraprabha Vati**, 2 pills twice daily.
3. **Kaishora Guggulu Vati**, 2 pills twice daily.

These three medicines can be used together.

Chapter 20: Diseases Of The Nerves (Snayukandara Roga)

Vata in its normal healthy state helps to maintain equilibrium in the different tissues and governing principles of the body, as well as maintaining balanced metabolism, balanced nervous system function and balanced sensory function. The aggravating factors that increase Vata and cause or worsen diseases of the nervous system in this chapter are listed on page 55.

General Medicines for Diseases of the Nerves

Diseases of the nerves benefit from the general Vata treatments discussed starting on page 56, including an emphasis upon warming foods and beverages, and an avoidance of cold foods and beverages. Of great importance is the general nerve Rasayana **Yogaraja Guggulu** that is applicable for use in many of the diseases in this chapter. Use of the variation called **Maha Yogaraja Guggulu**, which contains purified minerals (Bhasmas), is also of great importance. Another highly effective nerve medicine is **Narayana Taila,** which can be used both as an external massage and as medicinal drops for the nose or ear.

Nakhabheda (Breaking of the Nail)

Nakhabheda relates to the non-congenital breaking of the nail, and is concerned with the aggravated function of the dorsal nerves of the hand (radial, ulnar and medial). It is treated with general treatments to balance Vata (page 56), including medicated oil massage with **Narayana Taila**.

Vipadika (Cracking of the Sole)

Vipadika relates to fissures and cracking of the sole of the foot, and is concerned with the aggravated function of the nervous system. It is treated with the regular Vata treatments (page 56) along with a plaster made from a fat such as Ghee mixed with beeswax.

Padashula (Pain in the Sole)

Padashula relates to pain in the sole of the foot, and is concerned with the aggravated function of the nervous system. It is treated with hot compress of salt water or oil massage with **Narayana Taila**.

Padabhramsha (Chronic ankle sprain)

Padabhramsha relates to chronic ankle sprain, and is caused by a weakness of the nervous system. The weak ankle creates a tendency to slip and fall, causing chronic pain due to repeated injury. It is treated with the regular Vata treatments (page 56), hot compress of salt water or oil massage with **Narayana Taila**.

Padasuptata (Foot neuropathy)

Padasuptata relates to numbness and tingling of the foot, and is concerned with the aggravated function of the nervous system. The patient will typically complain of poor circulation and coldness. It is treated with oil massage with **Narayana Taila** and hot compress of salt water.

Pindikodvestanam (Spasm of the calf)

Pindikodvestanam relates to the spasm of the calf muscle, and is concerned with the aggravated function of the nervous system. It is treated with a hot compress of salt water, oil massage with **Narayana Taila**, and Rasayanas such as **Yogaraja Guggulu**, 2 pills twice daily.

Gridhrasi (Sciatica)

Gridhrasi is correlated with the aggravated function of the sciatic nerve. It is divided into two categories: one concerned with the character of Vata and the other related to the character of Vata-Kapha. Gridhrasi with the character of Vata is treated with general therapies to reduce Vata (page 56) along with hot salt water compress (to stimulate circulation), venesection between the toes and specific remedies depending on the presenting signs and symptoms. Gridhrasi with the character of Vata-Kapha is treated with digestive and appetizing herbs (page 173) along with the general medicines including **Kaishora Guggulu** (2 pills twice daily), **Yogaraja Guggulu** (2 pills twice daily) and **Narayana Taila**.

Gulphagraha (Swelling of the ankles)

Gulphagraha is swelling of the ankles caused by the aggravated function of the nerves in the legs. It is treated with general therapies to reduce Vata (page 56) along with hot compress and oil massage with **Narayana Taila**.

Janlivishlesa (Dislocation of the kneecap)

Janlivishlesa is the dislocation of the kneecap caused by the aggravated functioning of the nervous system. It is treated with a bandage oiled with **Narayana Taila** placed so as to hold the kneecap in place.

Urustambha (Paralysis of the thigh)

Urustambha is concerned with the aggravated function of the femoral artery and nervous system, causing the paralysis of the thigh. It is treated with therapies to reduce Vata-Kapha (page 81), along with warming and astringent plasters and poultices for external use, as well as enema, laxative and emetic remedies (pages 174 and 175). Specific remedies are chosen on the basis based of the presenting signs and symptoms, as well as the stage of the disease. General remedies used in urustambha include **Kaishora Guggulu** (2 pills twice daily), **Yogaraja Guggulu** (2 pills twice daily). For external application, a plaster can be made from **Karanja bark** (Indian beech / *Pongamia pinnata)*, or **Devadaru wood** (Himalayan cedar / *Cedrus deodara)* or **Arka** (milkweed / *Calotropis gigantea)*.

Treatment for urustambha can also be used for diseases that lead to progressive paralysis, such as multiple sclerosis and ALS (Amyotrophic lateral sclerosis). However, the application and use of these herbs requires close supervision by the physician, with additional treatments used as necessary. The progress of healing is often very slow.

Shronibheda (Hip pain)

Shronibheda relates to hip pain, and is concerned with the aggravated function of the nervous system. It is treated with the regular Vata treatments (page 56) along with hot compress and medicated oil massage. Specific treatment is differentiated on the basis of causation, which in men may include urinary disorders, and in women, issues related to uterine health.

Trikagraha (Back pain / Lumbago)

Trikagraha relates to lower back pain or lumbago, and is concerned with the aggravated function of the nervous system. It is treated with the general treatments to reduce Vata, medicated oil massage, hot compress. Specific medicines are chosen on the basis of the signs and symptoms and the causative factors.

Pristhagraha (Spondylitis)

Pristhagraha relates to spondylitis, and is caused by the aggravation of the nervous system. It is treated with therapies to reduce Vata (page 56) including medicated oil massage, hot compress, and hot fomentations prepared with a decoction of herbs that are used in the treatments of nerve diseases. General remedies for Pristhagraha include **Kaishora Guggulu** (2 pills twice daily), **Yogaraja Guggulu** (2 pills twice daily) and **Narayana Taila**.

Parswavamarda (Spasm of the chest or diaphragm)

Parswavamarda relates to an acute painful spasm of the chest or diaphragm, and is concerned with the imbalance of the nervous system. It is treated with general therapies to reduce Vata treatments (page 56) including medicated oil massage, hot compress and specific remedies based on the case history. One general remedy in parswavamarda is **Sudarshana Churna/Vati** taken with purified **Sarjikakshara**(sodium bicarbonate), one gram each 2-3 times daily, taken with carminative herbs (page 175).

Angasamshosa (Neurological atrophy)

Angasamshosa relates to neurological atrophy, caused by the aggravated function of the related nerve system, which in turn causes an imbalance of the arterial system. It is treated with general therapies to reduce Vata (page 56) along with the application of medicated steam, enema, medicated oil massage, general Rasayanas and specific remedies. Specific remedies to treat angasamshosa include **Kaishora Guggulu** (2 pills twice daily), **Yogaraja Guggulu** (2 pills twice daily). These can be used with **Ashwagandha root** (*Convolvulus arvensis / Withania somnifera*), **Kapikacchu seeds** (cowhage / *Mucuna pruriens*) and/or **Bala plant** (country mallow / *Sida cordifolia*), taken with milk. For external massage over the affected area, the standard compound **Narayana Taila** is used.

Grivastambha (Paralysis of the neck / Torticollis)

Grivastambha relates to paralysis of the neck or torticollis, and is concerned with the aggravated function of the related nerve and arterial system causing spasm. It is treated with the general treatments to reduce Vata and Kapha (page 81) along with application of steam, medicated oil massage, and medicated nasal snuff.

Hanustambha (Lockjaw / Trismus)

Hanustambha relates to lockjaw or trismus, and is concerned with the aggravation of the nerves that supply the masseter muscle, causing severe stiffness. It is treated with the general therapies to reduce Vata (page 56) along with the application of medicated oil massage, steam, and medicated nasal snuff.

Pakshavata (Paralysis)

Pakshavata is related to paralysis, including hemiplegia, and is concerned with the aggravated function of the nervous system. Causes include vascular problems such as stroke, or neurological disorders such as multiple sclerosis. Pakshavata is classified into four categories, related to Vata, Vata-Pitta, Vata-Kapha and Dhatukshaya ('tissue wasting'). Pakshavata is treated with specific remedies along with external applications. These medicines include both medicines for Vata restoratives and Rasayanas (page 140), as well as massage, external applications (to open blockages and soothe the nerves), laxatives (page 174) and enemas. Although the use of laxative remedies in Vata disorders is usually prohibited, this does not apply in the treatment of Pakshavata. Some general remedies used in Pakshavata include **Kaishora Guggulu** (2 pills twice daily) and **Yogaraja Guggulu** (2 pills twice daily). These two medicines are used along with the standard formula **Shulanirmulanarasa Vati** (2 pills twice daily) and other medicines based upon specific signs and symptoms. For external massage either **Narayana Taila** or **Vishatinduka Taila** (medicated purified nux vomica oil) is used.

Vata paksavata

Pakshavata with the character of Vata is treated with general therapies to reduce Vata (page 56), along with the general therapies to treat paksavata, in addition to specific remedies based on the presenting signs and symptoms. Vata paksavata is very difficult to cure.

Vata-Pitta paksavata

Pakshavata with the character of Vata-Pitta, with symptoms such as fainting and heat sensations, is curable with the use of treatments to reduce Vata-Pitta (page 81), along with the general therapies to treat Pakshavata, and specific therapies to address the presenting signs and symptoms.

Vata-Kapha paksavata

Pakshavata with the character of Vata-Kapha, with symptoms including edema, is curable with general treatments to reduce Vata-Kapha (page 81), along with the general therapies to treat Pakshavata, and specific therapies to address the presenting signs and symptoms.

Dhatukshaya paksavata

Pakshavata with the character of Dhatukshaya, caused by traumatic bleeding or injury is not curable.

Arditam (Facial paralysis)

Arditam relates to facial paralysis, and is concerned with the aggravated function of the related nerve system. It is treated with general therapies to reduce Vata (page 56), along with a medicated nasal snuff, medicated oil massage of the head, application of steam, poultice, eyewash, and specific remedies. Symptomatic treatments (such as for high blood pressure) are also used. General remedies used in arditam include **Kaishora Guggulu** (2 pills twice daily) and **Yogaraja Guggulu** (2 pills twice daily). These can be given along with the standard formula **Shulanirmulanarasa Vati**, 2-3 pills twice daily. For external application the medicated oils mentioned under Pakshavata are also used.

Dhanustambha (Tetanus)

Dhanustambha is correlated with tetanus, and is concerned with the aggravated function of the spinal cord. Dhanustambha with the forward flexure of the spine called Abhyantarayama is considered curable, and is treated with general therapies to reduce Vata (page 56) along with enema, application of medicated 'oil massage' (Abhyanga), steam, and specific remedies based on the presenting signs and symptoms. Tetanus with the backward flexure of the spine (opisthotonus) is not curable, but can be treated palliatively with the same treatments as dhanustambha with the forward flexure.

Viswachi (Arthritis of the hand)

Viswachi is correlated with arthritis of the hand, and is related to an aggravation of the related nerves. It is treated with the general therapies to reduce Vata (page 56) along with medicated oil massage, application of steam, venesection and specific remedies based on the presenting signs and symptoms. Although venesection practices are prohibited for most nerve diseases, this rule does not follow for treatment of Viswachi.

General remedies for Viswachi include **Maha Yogaraja Guggulu** (2 pills twice daily), **Kaishora Guggulu** (2 pills twice daily) and **Ajamodadi Churna** (1-2 grams twice daily). Topically, **Narayana Taila** can be applied.

Krostukashirsa (Arthritis of the knee)

Krostukashira is correlated with arthritis of the knee along with indications of overt inflammation, and is concerned with the aggravated nerve system and venous system. It is treated with general therapies to reduce Vata (page 56) along with venesection practices and the same remedies used for Viswachi (arthritis of the hand). A medicated plaster can be prepared with **Dhattura leaf** (jimson weed / *Datura stramonium)* and purified **Shilajatu**.

Khanja (Lameness of one leg)

Khanja is correlated with lameness affecting one leg, caused by damage to the related nerves of the lumbar area. It is treated with general therapies to reduce Vata (page 56) along with medicated oil massage, application of steam and the same remedies used for Viswachi (arthritis of the hand).

Pangu (Paraplegia / Lameness affecting both legs)

Pangu is correlated with paraplegia, and is caused by damage to the related nerves of the lumbar area, affecting both legs. It is treated with general therapies to reduce Vata (page 56) along with medicated oil massage, application of steam and the same remedies used for Viswachi (arthritis of the hand). Pangu caused by trauma is not curable.

Kalayakhanja (Loss of coordination of the back)

Kalayakhanja is correlated with a loss of coordination of the back, and is found in conditions like multiple sclerosis, birth defects, trauma, and some bone marrow diseases. It is caused by weakness in the related nerve system. It is treated with general therapies to reduce Vata along with application of medicated 'oil massage' (Abhyanga), 'steam bath' (Swedana) and the same remedies used for Viswachi (arthritis of the hand).

Vatakantaka (Sprained ankle)

Sprain ankle is concerned with the damage of ligaments. It is treated with general therapies to reduce Vata (page 56) along with medicated oil massage.

Amsashosa (Osteoarthritis of the shoulder)

Amsashosa is correlated with osteoarthritis of the shoulder, and is concerned with the degeneration of the shoulder joint. It is treated with general therapies to reduce Vata (page 56) along with medicated oil massage, general rasayanas, and the same remedies used for Viswachi (arthritis of the hand) (page 232). It is very difficult to cure.

Apabahuka (Atrophy of the arm)

Apabahuka is correlated with atrophy of the arm, and is concerned with the aggravated function of the related nerve system that causes poor circulation and dryness. It is treated with general therapies to reduce Vata (page 56) along with general rasayanas, medicated oil massage, application of steam, and general remedies used to treat nerve (Vata) disorders.

Khalli (Degenerative Arthritis)

Khalli is correlated with degenerative arthritis of the joint of the hand or leg. It is treated with general therapies to reduce Vata (page 56) along with application of hot poultice, medicated oil massage, application of steam, and general remedies described under Viswachi (arthritis of the hand) (page 232). Also used are venesection (page 92), laxatives (page 174), diuretics (page 195) and antacids (page 160).

Amavata (Joint swelling / Rheumatoid arthritis)

Amavata is correlated with severe joint swelling or rheumatoid arthritis, caused by undigested foods that promote the accumulation of 'toxins' (Ama) in the blood. These toxins in turn cause toxic gasses and secretions to accumulate in the joints that attack the structure of the joint. Amavata is a complex (Sannipataja) disease. Amavata is treated with diuretics (page 195), laxatives (page 174), antacids (page 160), medicated plasters, and general treatments described under Viswachi (arthritis of the hand) (page 232).

Nidranasha (Insomnia)

Nidranasha is correlated with insomnia, and is considered to be a symptom of an underlying mental/emotional disorder. Nidranasha can be delineated into five categories: Vataja, Pittaja, Manastapaja, Kshayaja and Abhighataja.

One general remedy to treat Nidranasha is a combination of equal parts powders of **Sarpagandha root** (*Rauwolfia serpentina*), **Jatamansi rhizome** (spikenard / *Valeriana jatamansi* / *Nardostachys jatamansi*), **Ashwagandha root** (*Convolvulus arvensis* / *Withania somnifera*) and **Chandanadi Churna** (standard compound). The dose is 500 mg taken before bed.

Vataja Nidranasha

The primary symptom is insomnia with a restless mind. Use the general formula described above along with general therapies to reduce Vata (page 56).

Pittaja Nidranasha

The primary symptom is insomnia with anger and irritation. Use the general formula described above along with mild laxatives (page 174).

Manastapaja Nidranasha

The primary symptom is insomnia caused by grief. Use the general formula described above.

Kshayaja Nidranasha

The primary symptom is insomnia caused by emaciation. Use the general formula described above along with medicines for gaining weight.

Aghighataja Nidranasha

The primary symptom is insomnia caused by trauma. Use the general formula described above along with treatment against the cause of the trauma.

Apasmara (Epilepsy)

Apasmara is correlated with epilepsy, and considered to be a form of brain defect with seizures and alteration in consciousness. Apasmara is divided into five types based upon causative factors and symptoms: Vataja, Pittaja, Kaphaja, Sannipataja and Aghantuja.

A general remedy for apasmara is the equal parts powders of **Vacha rhizome** (acorus / *Acorus calamus*) and **Shatavariyoga** (standard compound), 500-1000 mg twice daily. This is given along with specific remedies based upon the causative factors and the presenting signs and symptoms.

Ardhavabhedaka (Migraine headache)

Ardhavabhedaka is correlated with migraine headaches, and is considered to be Vata-Kaphaja disease, caused by the congestion and blockage of the cranial blood vessels. Treatment is based upon use of medicines that resolve this congestion and blockage. One useful remedy is 2-3 parts **Guggulu gum resin** (*Commiphora wightii*) mixed with one part **Vacha rhizome** (acorus / *Acorus calamus*), prepared as pills, taken in doses of 2 pills twice daily. **Shadbindu Taila** can be used as a medicated nasal snuff for general use. Another medicated nasal snuff can be made from **Vacha rhizome** and **Pippali fruit** (long pepper / *Piper longum*) to relieve headache pain.

Chapter 21: Diseases of the Skin (Charma Roga)

While skin diseases have many different causes, in general they are the result of the habitual intake of unhealthy or incompatible foods (e.g. fish with milk, meat with honey, etc.), an excessive reliance upon certain tastes or qualities in food (e.g. excessively greasy, sour or heavy foods), improperly cooked foods, eating too often, poor digestion, suppression of the urge to vomit and irregular sleep. Habits such as these vitiate the three Doshas and affect the quality of blood and lymph, thereby producing toxic materials that initiate skin disorders.

General Treatment of Skin Diseases

Treated at their early stage of manifestation, skin diseases will respond well to simple methods of treatment. For example, Vataja skin diseases in the early stages can be treated with intake of **Ghrita** (Ghee), Pittaja skin diseases with venesection (see page 92) along with purgation, and Kaphaja skin diseases with emesis. After such detoxification measures, external remedies act quickly.

Purgation can be induced with equal parts **Trivrit root** (Indian rhubarb /Operculina turpethum), **Danti seed** *(Baliospermum montanum)* and **Triphala** *(Phyllanthus emblica / Terminalia belerica / Terminalia chebula)*, in doses of 2-3 grams.

Emesis can be induced with a decoction of equal parts **Vacha rhizome** (acorus / Acorus calamus), **Vasaka leaf** (Malabar nut / Adhatoda vasica), **Patola fruit** *(Trichosanthes dioica)*, **Nimba leaf** (neem / Azadirachta indica) and **Priyangu seed** *(Prunus mahaleb)* with honey, in doses of 2-3 grams.

A simple external application for simple dermatitis (Charmasotha) is a plaster of a paste made from **Khadira extract** (catechu / Acacia catechu, white). Another external application is a plaster made from **Chandanam wood** (white sandalwood / Santalum album) and **Tankana Bhasma** (purified borax).

Kustham (Leprosy)

Kustham is correlated with the disease of leprosy, and in general, is caused by pathogenic defects of the blood (see page 255) that causes the blood to turn blackish. Ayurveda divides kustham into seven different forms known as Kapala, Udumbara, Mandala, Risyajihwa, Pundarika, Kakanam, and Dadrukustham. All types of leprosy are very difficult to cure, and is incurable in the advanced stage.

One general treatment for leprosy is equal parts **Vakuchi seed** *(Psoralea corylifolia)*, **Khadira extract** *(Acacia catechu*, white), **Nimba leaf** (neem / Azadirachta indica) and **Haritaki fruit** *(Terminalia chebula)*, taken in doses of 1-2 grams, twice daily. Another simple remedy for leprosy is **Kaishora Guggulu** (page 67), taken in doses of two pills twice daily.

For external use, a paste can be made from **Karanja seed oil** (Indian beech / *Pongamia pinnata)*, **Chakramarda seed/leaf** (taper / *Cassia tora)*, **Kustha root** *(Saussurea lappa)* and **Goumutra** (cow urine).

Kapala Kustham

Kapala kustham is a form of kustham caused by the aggravated function of the nerves along with blood defects. It is treated with general therapies to reduce Vata (page 56) along with venesection (see page 92), oily plasters, the general measures described for leprosy and specific remedies. These methods can also be used for neurodermatitis.

One specific remedy to treat kapala kustham is equal parts **Ela fruit** (greater cardamon / *Amomum subulatum)*, **Kustha root** *(Saussurea lappa)*, **Darvi root** *(Berberis asiatica)*, **Daruharidra bark/extract** (barberry / *Berberis nepalensis)* and **Shala resin** (sal tree / *Shorea robusta)*, taken in doses of 1-2 grams twice daily. Other remedies include **Kanakabindwaristam** or **Abhayarista**, either of which is taken after meals, in doses of 12-24 mL after meals, twice daily.

Udumbara Kustham

Udumbara kustham involves the aggravated function of the veins along with blood defects. It is treated with general measures to reduce Pitta (page 67) along with venesection (see page 92), cooling plasters, laxatives (page 174), and the general remedies for leprosy.

Mandala Kustham

Mandala kustham is caused by the aggravated function of the arteries along with blood defects. It is treated with general measures to reduce Kapha (page 77) together with venesection (see page 92), warming plasters, emetics (see page 175), and the general remedies for leprosy.

Risyajihwa Kustham

Risyajihwa kustham is caused by the aggravated function of the nerves and veins along with blood defects. It is treated with general measures to reduce Vata-Pitta (page 81), with venesection (see page 92), plasters, and the general remedies for leprosy.

Pundarika Kustham

Pundarika kustham is caused by the aggravated function of the veins and the arteries along with blood defects. It is treated with general measures to reduce Pitta-Kapha, along together with venesection (see page 92), plasters, and the general remedies for leprosy.

Kakanam

Kakanam involves complicated (Sannipata) symptoms involving the nervous, venous, and arterial systems, along with blood defects. Although it is considered incurable, the general measures described for leprosy can be used as a palliative measure.

Dadrukustham

Dadrukustham is a form of leprosy that resembles ringworm, and is caused by the aggravated function of the arteries along with blood defects. It is treated with the remedies used for mandala kustham.

Sidhma (Tinea versicolor)

Sidhma is correlated with *Tinea versicolor* infection, and involves the aggravated function of the nerves and arteries along with blood defects. It is treated with the general measures described for reducing Vata-Kapha (page 81), along with specific medicines, including **Kaishora Guggulu** (2 pills twice daily) and **Nimbadi** (2 pills twice daily). External therapies include a preparation made from one part **Rasakarpura** (white crystal of mercury sulfide / mineral camphor), one part **Yashada Bhasma** (purified zinc oxide) and three to four parts **Sphutikarika** (purified alum).

Dusivisha Kustham (Psoriasis)

Dusivisha kustham is correlated with the disease of psoriasis, and is considered to be caused by the accumulation of toxic material or 'poison' (Dusiviha) in the skin. Three types are described, including Ekakustham, Charmakhyam and Kitibha. Psoriasis of all three types is treated with the general therapies to reduce Vata-Kapha (page 81) together with the general remedies described under kustham (page 235). Some commonly used internal medicines for psoriasis include **Gandhakarasayana** (2 pills twice daily), **Vakuchyadi Vati** (2 pills twice daily) and **Kaishora Guggulu** (2 pills twice daily). External applications include powders of **Vakuchi seed** *(Psoralia corylifolia)* and **Khadira extract** (catechu, white / *Acacia catechu)*, mixed with unsalted butter, Ghee or coconut oil. Another remedy is a paste prepared by grinding the leaves of **Rajavriksha** (Indian laburnum / *Cassia fistula)* with vinegar. Another paste uses the seeds of **Chakramarda** *(Cassia tora)* ground with cow urine and the milk of **Snuhi cactus** *(Euphorbia nerifolia)*.

Ekakustham (Psoriasis with white scales)

Ekakustham is correlated with a form of psoriasis manifesting large patches of white scales, and is caused by the aggravated function of the nerves and arteries along with blood defects. The general treatments used are those for blood defects (see page 255), including **Kaishora Guggulu**.

Charmakhyam (Psoriasis with papules)

Charmakhyam is correlated with a form of psoriasis manifesting thick scaling papules, and is caused by aggravated functions of the nerves and arteries along with blood defects. Treatment consists of the same measures described under Dusivisham kustham.

Kitibha (Psoriasis with bright red or blue scales)

Kitibha is correlated with psoriasis manifesting with bright red or bluish colored scales, and is caused by the aggravated function of the nerves and arteries along with blood defects. Treatment consists of the general remedies described under Dusivisham kustham.

Vaipadikam (Rhagades)

Vaipadikam is correlated with painful fissures of the skin in the hand and/or leg. It is caused by the aggravated function of the nerves and arteries along with blood toxicity. It is treated with the general measures to reduce Vata-Kapha (page 81), along with the general remedies described under leprosy (see page 235). Useful remedies include **Kaishora Guggulu** (2 pills twice daily) and **Alarasayana** (2 pills twice daily).

Dadru (Ringworm)

Dadru is correlated with ringworm, and is caused by the aggravated function of the veins and arteries along with blood defects. For external use the standard compound **Dadruharalepa** is used as a plaster. It is made from one part each of **Shala resin** (sal tree /*Shorea robusta)*, **Gandhaka Bhasma** (purified sulfur oxide), **Tankana Bhasma** (purified borax), and **Sphutikarika** (purified alum). In serious cases, general treatments are used to reduce Pitta-Kapha (page 81) along with the general remedies described under leprosy (see page 235).

Charmadala (Candidiasis)

Charmadala is correlated with candidiasis, and is caused by the aggravated function of the veins and arteries along with blood defects. It is treated with the general measures described to reduce Pitta-Kapha (page 81) along with the general remedies described for leprosy (see page 235). If there is pruritus (anal itching) **Nimba leaf** (neem / *Azadirachta indica)* is taken internally in doses of 1-2 grams twice daily, or **Nimbadi** is used instead.

Pama (Eczema)

Pama is correlated with eczema, and is caused by the aggravated function of the veins and arteries along with blood defects. It is treated with general measures to reduce Pitta-Kapha (page 81) along with venesection (see page 92), and the general remedies described leprosy (see page 235). Useful remedies include **Kaishora**

Guggulu and **Alarasayana**. For external use, a combination of one part **Gandhaka Bhasma** (purified sulfur oxide) and two parts **Sphutikarika** (purified alum) is mixed with 50 parts **Narikela oil** (coconut / *Cocos nucifera*).

Kachchu (Pustular eczema)

Kachchu is correlated with the pustular form of eczema, and is caused by the aggravated function of the veins and arteries along with blood defects. It is treated with the general measures to reduce Pitta-Kapha (page 81), together with the general remedies described under leprosy (page 235) and eczema.

Vishpota (Pemphigus)

Vishpota refers to any skin disease characterized by the appearance of blisters. The non-infectious Kaphaja variety is correlated with pemphigus, whereas the Pitta-type can be linked to impetigo (page 242). Vishpota is caused by the aggravated function of the veins and arteries along with blood defects. It is treated with the same remedies used for eczema and leprosy (page 235).

Shataru (Flexural eczema)

Shataru is correlated with eczema found in the joint areas, typically manifesting along with ulcerated boils, and is caused by aggravated functions of the veins and arteries along with blood defects. It is treated with the same remedies used for eczema and leprosy (page 235).

Vicharchika (Scabies)

Vicharchika is correlated with scabies infection, and is caused by the aggravated function of the arterial system along with blood defects. It is treated with the general measures to reduce Kapha (page 77) along with the general remedies described under leprosy (see page 235). In particular, Vicharchika benefits from the external application of **Sphutikarika** (purified alum), prepared as an ointment.

Switram (Leucoderma / Vitiligo)

Switram is correlated with leucoderma/vitiligo, and is divided into three categories with the characters of Vataja, Pittaja and Kaphaja. The general internal medicines for switram are the same as used for leprosy (page 235), especially **Kaishora Guggulu** and **Vakuchi seed** *(Psoralia corylifolia)*. Also used internally is the standard formula **Vakuchyadi Vati**. Externally remedies made with **Vakuchi seed** *(Psoralia corylifolia)* are also used, including the standard compound **Vakuchyadi paste**, made from **Vakuchi seed** *(Psoralia corylifolia)* mixed with **Haritala Bhasma** (orpiment / purified yellow arsenic trisulfide) and **Goumutra** (cow urine) to make a paste. Another external remedy used is **Switrahara paste**, made with **Chitraka root** *(Plumbago zeylanica)*.

Vataja Leucoderma (Arunam)

Leucoderma with the character of Vata (slightly pink patches) is caused by aggravated function of related nervous system along with blood defects. It is easy to cure and treated with the general Vata treatments (page 56) along with the general remedies for leucoderma mentioned above.

Pittaja Leucoderma (Darunam)

Leucoderma with the character of Pitta (copper patches) is caused by aggravated function of related venous system along with blood defects. It is curable with and is treated with the general Pitta treatments (page 67) together with the general remedies for leucoderma.

Kaphaja Leucoderma (Switram)

Leucoderma with the character of Kapha (white patches) is caused by aggravated function of related arteries system along with blood defects. It is very difficult to cure and is treated with the general Kapha treatments (page 77) and the remedies for leucoderma.

Shitapittam (Urticaria / Hives)

Shitapittam is correlated with urticaria, and is divided into two categories, one with the character of Vata and another with the character of Kapha. The general treatment is internal use of equal parts powders of **Yavani seed** (wild omum / *Trachyspermum ammi)* and **Nimba leaf extract** (neem / *Azadirachta indica)*, 1-2 grams twice daily. For external use, pure alcohol can be applied to the raised patches to stop the itching.

Kaphaja Urticaria (Udara)

Urticaria with the character of Kapha is caused by aggravated function of the arterial system. It is treated with the general Kapha treatments (page 77) along with the general treatments for urticaria.

Vataja Urticaria

Urticaria with the character of Vata is caused by aggravated function of the related nervous system. It is treated with the general Vata treatments (page 56) together the general treatments for urticaria.

Kotha / Utkotha (Allergic rash)

Kotha or allergic rashes have the same etiology as urticaria and are treated with the same general remedies.

Visharpa (Erysipelas)

Visharpa is correlated with erysipelas and is usually caused by pathogenic defects of the blood (see definition and treatment on page 255). It is classified into seven categories, with the characters of Vata, Pitta, Kapha, Sannipata, Vata-Pitta, Vata-Kapha or Pitta-Kapha. For general internal treatment, 1-2 grams of **Trivrit root** (Indian rhubarb /*Operculina turpethum)* are taken with 30 mL of **Triphala decoction**, and 2 pills of **Kaishora Guggulu**, twice daily. Externally **Shukti Bhasma** (oyster shell ash /*Ostrea gigas)* can be applied.

Erysipelas caused by Vata, Pitta or Kapha

Erysipelas with the character of Vata or Pitta or Kapha is curable. In general, it is treated with venesection (see page 92), purgative remedies (page 174), fasting, bitter remedies and the specific remedies mentioned, along with the general treatments for the specific imbalance encountered.

Sannipataja Erysipelas

Erysipelas with the character of Sannipata, with complicated symptoms, is not curable.

Granthi Visharpa (Adenoma / Adenocarcinoma)

Adenoma is considered by Ayurveda to be visharpa (erysipelas) with the character of Vata-Kapha. It is concerned with aggravated functioning of the nerves, arteries and the lymphatic glands. It is treated with the general Vata and Kapha treatments (page 81) along with venesection (see page 92), fasting, purgative remedies (page 174), bitter remedies and the specific remedies against erysipelas. In the chronic state, if the abnormal growth becomes hard it has to be treated with surgery. Metastatic adenocarcinoma is complex (Sannipataja) and is not curable.

Agni Visharpa (Cellulitis)

Cellulitis is considered by Ayurveda to be visharpa (erysipelas) with the character of Vata-Pitta. It is caused by aggravated functions of the nerves and veins. It is difficult to cure, and is treated with general measures to reduce Vata and Pitta (page 81) along with general remedies for erysipelas along with venesection (see page 92).

Kardama Visharpa (Gangrenous cellulitis)

Gangrenous cellulitis is considered as a form of visharpa (erysipelas) with the character of Kapha-Pitta, caused by aggravated functions of the arteries and veins. It is not curable. It can be maintained however with the general Kapha and Pitta treatments (page 81) along with the general remedies for erysipelas (above), venesection (see page 92) and fasting.

Vishpota (Impetigo)

Vishpota refers to any skin disease characterized by the appearance of blisters. The infectious Pitta variety of Vishpota is correlated with impetigo and is caused by aggravated function of the veins along with blood defects. It is treated with the remedies used for erysipelas (above). In severe cases the lesions may have to be cleansed surgically.

Yavaprakshya (Keloid)

Yavaprakshya is correlated with keloid and is caused by aggravated functions of the nerves and arteries (epithelium). It is treated with a hot plaster of **Haritala Bhasma** (orpiment / purified yellow arsenic trisulfide). **Kaishora Guggulu** can be used internally, in doses of 2 pills twice daily. If it is infected has to be treated with surgery.

Andhalagi (Keloid folliculitis)

Andhalagi is correlated with keloid folliculitis and is caused by aggravated functions of the nerves and arteries. It is treated with the same remedy used for Keloid.

Vivrita (Cutaneous leishmaniasis)

Vivrita is correlated with cutaneous leishmaniasis, and involves an aggravated venous system that causes boils which enlarges to a nodule creating large holes. It is treated with general remedies for erysipelas (page 241). If it is infected has to be surgically cleansed.

Kachchapika (Carbuncle)

Kachchapika is correlated with carbuncle, and is caused by aggravated functions of the arteries and nerves. It is treated with the same remedies used for Keloid.

Balmika (Skin neoplasm with holes)

Balmika is correlated with a neoplasm of the skin that manifests with numerous holes is caused by complicated combined symptoms of the nervous, vein and arterial systems (Sannipataja). It is very difficult to cure and is treated with specific remedies against neoplasm (page 248) and surgery.

Indraviddha (Comedo)

Indraviddha is correlated with comedo, and is caused by aggravated function of the nerves and veins that cause a dilation of the hair follicle. It is treated with the same remedies used for erysipelas (page 241). If it is infected has to be treated with surgery.

Gardhabhika (Boil with pimples)

Gardhabhika is correlated with boil that manifests with pimples, and is caused by aggravated functions of the nerves and veins. It is treated with the same remedies used for erysipelas (page 241). If it is infected has to be treated with surgery.

Pashanagardhabha (Mumps)

Pashanagardhabha is correlated with mumps, and is caused by aggravated functions of the related nerves and arteries. Two helpful remedies include **Kaishora Guggulu** (2 pills twice daily) or **Mrityunjayarasa Vati** (2 pills twice daily). For external use, a plaster can be made from **Shilajatu Rasayana**, or from the combination of **Devadaru wood** (Himalayan cedar / *Cedrus deodara)*, **Manashila Bhasma** (purified realgar) and **Kustha root** *(Saussurea lappa).*

Jalagardhabha (Neuralgia)

Jalagardhabha is a kind of neuralgia that involves aggravated functions of the veins, causing inflammation of the nerves. It is treated with the methods used for erysipelas (page 241). If there is infection causing the nerve pain, it has to be treated with surgery. A simple internal treatment for neuralgia is a powder made from equal parts **Maricham seed** (black pepper / *Piper nigrum)*, **Nagaram rhizome** (Indian cyperus / *Cyperus pertenuis)* and **Yavakshara alkaline ash** (barley plant / *Hordeum vulgare)*, taken in doses of one gram with honey.

Kaksha (Herpes zoster)

Kaksha is correlated with Herpes zoster (shingles), and displays an aggravated functioning of the veins. It is treated with the same remedies used for erysipelas (page 241). If it is infected has to be treated with surgery.

Agnirohini (Bubonic Plague)

Agnirohini is correlated with bubonic plague, and is caused by complicated symptoms involving the nerves, veins and arteries (Sannipataja) that causes a very painful inflammation of the lymphatic glands of the armpit. It is considered incurable and fatal.

Chippam (Paronychia)

Chippam relates to paronychia, a soft tissue infection around the fingernail or toenail, and has the character of Vata and Pitta. It is treated with hot compress and surgical cleaning.

Kunakham (Tinea inguinalis)

Kunakham is correlated with *Tinea inguinalis*, a fungal infection of the inguinal region, and has the character of Vata and Pitta. It is treated with the same methods used for paronychia.

Anushayi (Tinea pedis)

Anushayi is correlated with *Tinea pedis*, a fungal infection of the feet, and has the character of Kapha. It is treated with the remedies used for abscess with the character of Kapha (page 246).

Vidarika (Inguinal bubo)

Vidarika is correlated with inguinal bubo, and has the character of Sannipata with complicated symptoms. It is treated with hot compress, massage, venesection (see page 92) and use of pressure to dissolve the swelling. If it is infected has to be treated with surgery.

Sharkararbuda (Ulcerative neoplasm of the skin)

Sharkararbuda is correlated with an ulcerative neoplasm of the skin, and has the character of Vata and Kapha. It is treated with the remedies used for lipoma (page 249) and the specific remedies against neoplasm, such as **Chandraprabha Vati** (2 pills twice daily) and **Kaishora Guggulu** (2 pills twice daily).

Kadara (Corn, Clavus)

Kadara or clavus has the character of Vata and Kapha. It is treated with surgery.

Alasam / Alasakam (Lichen simplex chronicus / Lichen planus)

Alasam is correlated with Lichen simplex chronicus, and generally has the character of Kapha along with blood defects. This disease is treated with venesection (see page 92), washing with vinegar, the use of plasters made of bitter and astringent remedies, as well as specific remedies based on signs and symptoms. The more advanced Lichen planus (alasakam) is caused by aggravated functions of the nerves and arteries along with blood defects. It is treated with the general Vata and Kapha treatments (page 81) together with general remedies for leprosy (see page 235) and specific internal remedies. Specific medicines for both alasam and alasakam include **Kaishora Guggulu** (2 pills twice daily), **Alarasayana** (2 pills twice daily) and **Nimbadi** (2 pills twice daily). For external use, use **Nimba leaf powder** (neem / *Azadirachta indica*) with **Sphutikarika** (purified alum).

Yuvanapidaka (Acne vulgaris)

Yuvanapidaka is correlated with Acne vulgaris, and has the character of Kapha and Vata along with blood defects. Padminikantaka is a term used to describe blackheads (open comedomes). It is treated with emetic remedies (see page 175) along with specific remedies for internal and external use. For internal use **Kaishora Guggulu** (2 pills twice daily) can be used to cleanse the blood. Externally **Shankha Bhasma** (purified conch shell ash, *Turbinella pyrum*) is commonly used as a plaster. Other external plasters include **Jatiphalam seed paste** (nutmeg / *Myristica fragrans*) and the powder of **Masura bean** (green lentil / *Lens esculenta*), which is fried in **Ghrita** (clarified butter / Ghee) and applied for ten to fifteen minutes.

Mashakam (Wart)

Masakam or wart has the character of Vata. It is treated with surgery. Blood cleaning medicines (page 255) can be used internally.

Tilakalaka (Freckle)

Tilakalaka is correlated with the appearance of freckles, and has the character of Pitta along with blood defects. It is treated with blood cleaning remedies together with specific remedies. Pills made from **Chandanam Churna** (white sandalwood / *Santalum album*) are often effective in reducing the number of lesions.

Nyachcham (Melanoma)

Nyachcham is correlated with melanoma, and has the character of Vata and Pitta. The terms vyanga relates to melanoma of the face, and nilika refers to a dark form of melanoma. All are treated with venesection (see page 92) and specific remedies. **Kaishora Guggulu** is typically used because it is valuable for both cancer and skin diseases, and is combined with with other internal medicines for cancer (page 248).

Shukaradamshtraka (Inflammatory ringworm)

Shukaradamshtraka relates to inflammatory ringworm, a form of ringworm that causes inflammatory masses that ooze pus and are studded with broken hairs. Shukaradamshtraka has the character of Sannipata and is treated with the remedies used for eczema (page 238).

Vidradhi (Abscess, external)

In general, the term vidradhi relates to external abscess, and is caused by blood defects or injury. It is divided into six categories: Vata, Kapha, Pitta, Sannipata, Kshataja and Raktaja. Whatever the cause, vidradhi has to be treated with venesection practices to remove the vitiated blood (page 92), and the specific remedies against internal abscess (see page 170).

Vataja Abscess

Abscess with the character of Vata is caused by aggravated function of the nervous system along with blood defects. It is treated with the application of steam, anti-inflammatory remedies in the form of plaster and poultice (page 155), venesection, and the specific remedies against abscess. If it is infected has to be cleaned with surgery.

Pittaja Abscess

Abscess with the character of Pitta is caused by aggravated function of the venous system along with blood defects. It is treated with the application of cold, anti-inflammatory remedies in the form of plaster and poultice (page 155), laxative remedies (page 174), venesection, and specific remedies. It has to be cleaned out with surgery if it is infected.

Kaphaja Abscess

Abscess with the character of Kapha is caused by aggravated function of the arterial system along with blood defects. It is treated with the application of warm anti-inflammatory remedies (page 155) in the form of steam, plaster, poultice and hot compress, emetic remedies (see page 175), venesection, and specific remedies. It has to be treated with surgery if it is infected.

Sannipataja Abscess

Abscess with the character of Sannipata has complicated symptoms. It is not curable. However it can be controlled with surgery and the specific remedies.

Kshataja Abscess

Abscess with the character of Ksataja is caused by traumatic condition. Abscess with the character of Raktaja is caused by pathogenic blood defects. They are treated with the same remedies used for abscess with the character of Pitta.

Pramehapidakas (Boils and pimples caused by Prameha)

There are many types of boils and pimples, some of which are caused by prameha, a group of urinary diseases that includes diabetes. Ayurveda counts ten as the most important, called Sharavika, Kacchapika, Jalini, Sarsapi, Alaji, Vinata, Vidradhika, Putrini, Masurika and Vidarika. In general, they have to be treated with surgery along with specific remedies. Some specific remedies against the pramehapidakas include **Pathadi Churna** (powdered root of *Stephania hernandifolia*, 1 gram twice daily), **Shilajatu Rasayana** (2 pills twice daily), **Pippalyadi decoction** (5 mL twice daily) and **Kaishora Guggulu** (2 pills twice daily). For external application **Khadiradi Churna** is helpful, which contains bitter **Nimba leaf** (neem / *Azadirachta indica*) along with astringents such as **Sphutikarika** (purified alum).

Sharavika (Furuncle), Kacchapika (Carbuncle) and Jalini (Painful carbuncle)

Sharavika, Kacchapika, and Jalini are three kinds of boils that have the character of Kapha, as well as fat defects, and are considered very difficult to cure. They can sometimes be controlled with the specific remedies and/or surgery.

Sharsapi (Herpes), Alaji (Erysipeloid), Vinata (Blue boil) and Vidradhika (Abscess-like boil)

Sarsapi, Alaji, Vinata, and Vidradhika are four kinds of boils and pimples that have the character of Pitta along with fat defects. They are easy to cure using the specific remedies against boils and pimples.

Putrini (Big carbuncle), Masurika (Chickenpox) and Vidarika (Bubo)

Putrini, Masurika and Vidarika are three kinds of boils that have the character of Vata along with fat defects. They are curable using the specific remedies mentioned.

Bhagandara (Fistula)

Fistula is generally caused by blood toxicity along with muscular tissue defects. It is divided into five categories: Vataja, Pittaja, Kaphaja, Sannipataja and Kshataja. A fistula with the character of Vata is called Shataponaka and is related to aggravated function of the nervous system. The fistula with the character of Pitta is called Ustragriva, and is related to aggravated function of the veins (inflammation). A fistula with the character of Kapha is called Parisravi and is related to aggravated function of the arterial system with presence of excess exudation. A fistula with the character of Sannipata is called Shambukavarta, which presents with complicated symptoms. The fistula with the character of Kshataja is called Unmargi, and is related to injury of the anus.

Fistula is treated with surgery followed by specific remedies for internal and external use. Fistulas with the character of Sannipata (complicated) and Kshataja (injury-related) are considered incurable. Internal medicine includes **Kaishora Guggulu**, given in doses of 2 pills twice daily. Externally a plaster can be applied made from equal parts tender leaf of **Vata** (banyan tree / *Ficus bengalensis)*, brick powder (water soaked), **Shunthi root** (dry ginger / *Zingiber officinalis),* **Gokshura fruit** *(Tribulus terrestris)* and **Punarnava plant** *(Boerhavia difusa).*

Galaganda (Goiter)

Galaganda is correlated with goiter and is caused by defects in the fatty tissues (meda) of the body. It is classified into three categories, with the character of Vataja, Kaphaja or Medoja. Goiter with the character of Vata shows painful swelling of the thyroid gland. Goiter with the character of Kapha presents with swelling of the thyroid gland with severe itching. Goiter with the character of Meda shows severe swelling of the thyroid gland with little itching. In general, galaganda is treated with venesection (see page 92), the application of steam, the use of general medicines according to character, along with specific remedies. Some specific medicines for goiter include **Hastikarnapalasa root** (bastard teak / *Butea monosperma)* taken with rice water in doses of 500 mg twice daily, and dried powder of **buffalo thyroid gland**, given in doses of 200 mg twice daily. If the goiter is infected, as is commonly the case in medoja goiter, it has to be treated with surgery.

Gandamala (Scrofula / Cervical tuberculous lymphadenitis)

Gandamala is correlated with scrofula, and has the character of Kapha along with fat defects (meda) that causes swelling of the lymphatic glands. It is treated with the general Kapha treatments (page 77) along with the application of burning practices, venesection (see page 92) and specific remedies for internal and external use. Some internal medicines used for scrofula are **Kanchanara Guggulu** (2 pills twice daily) and 1-2 g of **Shunthi root** (ginger / *Zingiber officinalis)* taken with a decoction of **Kanchanara bark** (mountain ebony / *Bauhinia tomentosa).* External medicines include a plaster made of **Rajavriksha root** (Indian laburnum /*Cassia fistula)* ground with rice water, and **Chhuchhundari oil.**

Apachi (Glandular tuberculosis)

Apachi is correlated with glandular tuberculosis and has the same etiology as scrofula. It is treated with surgery along with the specific anti-TB remedies used both internally and externally (see page 184). Glandular TB with the all the symptoms of pulmonary tuberculosis is considered incurable.

Granthi (Small neoplasm)

Granthi is a kind of neoplasm, either small or large, caused by the abnormal growth of epithelial tissues. Ayurveda divides neoplasms into six categories: Vataja, Pittaja, Kaphaja, Siraja, Medoja and Mansaja.

Treatment of Small Neoplasm

Small neoplasms, if not ulcerated, can be cured with proper and timely treatment. However, it takes significant time, often months and even years. Using surgical operations to take out abnormal growths is beneficial to prescribe in any condition, and often has good results for quick cure. If the operation is not properly performed, however, any abnormal cells that remain can grow again and spread (metastasize). Metastatic conditions have to be treated as soon as possible using the treatment for erysipelas (page 241), along with the general cancer treatments and venesection (see page 92). Some specific medicines against neoplasms include **Kanchanara Guggulu** (2 pills twice daily), **Chandraprabha Vati** (2 pills twice daily), **Kaishora Guggulu** (2 pills twice daily), **Lavangadyam Churna** (1 gram twice daily) and **Abhaya arista** (12-24 mL twice daily). Externally, a poultice can be made from equal parts **Shunthi root** (ginger / *Zingiber officinalis*), **Gandhaka Bhasma** (purified sulfur oxide), **Yavakshara alkaline ash** (barley plant / *Hordeum vulgare)*, **Vidanga seeds** *(Embelia ribes)*, and **Nagaram rhizome** (Indian cyperus / *Cyperus pertenuis)* mixed with **Anjanaki blood** (lizard blood). Another poultice for skin tumors can be made from the fresh leaf of **Upodaki plant** *(Basella rubra)*.

Vataja Neoplasm

A small neoplasm with the character of Vata appears as a cyst-like abnormal growth. It is treated with the general Vata treatments (page 56) along with anti-swelling remedies (page 257), massage dissolving techniques and the specific anti-cancer remedies for internal and external uses. It has to be treated with surgery if it is ulcerated.

Pittaja Neoplasm

A small neoplasm with the character of Pitta presents as an inflammatory abnormal growth.

It is treated with the general Pitta treatments (page 67) along with anti-inflammatory remedies (page 155), venesection (see page 92), and the specific remedies for internal and external uses. It has to be treated with surgery if it is ulcerated.

Kaphaja Neoplasm

A small neoplasm with the character of Kapha develops as a hard edema-like abnormal growth. It is treated with the general Kapha treatments (page 77) along with anti-edema remedies (page 257), massage dissolving techniques and the specific anti-cancer remedies for internal and external uses. It has to be treated with surgery if it is ulcerated.

Siraja Granthi (Angioma)

A small neoplasm with the character of Siraja is caused by abnormal growth of blood vessels. It is treated with the same principle of neoplasm with the character of Pitta. However, it is considered very difficult to cure.

Medoja Granthi (Lipoma)

The small neoplasm with the character of Medoja develops as a fatty abnormal growth. It is treated with the surgery, burning practices, and the specific anti-cancer remedies for internal and external uses.

Mansaja Granthi (Myoma)

The small neoplasm with the character of Mansaja is caused by abnormal growth of muscular tissues. It is treated with surgery, followed by the specific medicines to prevent recurrence.

Arbuda (Large neoplasm)

Arbuda or large neoplasms are divided into six categories just like the smaller neoplasms, with the same etiology and symptoms, with the characters of Vata, Pitta, Kapha, Medoja, Raktaja and Mansaja. Large neoplasms are in general treated with the same remedies used for small neoplasms, however they are more difficult to cure due to their size and advanced nature. Large neoplasms with the character of Raktaja (angioma) and Mansaja (Myoma) are considered to be incurable. Use of surgical operations is more dangerous for larger tumors, because there is a greater likelihood of metastasis. For this reason, two less dangerous methods are used. The first is surgery using an alkali thread, called Ksharasutra Chikitsa, binds the root of the tumor with a thread prepared with lime until it detaches. The second method is maggot treatments. In this treatment, a plaster of food is applied to the tumor and the maggots are allowed to develop and eat the neoplasm.

Shwetaraktarbuda (Adult Leukemia)

Shwetaraktarbuda is adult leukemia, and is a complicated (Sannipataja) disease. If treated early enough, it can be cured by medicine. At the beginning of treatment, combine the standard treatment with the remedies used for hemorrhage (page 258). Some specific remedies for leukemia include **Chandraprabha Vati** (2 pills twice daily), **Kaishora Guggulu** (2 pills twice daily) and **Chandanadi Churna** (1-2 g twice daily).

Slipada (Elephantiasis / Filariasis)

Slipada relates to filariasis, resulting in lymphatic blockage that causes severe leg edema. It is divided into three categories: Vataja, Pittaja and Kaphaja. The aggravated function of the lymphatic duct system (Kapha) has to be treated side by side with the remedies prescribed for the filiariasis. An external treatment is to grind **Arka root** (milkweed / *Calotropis gigantea)* with vinegar to plaster on the affected area. Alternatively, the powder or either **Vacha rhizome** (acorus / *Acorus calamus)*, **Chitraka root** (Leadwort, white flower / *Plumbago zeylanica)*, or **Devadaru wood** (Himalayan cedar / *Cedrus deodara)* can be ground with **Goumutra** (cow urine) and used as a plaster. Internally **Kaishora Guggulu** (2 pills twice daily) is taken along with pills made from five parts **Ajamoda seed** (wild celery / *Carum roxburghianum)* and one part **Yavakshara alkaline ash** (barley plant / *Hordeum vulgare)*, in doses of 1 gram twice daily. These remedies are only efficacious in the beginning stage.

Vataja Filiariasis

Filariasis with the character of Vata presents with painful edema. It is treated with the general Vata treatments (page 56) along with venesection (see page 92), burning with heated instruments and the specific remedies for internal and external uses.

Pittaja Filiariasis

Filariasis with the character of Pitta has the symptoms of burning and sensitive edema. It is treated with the general Pitta treatments (page 67) along with venesection (see page 92), the remedies used for large Pittaja neoplasm (page 250) and the specific remedies mentioned.

Kaphaja Filiariasis

Filariasis with the character of Kapha results in heavy edema. It is treated with the general Kapha treatments (page 77) along with venesection (see page 92) and the specific remedies mentioned previously.

Chapter 22: Diseases of Tissue Metabolism (Saptadhatu Roga)

Ayurveda classifies the major components of the body as plasma (Rasa), blood (Rakta), flesh (Mansa), fat (Medas), bone (Asthi), marrow (Majja) and semen (Shukra), collectively called the Sapta (seven) Dhatus (tissue elements). It is important to note that these are broad categories, and each Dhatu includes several different tissue types. For example, the tissue element of flesh (Mansa) includes the nerves, skin, tendons, membranes and glands.

In general, the body is said to contain ten handfuls of water, nine handfuls of plasma, eight handfuls of blood, five handfuls of fat, one handful of marrow and a half handful of semen. Besides these ingredients, the body also has quantities of by-products such as bile and the two types of Ojas (vital water), all of which should be in proportion. If the Dhatus and its component parts become unhealthy it can be a cause for many diseases including anemia, weight loss, thrombosis, arteriosclerosis, obesity, edema, varicosis, osteoporosis, impotence, and sterility.

The Concept of Metabolism in Ayurveda

Plasma (Rasa) is the essence of digested food. It goes to the liver through the portal vein of the gastrointestinal system, and from there to the heart where it circulates through the arteries for the nourishment of the bodily tissues. Ayurveda states that the bodily fire (Agni) causes the food nutrients to change their physical properties over the course of a thirty day cycle in order to nourish each part of the body. To understand this process it is important to remember that the nutrients extracted from food are understood not by their biochemical forms, but by their physical properties as defined by Ayurveda.

The physical properties of plasma are first active for five days in the blood. Then the blood (Rakta) mixed with nutritive plasma separates out nutrients with the physical properties of flesh (Mansa) so it can nourish the muscular tissues. The nutrients with the physical properties of flesh (Mansa) are active for five days, after which the greasy properties of the flesh starts to separate out and begins to nourish the fatty tissues (Medas) of the body. The activity of the nutrients with greasy properties continues for five days and then begins to nourish the bone (Asthi), with the cartilage especially absorbing the greasy elements. After five more days the greasy elements gradually change physical properties and begin to nourish the oily marrow (Majja). Then, after another five days the essence of the oily marrow converts to help generate semen (Shukra) and then Ojas (vital water), which spreads throughout the whole body. Thus over the course of 30 days the digested food is converted from one form into another to nourish all of the bodily tissues (Dhatus).

As the plasma begins to enter the tissues mucus forms as a byproduct. If the digestive process and the foods consumed are healthy, the mucus is sweet in taste and contains nutrients useable by the body. Healthy mucus coats and moistens the tissues. If the digestive process is unhealthy, the mucus becomes salty in taste and is excreted from the body. In the same way bile is the by-product of blood, which in a healthy state is pungent in taste and promotes the heat required for metabolism. In the unhealthy state bile is bitter and acid in taste and is excreted from the body. The by-product of semen (Shukra) is the vital water (Ojas) that is necessary for the proper functioning of the nervous system, brain and heart. Ayurveda distinguishes between two types of Ojas: one which is intrinsic to life and remains in the heart without change (Para Ojas), and one which fluctuates depending on dietary and lifestyle habits (Apara Ojas). The intrinsic Ojas of the heart is measured as eight drops which are yellow in color, whereas the circulating Ojas is measured as one half handful and is white in color.

Rasadosha (Pathogenic defects of plasma)

The plasma becomes pathogenic if its properties change making it too greasy, heavy or cold. In this state many physical problems can develop, including loss of appetite, loss of sense of taste on the tongue, nausea, heaviness, drowsiness, body ache, fever, blurred vision, anemia, blockage in the duct system, heart attack, impotency, weakness, loss of weight, indigestion, grey hair and wrinkling of the skin.

Pathogenic defects of the plasma are generally treated with the timely application of emetic remedies (page 175), enema, laxative remedies (page 174), a medicated nasal snuff made from **Katphalam bark** (box myrtle / *Myrica nagi)*, regulation of water consumption, exposure to windy and sunny places, digestive remedies (page 173), fasting and exercise. Foods or remedies that are heavy to digest, constrictitory or greasy in property have to be strictly prohibited.

Rasakshaya (Deficiency of plasma or plasma)

Deficiency of plasma or plasma is caused by weak function of the arterial system and the heart that causes physical and mental weakness. It is treated with digestive remedies (page 173) and general Rasayanas, with specific remedies chosen on the basis of the presenting signs and symptoms.

Rasavriddhi (Excess of plasma or plasma)

Excessive amount of plasma or plasma in the blood causes the symptoms of nausea and watery mouth. It is treated with the same methods used for pathogenic defects of plasma. In ancient times venesection and leeches were also used.

Raktadosha (Pathogenic defects of blood)

Pathogenic defects of blood exist when the properties of blood become imbalanced and excessively acid, greasy, hot or liquid. In this state many diseases can develop, including stomatitis, red eyes, hematorrhea, bloody smell of mouth and nose, erysipelas, abscess, hematuria, gout, menorrhagia, hot sensations, headache, weakness, acidity, anger, delusion, intoxication, drowsiness, blurred vision, skin diseases, leprosy, boils and pimples, and liver and spleen diseases.

Pathogenic defects of blood in general, are treated with timely application of laxative remedies (page 174), fasting, venesection (see page 92), and the remedies for hematorrhea (page 255). It is also necessary to strictly prohibit foods or remedies that are acidic or increase acidity, greasy, dilatory in effect (increasing heat in the circulation), and excessively liquid in nature. Some specific medicines for blood defects include:

1. **Atirasa root/plant** (dandelion / *Taraxacum officinalis).*
2. **Brahmi leaf/root** (gotu kola / *Hydrocotyle asiatica / Centella asiatica).*
3. **Chandanam wood** (white sandalwood / *Santalum album).*
4. **Chandraprabha Vati.**
5. **Gandhaka Bhasma** (purified sulfur oxide).
6. **Guduchi stem** *(Tinospora cordifolia).*
7. **Haridra Amalirasena.**
8. **Haritala Bhasma** (orpiment / purified yellow arsenic trisulphide).
9. **Kanchanara bark** (mountain ebony / *Bauhinia tomentosa).*
10. **Kharjura fruit decoction** (date / *Phoenix dactylifera).*
11. **Lauhasava.**
12. **Manashila Bhasma** (purified realgar).
13. **Mandura Bhasma** (purified iron ore oxide).
14. **Nilotpalam flower** (blue lotus / *Iris nepalensis).*
15. **Nimba leaf** (neem / *Azadirachta indica).*
16. **Nirgundi plant** *(Vitex negundo,* white).
17. **Punnaga bark** (Itching tree / *Schima wallichii).*
18. **Rakta Chandanam wood** (red sandalwood / *Pterocarpus santalinus).*
19. **Sanapushpi seeds** (rattle-box / *Crotolaria juncea).*
20. **Shilajatu.**
21. **Tinduksthi Kashmarya.**
22. **Triphala** *(Phyllanthus emblica / Terminalia belerica / Terminalia chebula).*
23. **Varuna bark** (Three-leaved caper / *Crataeva religiosa).*
24. **Vasaka leaf** (Malabar nut / *Adhatoda vasica).*

A reliable formula for raktadosha is the standard compound **Avipattikara Churna**.

Raktavriddhi (Excess blood)

An excessive amount of blood is caused by pathogenic defects of blood and promotes the same sorts of problems. It is treated with the same methods used for pathogenic defects of the blood (Raktadosha).

Raktakshaya (Deficiency of blood)

Deficiency of blood can be caused by poor digestion, toxins that kill red blood cells, blood loss or other reasons. This generally causes a weakness in the functioning of the venous system, promoting a desire for sour foods and a cooling environment. The blood can be restored with digestive remedies (page 173), blood restoratives such as **Dadimadi Churna**, **Bhallataka Rasayana** and iron compounds such as **Mandura Bhasma** (purified iron rust oxide). If untreated blood deficiency can lead to Pandu (anemia, see below).

Pandu (Anemia)

Pandu is correlated with anemia, and is caused by deficiency of blood. It is divided into five categories: anemia with the character of Vata, Pitta, Kapha, Sannipata and Mridbhakshana. The general treatment for anemia includes treatments to balance Pitta (page 67), to inhibit red blood cell destruction, as well as remedies to restore the blood including **Dadimadi Churna** (1-2 g twice daily), **Bhallataka Rasayana** (2 pills twice daily), **Mandura Bhasma** (purified iron rust oxide) (200 mg twice daily), **Triphala Guggulu** (2 pills twice daily), and **Shilajatu Rasayana** (2 pills twice daily).

Vataja Anemia (chronic anemia)

Anemia with the character of Vata is related to the tendency to be chronically anemic and weak. It is treated with the general Vata treatments (page 56) along with the general remedies for anemia.

Pittaja Anemia

Anemia with the character of Pitta is caused by bile accumulation in the blood. It is treated with the general remedies for anemia with the addition of general remedies to reduce Pitta (page 67).

Kaphaja Anemia

Anemia with the character of Kapha is caused by lack of red pigment of the blood. It is treated with the general Kapha treatments (page 77) along with the general remedies for anemia.

Sannipataja Pandu (Pernicious anemia)

Anemia with the character of Sannipata is advanced with complicated symptoms. It is very difficult to cure, and is treated with the general remedies for anemia and palliative treatment based upon signs and symptoms.

Mridbhakshanaja anemia (Clay-eating anemia)

Anemia with the character of Mridbhakshanaja is caused either by the contamination of food with clay or by directly eating clay, both of which inhibits nutrient absorption and weakens the blood. It is treated with strong purgative (page 174) and diuretics (page 195), along with the general remedies for anemia.

Swayathu (Edema / Swelling)

Swayathu is correlated with edema, and is caused either by deficiency of blood (Pandu, anemia) or blockage in the subcutaneous blood vessels. It is divided into nine categories: edema with the character of Vata, Pitta, Kapha, Vata-Pitta, Vata-Kapha, Pitta-Kapha, Sannipata, Aghata and Visha.

A general remedy for edema is **Punarnava plant/root** *(Boerhavia difusa)*, given in doses of 2-3 grams, two or three times a day with water. This remedy is more effective if prescribed with 200 mg of **Mandura Bhasma** (purified iron rust oxide). Other general remedies for edema include **Ajamodadi Churna** (2-3 grams twice daily), or **Shilajatu Rasayana** (2 pills twice daily) given with a decoction of **Triphala** (30-60 mL twice daily). If the swelling is localized to a single organ, treatment is differentiated based upon specific signs and symptoms.

Vataja Edema

Edema with the character of Vata is non-pitting, with an increase in swelling during the daytime. It is treated with the general Vata treatments (page 56) along with laxative (page 174) and diuretics (page 195), hot compress, oil massage and general remedies for edema.

Pittaja Edema

Edema with the character of Pitta presents with burning sensitive swelling. It is treated with the general treatments to reduce Pitta (page 67) along with purgatives (page 174) and diuretics (page 195), as well as the general remedies for edema.

Kaphaja Edema

Edema with character of Kapha is pitting edema that gets worse at night. It is treated with the general treatments to reduce Kapha (page 77) along with purgatives (page 174) and diuretics (page 195), as well as the general remedies for edema. In the early stages it can be treated with **Haritaki fruit** *(Terminalia chebula)* taken in doses of 1-2 grams with **Goumutra** (cow urine).

Samsarga Edema

Edema with the character two Doshas in combination (Samsarga) presents with combined symptoms. These have to be treated with combined approaches to reduce the particular combination of the Doshas, i.e. Vata-Pitta, Vata-Kapha Pitta-Kapha (page 81), along with general remedies for edema.

Sannipataja Edema

Edema with the character of Sannipata is very difficult to cure. It can be controlled however with the general remedies for edema as well as symptomatic measures. One useful formula is five parts each **Ajamodadi Churna** and **Punarnavadiyoga**, taken with two parts **Yavakshara alkaline ash** (barley plant / *Hordeum vulgare)* and one part **Mandura Bhasma** (purified iron rust oxide), given in doses of 1-2 grams twice daily. This remedy can also be used for kidney failure. Another helpful remedy for Sannipataja edema is **Chandraprabha Vati** (2 pills twice daily).

Aghataja Edema

Edema with the character of Aghataja is caused by injury or trauma. It is treated with the general Vata treatment (page 56) along with the remedies used for erysipelas (page 241) and the general remedies for edema.

Vishaja Edema

Edema with the character of Vishaja is caused by allergy or toxins. It is treated with antitoxin remedies (page 155) along with the general remedies for edema.

Raktapitta (Hematorrhea / Hemorrhage)

Raktapitta is correlated with both hematorrhea and passive hemorrhage, and is caused by the excess volume of blood with an additional accumulation of bile in the plasma that causes bleeding. It is divided into five categories: hematorrhea with the character of Vata, Pitta, Kapha, Sannipata and Vata-Kapha.

While treating raktapitta remedies with very strong astringent and hemostatic properties should never be prescribed at the very beginning as this can increase the chance of abdominal tumors, leucoderma, painful urination, fever, liver enlargement, splenitis, hemorrhoids and other disorders. During treatment the strength and stamina of patient is carefully observed, and when the flow of vitiated blood begins to diminish then specific astringent remedies are prescribed to stop bleeding. Some remedies however can be used at the outset, including the mildly astringent **Vasaka leaf** (Malabar nut / *Adhatoda vasica)*, given in doses of 1-2 grams twice daily. Another useful formula that can be used at the outset is **Chandanadi Churna**, given in dose of 1-2 grams twice daily. Strong astringents that can be added later include **Sauvira Bhasma** (purified antimony sulfide) given with equal parts with **Laksha** (lac / *Coccus lacca)* in doses of 500 mg twice daily, taken with milk. For external application the area can be washed with **Sphutikarika** (purified alum) and water. Once the bleeding is resolved measures are undertaken to build up the blood by taking blood restoratives such as **Dadimadi Churna**, given in doses of 1-2 grams twice daily.

Vataja Raktapitta

The symptoms of hematorrhea with the character of Vata are bleeding from the urinary tract and intestine. It is treated with emetic remedies (see page 175), fasting, sweet, bitter and astringent remedies and foods, and the specific remedies against hematorrhea.

Pittaja Raktapitta

The symptoms of hematorrhea with the character of Pitta are heavy bleeding from any part of the body. It is treated with the general treatments to reduce Pitta (page 67) along with purgative remedies (page 174), fasting, sweet, bitter, and astringent remedies and foods, and the specific remedies against hematorrhea.

Kaphaja Hematorrhea

The symptoms of hematorrhea with the character of Kapha are bleeding from the mouth and nose, etc. It is treated with purgative remedies (page 174), the general Pitta treatments (page 67), and fasting. Sweet, bitter and astringent remedies and foods can be used, along with the specific remedies against hematorrhea.

Sannipataja Hematorrhea

Hematorrhea with the character of Sannipata relates to severe bleeding combined with complicated symptoms, such as the rupture of a tumor. It is not curable.

Vata-Kapha Hematorrhea

Hematorrhea with the character of Vata-Kapha has bleeding from both the upper and lower parts of the body. It is very difficult to cure. However is treated by combining the methods used for Vataja and Kaphaja hematorrhea.

Vatarakta (Gout)

Vatarakta is correlated with gout, and is generally caused by acid blood derived from poorly digested or contradictory foods, or exposure to toxins. This causes an aggravation of the nervous system (Vata), leading to arthritis and skin diseases. It is treated with the general measures to reduce Vata (page 56) along with medicated plaster, oil massage, laxative remedies (page 174), enema, venesection (see page 92) and Rasayanas (page 140). Specific remedies for Vatarakta includes a decoction of **Guduchi stem** *(Tinospora cordifolia)* (90-120 mL twice daily) and the standard formula **Kaishora Guggulu** (2 pills twice daily). Both these remedies become more effective if taken with a mild laxative. External applications include a paste of **Tila seed** (sesame / *Sesamum indicum*), ground in milk and applied as a plaster.

Vatarakta, advanced / Gambhira (Systematic lupus erythematosus)

The advanced form of Vatarakta can be correlated with systematic lupus erythematosus (SLE), with acidic blood and the aggravated function of the nervous system. It is treated with the general measures to reduce Vata (page 56), along with laxative remedies (page 174), diuretics (page 195), the remedies used for kidney failure and edema (page 257), enemas, venesection, and symptomatic treatments based upon signs and symptoms and specific remedies. One useful remedy for SLE is **Kaishora Guggulu**, given in doses of 2 pills twice daily.

Daha (Hot sensation)

Daha relates to a feeling of excess heat or burning sensations, and is as a symptom is caused by fluid imbalance or blood defects. Treatment is thus directed to the cause. For example, hot sensation caused by blood defects is treated with venesection (see page 92) and fasting, and/or the remedies for blood defects (see page 255). Hot sensation caused by dehydration is treated with sugar cane juice or sugar water. Hot sensation caused by deficiency of blood or plasma is treated with the remedies used for hematorrhea (see page 258) or the oily remedies typically prescribed for balancing Vata (page 56).

Mansadosha (Pathogenic defects of muscular tissues)

Mansadosha refers to pathogenic defects in muscle tissues caused by the exudation and infiltration of defects derived from plasma and blood into the muscular structures. This condition can cause many physical problems to develop, including neoplasm, glandular diseases, throat swelling and abnormal muscular growth. Pathogenic defects of the muscular tissues are generally treated with laxatives (page 174), enema, emetics (page 175), diuretics (page 195), medicated nasal snuff, and surgery. In some conditions these treatments are combined with surgical measures such as cauterization or the external application of alkali remedies (page 171) to burn away the abnormal tissue.

Mansakshaya (Muscular atrophy)

Muscular atrophy is caused by the aggravated function of the nervous system, causing a corresponding imbalance in the arterial supply of nutrients. It is treated with the general measures to reduce Vata (page 56) along with oil massage and Rasayanas (page 140), as well as foods and medicines that increase weight.

Weight-increasing foods and medicines include:

1. **Ashwagandha root** *(Convolvulus arvensis / Withania somnifera)*.
2. **Milk products**, including **Ghrita** (Ghee).
3. **Narikela** (coconut / *Cocos nucifera*).
4. **Kharjura fruit** (date / *Phoenix dactylifera*).

5. **Karkata nut** (pistachio / *Pistacia vera*).
6. **Akshota nut** (walnut / *Juglans regia*).
7. **Shilajatu Rasayana**.
8. **Hastanjali tuber** *(Orchid incarnata)*.
9. **Musali tuber** *(Curculigo orchioides)*.
10. **Gokshura fruit** *(Tribulus terrestris)*.
11. **Kapikacchu seeds** (cowhage / *Mucuna pruriens*).
12. **Dadima rind** (pomegranate / *Punica granatum*).

Medodosha (Pathogenic defects of fat)

Medodosha refers to pathogenic defects of fatty tissue that typically occurs as fat increases in the body. The excess fat causes many physical problems such as obesity, early symptoms known to lead to urinary diseases such as prameha, strong appetite, body odor, weakness and thirst. Pathogenic defects of fat are treated with fasting, exercise, increase in mental activity, reduction in sleep, and indulgence in sex. There are also herbal remedies that can be used to lose weight, mentioned under the treatment of obesity (Medovriddhi).

Medokshaya (Weight loss / Cachexia)

Medokshaya refers to a loss of body fat and general weight loss, usually caused by the aggravated function of the nervous system. It is treated with general measures to reduce Vata (page 56) along with digestive remedies (see page 173) and the remedies for gaining weight (see page 260). Patients are also recommended to spend time in a peaceful atmosphere to balance the nervous system.

Medovriddhi (Obesity)

Medovriddhi relates to obesity, and is typically caused by a strong appetite combined with strong digestive functions, which gradually causes more and more fat to accumulate. It is treated with fasting, increased exercise, increased mental activity, less sleep, and increased indulgence in sex. Enemas can be prepared with remedies that increase dryness and heat. Bitter and pungent remedies are also used, along with specific remedies for losing weight, including:

1. Equal parts **Shilajatu Rasayana** with **Agnimantha bark extract** *(Premna integrifolia)*, taken in doses of 1 gram twice daily.
2. **Lauha Bhasma** (purified iron oxide), 200 mg twice daily with honey.
3. **Triphala,** 1-2 grams twice daily.
4. Equal parts **Guduchi stem** *(Tinospora cordifolia)* and **Musta tuber** *(Cyperus rotundus)*, taken in doses of 1-2 grams twice daily.
5. One part **Vidanga seeds** *(Embelia ribes)* with two parts **Nagaram rhizome** (Indian cyperus / *Cyperus pertenuis)*, taken in doses of 1 gram twice daily.

6. **Madhu** (honey) mixed into cold water before meals can help to suppress the appetite.

Asthidosha (Pathogenic defects of bone)

Ashtidosha relates to pathogenic defects of bone caused primarily by an irritation of the nervous system. This can cause many problems including degeneration of the bone, abnormal growth of the bone or cartilage, tuberculosis of bone, alopecia or poor quality hair, and problems with the teeth and nails. It is treated with the general measures to reduce Vata (page 56), as well as medicated enema, milk and Ghee preparations with bitter remedies, and specific remedies based upon signs and symptoms. Some specific medicines for bone defects include **Yogaraja Guggulu** (2 pills twice daily), **Manduravataka** (2 pills twice daily) and **Shringaputa** (deer horn ash / *Cervus nippon)* (200 mg twice daily). A simple remedy for hair loss (alopecia) is to lightly scratch the affected area and gently rub on powder of **Maricham seed** (black pepper / *Piper nigrum).*

Majjadosha (Pathogenic defects of the marrow)

Majjadosha relates to pathogenic defects in the marrow, and is caused by the exudation and infiltration of metabolic defects into the marrow tissue. Majjadosha is associated with many problems including fainting, dizziness, blurred vision, joint pain, and soreness of the joints. It is treated with sweet and bitter remedies such as **Dadimadi Ghritam** (3-6 g twice daily).

Majjakshaya (Deficiency of marrow)

Majjakshaya relates to a deficiency of marrow caused by aggravated function of the nervous system, which weakens the entire body. Majjakshaya causes many physical problems but especially involves diseases of the nerves. It is treated with general measures to reduce Vata (page 56), along with the standard compound **Dadimadi Ghritam**, given in doses of 3-6 grams twice daily.

Ojakshaya (Vital deficiency)

Ojakshaya is a Vataja disease that relates to a deficiency of Ojas (vital energy), and manifests with a number of symptoms including hypoglycemia, low blood pressure and chronic fatigue, caused by a deficiency of plasma (Rasa) and/or blood sugar. Ojakshaya is treated with digestive (page 173) and aphrodisiac remedies (page 211), along with Rasayanas (page 140) and nourishing greasy foods such as meat, Ghee and cooked fruit. Spending time in a peaceful atmosphere is also prescribed, as well as oil massage. Some specific medicines used in Ojakshaya include **Karpurasava** (10 drops 2-3 times daily), **Trikaturasayana** (2-3 pills twice daily) taken with **Chyavanaprasha paste** (2-3 grams twice daily), and **Shulanirmulanarasa Vati** (2 pills twice daily).

While treating Ojakshaya it is very important that treatment also be given to the underlying cause of the Ojas deficiency, including anemia, chronic diarrhea, menorrhagia, hepatitis, and malnutrition. The treatments used for Ojakshaya are also used to maintain health and promote weight gain in acquired immunodeficiency syndrome (AIDS).

Chapter 23: Diseases of Pregnancy and Delivery (Garbha Roga)

There are many factors that can affect pregnancy and delivery or damage the fetus. Injury, excessive vibrations, incorrect postures, lack of sleep, emotional distress (quarrels and fights), poor digestion, poor diet and defects in the paternal semen are examples. Management of a pregnant woman requires caution. As much as possible, diseases of pregnant women should be managed with a soft, sweet diet and pleasant surroundings. Strong measures like emesis or venesection are used only in emergencies.

Raktasrava (Bleeding during pregnancy / Miscarriage)

Raktasrava refers to bleeding during pregnancy, and usually signifies miscarriage. It has the character of Pitta and Vata along with blood defects. It is treated with the general Pitta and Vata treatment together with blood cleansing remedies (page 255). Additional medicines include cold compress, cooling medicated plasters or pessary and remedies against menorrhagia (page 219). Specific remedies for raktasrava are chosen from the **Kakolyadigana** group of herbs mentioned in the *Sushruta Samhita*, usually given with milk. These include:

1. **Kakoli bulb** *(Fritillaria cirrhosa)*.
2. **Jivaka bulb** (wild garlic / *Allium wallichii*, small).
3. **Mudgaparni** *(Phaseolus trilobus)*.
4. **Masaparni** *(Teramnus labialis)*.
5. **Guduchi stem** *(Tinospora cordifolia)*.
6. **Karkatashringi fruit gall** *(Pistacia intergerrima* / Insect gall).
7. **Vamshalochana** (Bamboo manna / *Bambusa breviflora*).
8. **Padmakam bark/fruit** *(Betula alnoides)*.
9. **Jivanti leaf** *(Leptadenia reticulata)*.

Garbhasrava (Miscarriage due to uterus dysfunction)

Garbhasrava refers to miscarriage, and is often caused by the diseases of the uterus. Prevention of this problem is possible by good general health and lifestyle practices prior to pregnancy, as well as specialized methods used for the purification of the uterus and semen (page 39). The woman who has a miscarriage has to be treated with the same methods used for puerperal diseases (see page 268).

Garbhasphuranam (Vibrational harm to the embryo)

Any unusual vibration during early pregnancy can harm the embryo and lead to miscarriage. For example, travelling in vehicles that vibrate roughly, shaking the mother, and rough sexual intercourse can all promote garbhasphuranam. This disease has the character of Pitta along with blood defects and/or circulatory defects. It is treated with the general measures to reduce Pitta (page 67) together with blood cleaning remedies (page 255). Herbs from the **Utpaladi** (lotus group) mentioned in the *Sushruta Samhita* are the primary remedies used, usually taken with milk. These include:

1. **Raktotpalam** (red lotus / *Nymphaea rubra*).
2. **Padmam flower** (white lotus / *Nelumbo nucifera*).
3. **Saugandhika** (good smelling lotus / *Nymphaea spp.*).
4. **Kuvalaya** (blue/white lotus / *Nymphaea spp.*).
5. **Nilotpalam flower** (blue lotus / *Iris nepalensis*).

Garbhaprashamsa (Ectopic pregnancy / Dislocation of embryo)

Garbhaprashamsa refers to ectopic pregnancy and has the character of Vata and Pitta, manifesting symptoms including anuria, tympanitis, back pain, and bleeding. Cooling and oily remedies are prescribed for both internal and external use. Specific measures for garbhaprashamsa include:

1. For anuria, use milk boiled with diuretic grasses from the **Darbhandigana** (sacrificial grass group), mentioned in the *Sushruta Samhita*.
2. For pain, use **Mahasahayoga**, made from equal parts **Mudgaparni** *(Phaseolus trilobus)* and **Masaparni** *(Teramnus labialis)*, 1-2 grams boiled with milk and taken twice daily.
3. For tympanitis, use **Hingu compound**, made by heating **Hingu gum** (asafoetida / *Ferula narthex)* in warm **Tila oil** (sesame seed / *Sesamum indicum)*, applied externally.
4. For bleeding, use hemostatics from the **Utpaladigana** (Lotus group) mentioned under Garbhasphuranam.

Garbhaprasupti (Motionless fetus)

A motionless fetus is the result of imbalances of the nervous system (Vata), and is a serious condition that can lead to death of the developing baby. It is treated with highly nutritive food taken with plenty of **Ghritam** (Ghee), and constant warm massage around the belly and the back.

Udavartavibandha (Constipation during pregnancy)

While constipation is a common occurrence in pregnancy, constipation in the eighth month of pregnancy is considered very serious. It should not be neglected as it can be the cause of death of the fetus, and in rare instances can cause the death of the mother as well. It has to be treated as soon as possible with special enema made of milk mixed with the decoction called **Viranadimulan** *(Charaka Samhita).*

Some of the roots used in this enema are:

1. **Ushira** *(Andropogon muricatum).*
2. **Dhanyam** (rice / *Oryza sativa).*
3. **Shastika** (variety of rice paddy / *Oryza sativa).*
4. **Kasa** *(Sacharum spontanum).*
5. **Vetasa** (cane sugar / *Saccharum officinarum).*
6. **Yavani seed** (wild omum / *Trachyspermum ammi).*
7. **Kashmari root** *(Gmelina arborea).*
8. **Parusaka fruit** *(Grewia asiatica).*

Garbhakandu (Itching during pregnancy)

Itching during the pregnancy is caused by greasy food. Byproducts of greasy foods can cause blockages (blood congestion) and allergic-like itching. According to Ayurveda, circulation to the chest area is increased in the seventh month, and so this problem is more prevalent at that time.

It is treated by rubbing the affected area with the **Rakta Chandanam wood** (red sandalwood / *Pterocarpus santalinus)* mixed with powder of **Lotus stem** (any variety). Also used is oil massage prepared with **Karavira leaf** (sweet-scented oleander / *Nerium indicum)*, and bathing with the decoction made of **Jati flower** (Jasmine / *Jasminum officinalis)* and **Madhukam root** (licorice / *Glycyrrhiza glabra).* Greasy food and salt have to be avoided in diet.

Aprapannapara (Fixation of placenta)

In general, the placenta has to come out right after delivery. Fixation of placenta is very harmful to the mother. If it does not come out as soon possible, it has to be taken out by pressing and making stirring motions on the stomach and the back.

Some countermeasures include:

1. Brushing or poking the palate and the throat with hair to cause strong nausea.
2. An incense can be made with **Bhurja tree bark** (Birch tree / *Betula bhojapatra)* and/or **Krishna sarpa slough** (the black snake is called **Krishna sarpa**, and the slough is called **Kanchuka**). The smoke wafted onto the vagina.

3.   Surgery is used in refractory cases.

Makalakashulam (Pain after delivery)

Colic pain after delivery is caused by aggravated function of the related nervous system. It is treated with **Yavakshara alkaline ash** (barley plant / *Hordeum vulgare)* or **Pippalyadi** (see page 157) with warm water.

Garbhasanga (late delivery caused by absence of labor)

Absence of labor necessary for delivery is caused by weakness of the uterine nervous system (Vata). In this case, the pregnant woman will not deliver on time, often the cause of serious complications. It is treated by wafting incense smoke made from **Kanchuka** (black snake slough) or **Madanam fruit** *(Randia dumetorum)* around the vagina for the purpose of stimulation.

Sutikaroga (Puerperal diseases)

Puerperal diseases in the weeks after delivery include fever, edema, arthritis, indigestion, etc. In these cases, first of all, the nervous system has to be controlled with the general Vata treatments (page 56) along with symptomatic treatments and specific remedies specific to each problem. Puerperal diseases require a strong effort by the physician to cure.

Kikkisha (Stretch marks)

Stretch marks during pregnancy are caused by belly enlargement stretching the skin. They are treated by first rubbing the affected area with cow dung, then applying **Varunapatram** (Ghee preparation - *Chakradatta)*, which is a plaster made of **Varuna leaf** (Three-leaved caper / *Crataeva religiosa*) pounded with water and mixed with **Ghritam** (Ghee).

Mudhagarbha (Difficult labor)

Difficult labor is caused by the baby being wrongly positioned for delivery. It is divided into four main categories:

1.   Kila is the position of a baby in which hands and legs are erect and the head is facing down causing delivery blockage.
2.   Pratikhura is the position of a baby in which hands, legs and head come out at the same time causing delivery blockage.
3.   Bijaka is the position in which the head comes out with the hands causing blockage of delivery.
4.   Parigha is the position in which the newborn's body stays horizontal instead of vertical, causing delivery blockage.

In some cases the baby can be repositioned for easy delivery, but this is not simple to accomplish with external manipulation. It can thus be a cause of death for the mother and the baby, and to save the life of the mother, the blocked newborn has to be delivered with surgery as soon as possible.

Stanaroga (Abscess of the breast)

Abscesses of the breast are very common during the breastfeeding period. They are treated with the same remedies used for external abscess (page 170), along with repeated removal of the breast milk.

Stanyadosha / Stanyadusti (Defects of Mother's Milk)

Defects of mother's milk are classified into seven categories that have been mentioned, along with their treatments, in the children's diseases chapter. See page 271.

Stanyanasha (Deficiency of Mother's Milk)

It is imperative to treat deficiencies of mother's milk. Increasing milk production will ensure the baby's full and proper development. Highly nutritive food, including milk, Rasayanas (page 140) and specific remedies that increase milk have to be prescribed. It is also important to maintain a loving, peaceful atmosphere for the mother, and to ensure that the mother's digestive system is healthy.

Some medicines that increase breast milk are:

1. **Ashwagandha root** *(Convolvulus arvensis / Withania somnifera).*
2. **Shatavari root** (asparagus / *Asparagus racemosus).*
3. **Dadima rind** (pomegranate / *Punica granatum).*
4. **Ghrita** (Ghee) with **Matsyandika** (molasses).

Chapter 24: Diseases of Childhood (Bala Roga)

Many children's diseases are caused by vitiation of breast milk. When vitiated milk is consumed, it will cause the corresponding disease in the nursing child. A simple method of detoxifying the milk is to give the mother **Haridra root** (turmeric / *Curcuma longa*).

Some types of childhood diseases are caused by unseen biological forces called Graha. In diseases of Graha the treatments based upon Tridosha siddhanta do not work. This makes these diseases difficult to cure using herbal therapies. Instead, spiritual healing is often used.

Mild diseases should be treated using simple methods. For example, bedwetting can be treated by feeding the child each day with one or two pieces of dried **Kharjura fruit** (date / *Phoenix dactylifera*).

Stanyadosha (Diseases of Breast Milk)

Milk that becomes homogenous when mixed with water (mixes evenly) is considered to be pure. Milk that does not mix evenly is vitiated, and must be purified.

Children diseases caused by defects of breast milk are classified into seven categories: Vata, Pitta, Kapha, Sannipata, Vata-Pitta, Vata-Kapha, and Pitta-Kapha. Different Doshas will cause different signs of vitiation. Combinations of more than one Dosha will cause a mixture of defects to appear in the milk.

General medicines to purify the milk are found in the **Mustadigna** or the **Aragwadhadi** group of herbs mentioned in the *Sushruta Samhita*. Some of these are emetics, an important method of purification. Choice of which herb to use requires a skilled physician.

In addition, it is important for women to pay attention to the swelling and pain in the breasts during menses. Normally this will be slight, and the breasts will return to normal condition quickly. Otherwise this indicates that there is blockage that must be corrected using hot compresses or hot fomentation to clean the duct systems to keep the breasts healthy. A combination of herbs that can be used as a paste are equal parts **Dhattura leaf** (downy datura /*Datura metal*), **Haridra root** (turmeric / *Curcuma longa*), **Ahiphenam seed** (poppy / *Papaver somniferum*) and **Shilajatu Rasayana**.

The Aragwadhadi group includes:

1. **Rajavriksha pulp** (Indian laburnum / aragwadha / *Cassia fistula*).
2. **Madanam fruit** (*Randia dumetorum*).

3. **Kutaja bark** *(Holarrhena antidysenterica).*
4. **Patha root** *(Stephania hernandifolia).*
5. **Kantakari herb** (Black nightshade / *Solanum xanthocarpum).*
6. **Patala root/bark** *(Stereospermum personatum).*
7. **Murva plant** *(Bauhinia vahlii).*
8. **Saptaparna bark** (dita bark / *Alstonia scholaris).*
9. **Nimba leaf** (neem / *Azadirachta indica).*
10. **Karanja bark/seed oil** (Indian beech / *Pongamia pinnata).*
11. **Patola fruit** *(Trichosanthes dioica).*
12. **Kiratatiktam plant** *(Swertia chirata).*
13. **Guduchi stem** *(Tinospora cordifolia).*
14. **Chitraka root** (leadwort, white flower / *Plumbago zeylanica).*

The Mustadigana group includes:

1. **Musta tuber** (nut grass / *Cyperus rotundus*, big).
2. **Haridra root** (turmeric / *Curcuma longa).*
3. **Daruharidra bark** (barberry / *Berberis nepalensis).*
4. **Haritaki fruit** *(Terminalia chebula).*
5. **Amalaki fruit** (Indian gooseberry / amla / *Phyllanthus emblica).*
6. **Kustha root** *(Saussurea lappa).*
7. **Patha root** *(Stephania hernandifolia).*
8. **Kutaki rhizome** (Indian gentian / *Picrorhiza kurroa).*
9. **Ativisha tuber, purified** (aconite / *Aconitum heterophyllum).*
10. **Bhallataka fruit/purified seeds** (marking nut tree / *Semecarpus anacardium).*
11. **Chitraka root** (leadwort, white flower / *Plumbago zeylanica).*

Vataja Milk Defects

Milk vitiated by Vata will be astringent, tasteless, frothy and dry, and if dropped in water will float. This kind of milk causes constipation, gas and weakness in the child. It is treated with the remedies for purification of milk along with general remedies for Vata. One useful formula is **Dashamula Churna** (powder), 1-2 grams of the powder with honey twice daily. This mixture is also given to infant by placing a little drop on the tongue.

Pittaja Milk Defects

Milk vitiated by Pitta will be hot, sour, pungent and yellowish. It will produce a yellow color if dropped into water. Such milk causes dysentery, jaundice, thirst and other characteristic symptoms in the child. It is treated with the remedies for purification of milk along with general remedies for Pitta (page 67), to be taken by both mother and baby.

Kaphaja Milk Defects

Milk which is vitiated by Kapha will be sticky, overly sweet, and thick. It will sink if dropped into water. Such milk will cause vomiting, swelling of the face, excessive salivation and sleepiness in the child. It is treated with the remedies for purification of milk along with general remedies for Kapha treatment (page 77), to be taken by both the mother and the baby.

Combined Dosha Milk Defects

Mother's milk defects with combined characters can be Vata-Pittaja, Vata-Kaphaja, or Pitta-Kaphaja. This kind of milk can be cause of entry of unseen biological forces (Grahas). Treatment of Graha-related disorders are mentioned below.

Sannipataja Milk Defects

Mother's milk with the character of Sannipata contains all the defects mentioned under Vata, Pitta, and Kapha. This kind of milk causes aphasia, poliomyelitis, etc. Treatments for these diseases are mentioned below.

Phakka (Beriberi / Polyneuritis)

Phakka corresponds with inflammation of the nerves and heart, which itself can be a symptom of Beriberi (vitamin B1/thiamine deficiency). The manifestation of the disease is divided into three categories, with the characters of Kshiraja, Garbhaja and Vyadhija. Longterm deficiency of this nutrient makes it very difficult to cure. Treatment includes usage of whole grains in preference to refined grains (which lack vitamin B1) in the diet, the use of nourishing foods rich in vitamin B1 (e.g. milk, eggs, meat), as well as internal medicines taken by both the mother and the baby.

Kshiraja Phakka

Phakka with the character of Kshiraja is caused by defects in the milk of the mother, and causes the child to become thin and unstable in standing and walking. It is treated with remedies to purify the milk of the mother, to be taken by the mother along with remedies for nerve diseases (general Vata treatments - page 56), oil massage, digestive remedies (page 173), Rasayanas (page 140) and a proper diet.

Garbhaja Phakka

Phakka with the character of Garbhaja is caused by the untimely stoppage of breast-feeding, due to pregnancy or other reasons. It is treated with digestive remedies (page 173), Rasayanas (page 140), massage and proper diet.

Vyadhija Phakka

Phakka with the character of Vyadhija is caused by long-term chronic disease in the child that causes a low weight, enlarged stomach and enlarged head. It is treated with digestive remedies (page 173), Rasayanas (page 140), massage and a proper nutritive diet.

Revatigraha Dosha (Epidemic cerebrospinal meningitis)

Revatigraha Dosha is associated with the epidemic form of cerebrospinal meningitis, caused by unseen biological forces (Graha). It is divided into twelve categories: meningitis with the character of Nanda, Sunanda, Putana, Mukhamandika, Kataputana, Shakunika, Sushkarevati, Aryaka, Sutika, Nirrita, Pilipicchaka, and Kalika. Meningitis of all types is very difficult to cure.

Regular medicine prescribed for the symptoms of meningitis usually cause a worsening of the symptoms. In light of this, traditional physicians investigated other methods of treatment, including spiritual healing and found that these were more effective. While performing this spiritual healing ritual a specific incense made from **Guggulu gum resin** *(Commiphora wightii)* and other herbs is burnt to pacify the Graha, with sweet, spicy odors. The different types of incense used in each condition are described in the *Chakradatta*.

The method of spiritual healing is different for each condition. For example, to treat Nanda salutation is first given to Lord Narayana. An idol is made by taking earth from both shores of a river and placed on a crossroads. An oblation is made to the idol at noon, facing in an eastern direction, using a variety of ritual objects, including cooked white rice, white flowers, seven white banners, seven earthen lamps, seven cakes of black gram, seven flatbreads fried in Ghee, seven preparations of steamed black gram, perfumes, flowers, betel leaf, fish, meat, and wine. The child is then bathed with herb-infused waters for purification, followed by the bathing the child in the smoke prepared from an incense of **Lashunam bulb** (garlic / *Allium sativum)*, **Sarshapi seed** (black mustard / *Sinapis juncea)*, **Nimba leaf** (neem / *Azadirachta indica)*, and **Bilwa fruit** (bael / *Aegle marmelos)*, followed by the recitation of the following mantra:

> *Om Namo Ravanaya Amukasya Vyadhim*
> *Han Han Muncha Muncha Hrim Phat Swaha*

This oblation is offered for three days, and on the fourth day food is offered to the attending priests. In this way, auspicious healing arises and the child returns to health.

Skandagraha Dosha (Poliomyelitis)

Skandagraha Dosha is correlated with poliomyelitis, and is caused by the unseen biological force called Skanda. Paralysis of the different organs are the primary symptoms of this Graha. It is treated with the principles of spiritual healing along with the general Vata treatments (page 56) but is considered very difficult to cure. Even after cure, the affected organs can remain permanently damaged.

Skandapasmaragraha Dosha (Aseptic meningitis)

Skandapasmaragraha Dosha is correlated with aseptic meningitis and is caused by the unseen biological force called Skandapasmara. It causes epilepsy-like symptoms. It is treated with the principles of spiritual healing along with the formula called **Surasadigana**.

Shakunigraha Dosha (Herpangina A type)

Shakunigraha Dosha is correlated with herpangina A type, and is caused by the unseen biological force called Shakuni. It causes lesions of the mouth and skin. It is treated with the principles of spiritual healing along with wound-healing remedies (page 89). For children, **Madhu** (honey) is an effective agent to heal wounds.

Revatigraha Dosha (Herpangina B type)

Revatigraha Dosha is correlated with herpangina B type caused by the unseen biological force called Revati. It causes lesions and diarrhea. It is treated with the principles of spiritual healing along with wound-healing remedies (page 89).

Putanagraha Dosha (Enterovirus gastritis A type)

Putanagraha Dosha is correlated with enterovirus gastritis A type, and is caused by the unseen biological force called Putana. Dysentery is the primary symptom. It is treated with the principles of spiritual healing along with the remedies against dysentery (page 164).

Andhaputanagraha Dosha (Enterovirus gastritis B type)

Andhaputanagraha Dosha is correlated with enterovirus gastritis B type, and is caused by the unseen biological force called Andhaputana. The primary symptom is dysentery. It is treated with the principles of spiritual healing along with the remedies against dysentery (page 164).

Shitaputanagraha Dosha (Enterovirus gastritis C type)

Shitaputanagraha Dosha is correlated with enterovirus gastritis C type, and is caused by the unseen biological force called Shitaputana. The primary symptom is dysentery. It is treated with the principles of spiritual healing along with the remedies against dysentery (page 164).

Mukhamandika (Renal cortical necrosis)

Mukhamandika is correlated with renal cortical necrosis, and is caused by the unseen biological force called Mukhamandika. Hemolysis is the main symptom, causing a bright red face, hands and legs. It is treated with the principles of spiritual healing along with Rasayanas (page 140).

Naigamesagraha Dosha (Hypocalcemic tetany)

Naigamesagraha Dosha is correlated with hypocalcemic tetany, and is caused by the unseen biological force called Naigamesa. Flexure of the back is the primary symptom. It is treated with the principles of spiritual healing along with nerve restoratives.

Balagraha Dosha Upadrava (Childhood leukemia)

Balagraha Dosha upadrava is correlated with childhood leukemia, and can be caused by any unseen biological force. It is considered to be a complicated symptom resulting from any disease caused by the unseen biological forces that attack children. It is not curable because it develops so rapidly, but is treated with the principles of spiritual healing.

Mastulungakshaya (Atrophy of the brain)

Mastulungakshaya is correlated with atrophy of the brain, and is caused by the aggravated function of entire nervous system. It is treated with the general treatments to reduce Vata (page 56) along with medicated oil massage on the top head where the skull bone of the infant is still soft. **Narayana Taila** is used for this purpose, or plain **Tila seed oil** (sesame / *Sesamum indicum).* In addition the mother should take nerve restoratives such as **Yogaraja Guggulu**, 2 pills twice daily.

Upashirsaka (Hydrocephalus)

Upashirsaka is correlated with hydrocephalus, and is caused by the aggravated function of the newborn's nervous system. The main symptom is that the head becomes disproportionately enlarged. It is treated with the general Vata treatments (page 56), to be taken by both the baby and mother. If it is infected it has to be treated with surgery followed by the treatments for abscess (page 170).

Karnasrava (Otorrhea)

Karnasrava is correlated with otorrhea, and is caused by aggravated function of the related nerves of the ear. It can also be caused by breast milk dripping into the ear while feeding. A discharge of the ear is the primary symptom. It is treated with the general treatments to reduce Vata (page 56) along with specific remedies, including eardrops made from **Narayana Taila** and **Sphutikarika** (purified alum). Also used in the ear canal for its drying effect is **Samudraphenam Churna** (sea foam / *Sepia species).* Other useful preparations for topical use include:

1. **Apamarga plant ash** *(Achyranthes aspera)* boiled with sesame oil and water.
2. **Daruharidra bark extract** (barberry / *Berberis nepalensis)* with sesame oil.
3. **Bhringaraja plant** *(Eclipta alba)* with sesame oil.

Putikarna (Purulent otitis media)

Putikarna is correlated with purulent otitis media, and is caused by the aggravated function of the related veins of the ear. Inflammation is the primary symptom. It is treated with the general Pitta treatments (page 67) along with anti-inflammatory remedies (page 155). The eardrops mentioned above for otorrhea can also be used.

Karnapaka (Aural infection)

Karnapaka is an infection of the outer ear, and is caused by aggravated function of the related vein. It is treated with the general Pitta treatments (page 67) along with anti-inflammatory remedies (page 155). The eardrops mentioned under otorrhea can also be used.

Utpata (Infection of earring hole)

Utpata is an infection of earring hole, and is caused by blood defects. It is treated with the same remedies used for aural infection.

Talukantaka (Polyp of the palate)

Talukantaka is a polyp of the palate, and is caused by aggravated function of the related arteries. Excrescence of the mucous membrane on the palate is the primary symptom. It is treated with the general Kapha treatments (page 77) along with specific remedies including a paste prepared **Khadira extract** (catechu / *Acacia catechu*, white) and **Sphutikarika** (purified alum). For internal use **Haritakiyoga** is used.

Rohini (Diphtheria)

Rohini is correlated with diphtheria, and presents with complicated symptoms of the aggravated nerves, veins and arteries. A thick fibrous abnormal growth forms around the throat area and must be treated as soon as possible otherwise it is fatal. Diphtheria is classified into five categories, with the character of Vata, Pitta, Kapha, Sannipata and Raktaja.

Vataja Diphtheria

Diphtheria with the character of Vata causes painful abnormal growth. It is curable with venesection (see page 92), rubbing the affected area with salt, constant gargling with warm oil, and use of emetic remedies (once or twice - see page 175) and a medicated nasal snuff made from **Bhringaraja plant** *(Eclipta alba)*.

Pittaja Diphtheria

Diphtheria with the character of Pitta has an inflammatory abnormal growth along with high fever. It is curable with venesection (see page 92), emetic remedies (see page 175), and a medicated nasal snuff. Additionally the affected area is rubbed with **Rakta Chandanam Churna** (red sandalwood / *Pterocarpus santalinus)* mixed together with sugar and honey. The patient is given a gargle with a decoction made from **Draksha fruit** (grapes / *Vitis vinifera).*

Kaphaja Diphtheria

Diphtheria with the character of Kapha has an edema-like abnormal growth. It is curable with venesection (see page 92), emetic remedies (see page 175), and a medicated nasal snuff. The affected area is rubbed with soot removed from a mustard or sesame oil lamp. Gargling is done with oil prepared with salt and anti-Kapha remedies such as **Vidanga seeds** *(Embelia ribes).*

Sannipataja Diphtheria

Diphtheria with the character of Sannipata manifests with serious complicated symptoms, and is not curable.

Raktaja Diphtheria

Diphtheria with the character of Raktaja has an abnormal growth around the throat with skin eruptions and high fever. It is not curable, but is treated with the methods used for diphtheria with the character of Pitta.

Dantajanma (Teething Sickness)

Fever, diarrhea and vomiting in a child at the time of the emergence of a new tooth (dentition) is called Dantajanma, or teething sickness. Treatment is usually not necessary as the sickness will disappear when the tooth breaks out from the gum. If required, specific symptoms including fever, diarrhea and vomiting can be treated with the regular remedies used for this purpose. Honey can be applied topically to the gum to relieve discomfort.

Sahajarsha (Congenital hemorrhoid)

Sahajarsha is correlated with congenital hemorrhoid, and is not curable. However it can be maintained with regular medicines used for hemorrhoid (page 170).

Ashmari (Bladderstone)

Treatment of bladderstone in children is mentioned in the urinary system disease section (page 200).

Kukunaka (Blepharitis)

Kukunaka is correlated with blepharitis, and is caused by aggravated function of the related arteries and pathogenic defects of blood. The main symptoms are inflammation in the eyelid margins. It is treated with the general Kapha treatments (page 77), blood cleansing remedies, and Anjanam (eye salves) including **Rasanjana** and **Krimighna Yoga**.

Masurika (Smallpox)

Masurika is correlated with smallpox, and is caused by an unseen biological force (graha) that causes pathogenic defects of blood. It is treated with the same remedies used for leprosy (see page 235), and the remedies for erysipelas with the character of Pitta-Kapha (page 241).

Pramehajanya (Chickenpox)

Pramehajanya is correlated with chickenpox, and is caused by pathogenic agents in the fat. It is treated with the same remedies used for leprosy (see page 235), or the remedies for erysipelas with the character of Pitta-Kapha (page 241).

Romantika (Measles)

Romantika is correlated with measles, and is caused by the aggravated function of both the arterial and venous systems. It is treated with the general treatments to reduce Kapha and Pitta (page 81). In general, measles does not need treatment because it usually resolves after one week. If the disease causes an imbalance in the venous system however this can cause a low temperature and result in a respiratory infection. In the same way, if there is an imbalance of the arterial system it can cause dysentery. To prevent these complications it is thus important to use the general measures to reduce Kapha and Pitta.

Ajagallika (Verruca plana juveniles)

Ajagallika is correlated with verruca plana juveniles, and is caused by the aggravated functions of the nervous and arterial systems of the skin. An abnormal wart-like growth is the main symptom. It is removed with burning treatments (cauterization), and has to be treated with surgery if it is infected.

Jatumani (Nevus)

Jatumani is correlated with nevus, and is caused by the aggravated function of the arterial system along with blood defects. The primary symptom is a small tumor-like growth on the skin, with or without hair. It is treated with surgery or gentle cauterization.

Ahiputana (Perianal candidiasis)

Ahiputana is correlated with perianal candidiasis, and is caused by the aggravated function of the arterial system along with blood defects. It is seen as a spreading infection found around the anus of children. It is treated with the general medicines to reduce Kapha (page 77) and blood defects (page 255), along with a plaster made from **Nimba leaf Churna** (neem / *Azadirachta indica*).

Charmadalakhya (Candidiasis)

Charmadalakhya is correlated with Candidiasis, and is caused by toxins or defects in the breast milk along with blood defects. A spreading infection in the moist areas of skin is the primary symptom. It is treated with the remedies mentioned above for perianal candidiasis.

Arumshika (Pediculosis)

Arumshika is correlated with pediculosis, and is caused by the aggravated function of the related artery along with blood defects. Ulcerative infection by lice is the cause. It is treated with venesection (see page 92) followed by bathing with **Nimba leaf decoction** (neem / *Azadirachta indica*), together with the external application of specific remedies such as a paste prepared with **Haritala Nisha Nimbakalka**.

Mahapadmavisharpa (Cellulitis)

Mahapadmavisharpa is correlated with cellulitis and is treated as a form of erysipelas. It is divided into two categories: one starts from the head and spreads towards the heart area, and the other starts from the heart area and spreads down to the bladder area. It is a serious disorder and is often fatal.

Parigarbhika (Pining sickness of children)

Parigarbhika is correlated with a pining sickness of children, caused by breast-feeding during pregnancy. Indigestion and wasting away are the primary symptoms. It is treated with digestive remedies (page 173) and Rasayanas (page 140) such as **Bilwa fruit** (*Aegle marmelos*), given as a powder with honey. Generally speaking a pregnant woman should avoid breastfeeding.

Muka (Aphasia)

Muka is correlated with aphasia, and is caused by congenital deafness and/or defects of the breast milk. It is treated with the stimulation of the ear and purification of the breast milk. The remedies for purification of breast milk are described on page 271.

Nabhipaka (Infection of the umbilicus)

Nabhipaka is correlated with an infection of the umbilicus, and relates to a vitiation of Pitta. It is treated with **Nishadi Taila**. A powder can also be applied, prepared from equal parts **Haridra root** (turmeric / *Curcuma longa*), **Lodhram**

bark *(Symplocos paniculata)*, **Priyangu seed** *(Prunus mahaleb)* and **Madhukam root** (licorice / *Glycyrrhiza glabra)*, sprinkled on the affected area.

Chapter 25: Diseases of the Mouth, Throat, Nose, and Ears

Diseases of the head including the mouth, throat, nose, ears and eyes are described under the Shalakya Tantra (page 37) division of Ayurveda. The following is a summary of these treatments with the exception of diseases of the eyes, which are discussed in the following chapter.

General Treatment of Mouth and Throat

Many diseases of the mouth and throat described in this chapter can be treated with general medicines such as **Pippalyadiyoga**, made from a selection of four or five spicy herbs such as **Maricham seed** (black pepper / *Piper nigrum*), **Jirakam seed** (cumin / *Cuminum cyminum*), and **Pippali fruit** (long pepper / *Piper longum*). This formula is chosen when the mouth disease is related to digestive problems, as is often the case. **Kasturadi Vati** is another medicine used as a specific against diseases of the mouth, throat and palate. This formula has an astringent property, and used to stop bleeding and reduce secretions. In addition, medicated 'nasal snuffs' (Nasya) are mentioned frequently, not only powders taken by nose, but also medicated oils. These are used to nourish and heal but also to stimulate nasal secretions and the removal of toxins.

Diseases of the Lips (Oshtharoga)

Diseases of the lips are classified into eight categories, with the characters of Vata, Pitta, Kapha, Sannipata, Raktaja, Mansaja, Medoja and Abhighataja. Many can often be treated with the remedies used for general disorders of the mouth, mentioned at the beginning of this chapter.

Vataja Lip Disease (painful, dry lips)

Disease of the lips with the character of Vata is caused by the aggravated function of the related nerves. Pain, dryness and cracking are the primary symptoms. It is treated with the general Vata treatments (page 56) along with the application of steam, medicated oil as a medicated nasal snuff, and medicated oily plasters and poultices. Powder of **Shrivestaka compound** can be used to rub onto the lips.

Pittaja Lip Disease (Cold sores / Herpes)

Disease of the lips with the character of Pitta is caused by the aggravated function of the related veins. The primary symptoms are blisters and inflammatory eruptions. It is treated with the remedies used for abscess with the character of Pitta (see page 246), along with venesection (see page 92).

Kaphaja Lip Disease

Disease of the lips with the character of Kapha is diagnosed when there are painless and colorless eruptions on the lips. It is treated with the general treatments to reduce Kapha (page 77) along with venesection (page 92), as well as the application of steam, a medicated 'nasal snuff' (Nasya), and gargling with anti-Kapha remedies. **Pratisarana Yoga** is a specific remedy for lip application.

Sannipataja Lip Disease

Disease of the lips with the character of Sannipata is diagnosed by complicated eruptions. Although it is not curable, it can be maintained with symptomatic treatments.

Raktaja Lip Disease

Disease of the lips with the character of Rakta is caused by pathogenic defects in the blood. Dark red lips and bleeding are the primary symptoms. It is treated with the remedies used for abscess with the character of Pitta (page 246) along with venesection (page 92).

Oshtharbuda (Cancer of the lips)

Oshtharbuda is correlated with cancer of the lips, and is caused by pathogenic defects of blood. In general, it develops after a persistent bleeding condition of the lips is left without proper treatment. This disease is counted as a form of raktaja lip disease, and is treated with the same methods.

Mansaja Lip Disease

Disease of the lips with the character of Mansaja is caused by pathogenic defects in the muscular tissues. Abnormal muscular growth is the primary symptom. Although it is not curable, it can be maintained with the treatments for muscular tissue defects (page 260).

Medoja Lip Disease

Disease of the lips with the character of Medoja is caused by pathogenic defect of fatty tissues. Lip torsion and copious white discharge are the main symptoms. It is treated with steam application, puncturing to let out the discharge, and cauterization. **Priyangu compound** is a specific remedy that can be used for external application.

Abhighataja Lip Disease

Disease of the lips with the character of Abhighataja is caused by trauma. A wound with coagulation of blood and itching are the main symptom. It is treated with the same process used for abscess with the character of Pitta (page 246), along with venesection (page 92).

Jalarbuda (Cancer of lips in the form of blisters)

Cancer of the lips taking the form blisters is related to a vitiation of both Vata and Kapha. It is an exceptional and rare disease, and so is generally not counted among the eight categories of diseases of the lips. It is treated with the general Vata-Kapha treatments (page 81) along with the specific remedies used against arbuda (page 250).

Diseases of the Mouth, Gums and Teeth (Mukha Roga)

Many diseases of the mouth, gums and teeth are caused by factors that aggravate Kapha. For example, excess sweet and sour (acid) foods are harmful to the teeth and gums. In the same way, bitter and astringent foods and medicines have a therapeutic value.

Sarvasara / Mukhapaka (Stomatitis)

Sarvasara / Mukhapaka relates to stomatitis, and is caused by blood defects. A vesicular inflammation of the mucous membrane of the mouth is the primary symptom. It is classified into four categories, with the character of Vataja, Pittaja, Kaphaja, and Raktaja. In order to avoid recurring infection venesection (see page 92) and blood cleansing remedies (page 255) are prescribed. Specific treatments include chewing on the new fresh leaves of **Jati** (Jasmine / *Jasminum officinalis*), and sucking on **Kasturadi Vati** as a lozenge.

Vataja stomatitis

Stomatitis with the character of Vata manifests as many painful vesicles. It is treated with the general measures to reduce Vata (page 56) along with plaster made of honey mixed with **Tankana Bhasma** (purified borax).

Pittaja stomatitis

Stomatitis with the character of Pitta manifests as small red vesicles with burning pain. It is treated with the general Pitta treatments (page 67) along with laxatives (page 174) and a plaster made from honey mixed with **Tankana Bhasma** (purified borax).

Kaphaja stomatitis

Stomatitis with the character of Kapha manifests as colorless itching vesicles. It is treated with the general measures to reduce Kapha (page 77) along with a plaster made from honey mixed with **Tankana Bhasma** (purified borax).

Raktaja stomatitis

Stomatitis with the character of Raktaja has the same etiology as Pittaja stomatitis, and is treated with the same remedies.

Dantapupputaka (Gingivitis)

Dantapupputaka is correlated with gingivitis, and is caused by Kapha defects along with blood defects. Painful swelling of the gums is the primary symptom. It is treated with venesection (see page 92), tooth powers made of salts and alkali remedies (page 171), and a medicated 'nasal snuff' (Nasya) with **Shadbindu Taila**. A simple tooth powder can be made from equal parts **Karpura leaf extract** (camphor / *Cinnamomum camphora*), **Kathini Bhasma** (white chalk / khari / calcium carbonate), **Arjaka leaf/extract** (white mint plant / *Mentha spp.)* and a small amount of **Sarjikakshara** (sodium bicarbonate). A plaster can also be used, made of equal parts **Lodhram bark** *(Symplocos paniculata)*, **Musta tuber** *(Cyperus rotundus)* and **Daruharidra bark extract** (barberry / *Berberis nepalensis)* mixed with honey.

Shitada (Pyorrhea)

Shitada is correlated with pyorrhea, and displays the symptoms of a Kapha imbalance along with blood defects. Bleeding with a purulent discharge around the gums and teeth are the primary symptoms. Useful remedies include:

1. Gargling with a decoction of **Nagara Yoga**.
2. The application of a paste made from **Jatiphalam seed/bark** (nutmeg / *Myristica fragrans)* is rubbed into the affected region.
3. **Narayana Taila** mixed with a small amount of **Saindhavam** (mineral salt), used as a mouth wash (Gandusha).
4. The application of a plaster applied to the gums made of **Priyangu compound**, **Musta tuber** (nut grass / *Cyperus rotundus*, big) and **Triphala,** cooked with **Ghrita** (Ghee).
5. **Triphala**, used as a powdered nasal snuff or put into water to wash, clean and nourish the gums.
6. Equal parts **Khadira extract** (catechu / *Acacia catechu*, white) and **Sphutikarika** (purified alum) can be applied directly, particularly if the bleeding is severe.

Upakusha (Periodontitis)

Upakusha is correlated with periodontitis, and is caused by Pitta Dosha along with blood defects. Inflammation and loose teeth are the main symptoms. It is treated with venesection (see page 92), tooth powder, gargles and a medicated nasal snuff. One useful tooth remedy prepared as a toothpowder is made from equal parts **Lavanapanchakam** (the five salts) and **Trikatu**, mixed with honey.

Vaidarbha (Traumatic swelling of the gums)

Vaidarbha refers to the traumatic swelling of the gums caused by injuries. It is treated with gargling and cold water, plasters made from cooling remedies (page 154), and application of alkali remedies (page 171) after cleaning.

Adhimansa (Wisdom tooth eruption)

Adhimansa refers to a painful swelling caused by the eruption of the wisdom teeth through the thickened gum tissue. It is treated with surgery to open and allow the tooth to emerge.

Dantanadi (Tooth/Gum abscess with sinus)

Dantanadi refers to an abscess in the gum causing the formation of a sinus. An abscessed tooth with sinus should be removed by surgery as soon as possible according the method described in the *Sushruta Samhita*, Chikitsthana, chapter 22.

Dalana (Pulpitis)

Dalana refers to a pulpitis (tooth pulp inflammation) caused by the aggravated function of the related nerves. Severe toothache is the main symptom. It is treated with general Vata treatments (page 56), and by applying a warm medicated plaster made from medicated oils such as **Narayana Taila** oil or from **Hingu gum** (asafoetida / *Ferula narthex)*. In addition, gargling with warm salt water or **Sphutikarika** (purified alum) is helpful.

Krimidanta (Tooth cavity)

Krimidanta refers to a cavity of the tooth, and is caused by aggravated function of the related nerves. The presence of a black spot on the tooth and pain are the main symptoms. It is treated with the general treatments to reduce Vata (page 56), warm oily gargle (Gandusha), and using **Hingu gum** (asafoetida / *Ferula narthex)* as a plaster. Venesection (see page 92) and medicated nasal snuff are also used. A tooth cavity at the beginning can be cured by the cauterization of the hole, but the tooth has to be taken out if the cavity causes degeneration and looseness of the tooth.

Bhanjanaka (Cracking of the tooth)

Bhanjanaka refers to the cracking of the tooth, and is caused aggravated function of the related nerves and arteries, gradually weakening the tooth until it easily breaks. It is not curable, and the damaged tooth can be taken out if the problem is serious. This problem can also be caused by accident (Abhighataja).

Dantaharsha (Tooth pain / Toothache)

Dantaharsha is correlated with tooth pain, and is caused by aggravation of the tooth nerve. It is treated with the general treatments to reduce Vata. Warm **Narayana Taila** is commonly used as a gargle (Gandusha), with **Bhringaraja Taila** (*Eclipta alba* oil) as a medicated nasal snuff. If the cause of the pain is infection or another condition these must be treated as well.

Other methods for reducing tooth pain include:

1. **Ahiphenasava** can be applied to the painful area.

2. A small piece of warmed **Hingu gum** (asafoetida / *Ferula narthex)* is applied to the painful area.

3. A tincture made from **Mundi flower** *(Sphaeranthus indicus)* is applied to the painful area.

Dantasharkara (Tartar of the tooth)

Dantasharkara is correlated with tartar formation on the tooth, and is caused by infection of the gum and aggravation of the related nerves. The tartar is removed by scratching very carefully without harming the gum, followed by rubbing the affected area with **Laksha powder** (lac / *Coccus lacca).*

Kapalika (Destructive tartar of the tooth)

Kapalika refers to a destructive tartar of the tooth, caused by same etiology as tartar of the teeth, and is treated in the same way. However, it is difficult to cure.

Shyavadantaka (Blue teeth)

Shyavadantaka refers to the appearance of blue-colored teeth, caused by internal hemorrhage. This condition is not curable.

Khalibardhana (Extra teeth)

Khalibardhana refers to extra teeth, and is caused by aggravation of the related nerves during tooth formation. Extra teeth have to be taken out and the socket cauterized.

Karala (Tooth degeneration)

Karala refers to the degeneration of the teeth, and is caused by a severe aggravation of the related nerves. Without prompt treatment it can destroy the jaw. It is not curable.

Hanumoksha (Dental facial paralysis)

Hanumoksha refers to dental facial paralysis, and is caused by an aggravation of the related nerves. It is treated with the same remedies used for facial paralysis (page 231).

Diseases of the Tongue (Jihwa Roga)

Jihwaroga / Kantaka (Glossitis)

Jihwaroga is correlated with glossitis, and is divided into three categories, each with the character of Vata, Pitta or Kapha. Glossitis with Vataja character causes symptoms of cracking and partial loss of sensation on the tongue. Glossitis with the character of Pitta causes symptoms of burning pain and redness of the tongue. Glossitis with the character of Kapha causes thickness, swelling and heaviness of the tongue. These three forms of glossitis are treated with the same remedies used for diseases of the lips differentiated by the characters of Vataja, Pittaja and Kaphaja.

Upajiwhaka

Upajiwhaka can be correlated with inflammation of the epiglottis, and is associated with Kapha (swelling) and blood defects. Inflammation and itching of the epiglottis are the main symptoms. It is treated with surgery.

Alasa/Ranula

Alasa (Ranula) is associated with a cystic tumor manifesting as a swollen area beneath the tongue. It is caused by Kapha and blood defects. Although incurable the swelling can be partially controlled somewhat with **Kasturadi Vati**.

Jihwastambha (Paralysis of the tongue)

Paralysis of the tongue is caused by Alasa and can be treated with the same way. An additional medicine is made from equal parts **Devadaru wood** (Himalayan cedar / *Cedrus deodara*), **Guggulu gum resin** *(Commiphora wightii)*, **Madhukam root** (licorice / *Glycyrrhiza glabra*), and **Shala resin** (sal tree /*Shorea robusta*). This medicine is rubbed over the tongue.

Diseases of the Palate (Talugata Roga)

Diseases of the palette are primarily treated with surgery. After surgery, specific post-surgical treatments can be applied:

1. If an ulcer erupts after surgery, it can be treated with a compound of equal parts **Maricham seed** (black pepper / *Piper nigrum*), **Ativisha tuber, purified** (aconite / *Aconitum heterophyllum*), **Patha root** *(Stephania hernandifolia)*, **Vacha rhizome** (acorus / *Acorus calamus*), **Kustha root** *(Saussurea lappa)*, and **Kutaja bark** *(Holarrhena antidysenterica)* mixed with **Madhu** (honey) and **Saindhavam** (mineral salt).

2. A gargle can be prepared from a decoction of equal parts **Vacha rhizome** (acorus / *Acorus calamus*), **Ativisha tuber, purified** (aconite / *Aconitum heterophyllum*), **Patha root** *(Stephania hernandifolia)*, **Rasna shrub** *(Vanda roxburghii)*, **Kutki rhizome** (Indian gentian / *Picrorhiza kurroa*) and **Nimba leaf** (neem / *Azadirachta indica*).

3. To subdue the deranged Kapha, **Vartis** (incense sticks) can be made from **Ingudi fat** *(Madhuka butyracea)*, **Apamarga herb** *(Achyranthes aspera)*, **Danti seed** *(Baliospermum montanum)*, **Sarala resin** (pine / *Pinus roxburghi*), and **Devadaru wood** (Himalayan cedar / *Cedrus deodara*). The incense sticks are burnt and the smoke is inhaled by the patient in the morning and in the evening.

Galashundika (Uvulitis)

Galashundika is correlated with uvulitis, and is caused by Kapha imbalance along with blood defects. Swelling of the uvula in the form of cystic lump is the primary symptom. It is treated with surgery followed by the post-surgical treatments above.

Tundikeri (Catarrhal croup)

Tundikeri relates to catarrhal croup, and is caused by symptom of Kapha along with blood defects. Inflammation around the uvula with a cystic lump is the primary symptom. It is treated with surgery followed by the post-surgical treatments mentioned above.

Adhrusa (Palatitis)

Adhrusa is correlated with inflammation of the palate (palatitis), and is caused by pathogenic defects of the blood. Severe inflammation of the palette with fever is the primary symptom. It is treated with surgery followed by the post-surgical mentioned treatments above.

Kachchapa (Palatal Polyp)

Kachchapa relates a polyp of the palate, and is caused by Kapha Dosha. Excrescence of the mucous membrane of the palate in the form of a round shape is the primary symptom. It is treated with surgery followed by the post-surgical treatments mentioned above.

Taluraktarbuda (Palatal angioma)

Taluraktarbuda is correlated with an angioma of the palate, and is caused by blood defects. A red lotus-like abnormal growth on the palate is the primary symptom. It is not curable.

Mansasanghata (Palatal myoma)

Mansasanghata relates to a myoma of the palate, and is caused by pathogenic defects in the muscular tissues. A painless tumor on the palate is the primary symptom. It is treated with surgery followed by the post-surgical treatments mentioned above.

Talupupputa (Palatal nodules)

Talupupputa can be correlated with nodules that arise on the palate, and are caused by Kapha Dosha along with pathogenic defects of the fatty tissues. Painless nodules on the palate are the main symptoms of it. It is treated with surgery followed by the post-surgical treatments above.

Talushosha (Atrophy of the palate)

Talushosha relates to atrophy of the palate, and is caused by symptom of Vata Dosha. It is treated with the general measures to reduce Vata (page 56).

Talupaka (Infection of the palate)

Talupaka relates to an infection of the palate, and is caused by Pitta Dosha. A purulent infection of the palate is the primary symptom. It is treated with the general measures to reduce Pitta (page 67) along with laxatives (page 174), medicinal plaster and the specific remedies against diseases of mouth (page 283).

Diseases of the Throat (Kantha Roga)

Swarabheda (Hoarseness / Laryngitis)

Swarabheda relates to hoarseness and laryngitis, and is caused by a Vata imbalance. This problem is treated with general measures to reduce Vata (page 56) in the form of remedies that are used either to suck on or to gargle with in a warmed solution. Either **Tankana Bhasma** (purified borax) or **Gunja leaves** (crab's eye / *Abrus precatorius)* can be used for this purpose. Intake of **Amalaki fruit** (Indian gooseberry / amla / *Phyllanthus emblica)* with milk can be used for internal use.

Galagraha (Pharyngitis)

Galagraha is correlated with pharyngitis, and is caused by an imbalance of Kapha and Pitta. An inflamed sore throat is the primary symptom. It is treated with general measures to balance Kapha and Pitta (page 81) along with **Mrityunjayarasa Vati** and gargling with a solution of **Sphutikarika** (purified alum).

Galaudha (Acute pharyngitis)

Galaudha is correlated with acute pharyngitis, and is caused by Kapha along with blood defects. Severe swelling with high fever are the primary symptoms. It can cause complete blockage of the gullet and windpipe, and is considered incurable. Palliative measures include laxative remedies (page 174), gargling with **Sphutikarika** (purified alum powder), along with **Pitaka Yoga, Kalaka Yoga**, or **Mrityunjayarasa Vati**.

Adhigihwa (Tonsillitis)

Adhigihwa relates to tonsillitis, and is caused by Kapha along with blood defects. Painful swelling of the tonsils is the primary symptom. Specific remedies include either **Pitaka Yoga** or **Kalaka Yoga**, taken twice daily and kept in mouth until dissolved. **Mrityunjayarasa Vati** can also be given, as well as gargling with a solution made with **Sphutikarika** (purified alum). In advanced or chronic cases, surgery is used.

Galayu (Pharyngeal nodule)

Galayu relates to a pharyngeal nodule, and is caused by Kapha along with blood defects. The primary symptom is a small nodule that resembles the seed of **Amalaki fruit** (Indian gooseberry / amla / *Phyllanthus emblica)*, which feels like something is stuck in the throat. It is curable only with surgery.

Kanthashaluka (Vocal cord nodule)

Kanthashaluka relates to a nodule of the vocal cord, and is caused by an aggravation of Kapha. A nodule in the throat that resembles **Badari fruit** (jujube / *Zizyphus jujube)* is the primary symptom. It is treated with surgery.

Ekavrinda (Cyst of the throat)

Ekavrinda relates to a cyst of the throat, and is caused by Kapha along with blood defects. It is treated with venesection (see page 92), laxatives (page 174) and emetics (page 175), along with **Pitaka Yoga** or **Kalaka Yoga**.

Vrinda (Acute cyst of the throat)

Vrinda relates to an acute cyst of the throat, and is caused by a Pitta imbalance along with blood defects. Severe burning sensation with high fever is the primary symptom. Although it is considered incurable palliative measures include **Pitaka Yoga** or **Kalaka Yoga**. A painful acute cyst of the throat is caused by aggravation of the related nerve (Vata).

Galavidradhi (Abscess of the throat)

Galavidradhi relates to an abscess of the throat and is a complicated (Sannipataja) disease. It is treated with surgery.

Swaraghna (Vocal cord paralysis)

Swaraghna can be correlated with vocal cord paralysis, and is caused by an aggravation of the related nerve (Vata). Hoarseness and dyspnea are the primary symptoms. Although it is considered incurable it can be treated with the same general remedies used for paralysis (page 230).

Balasha (Croup)

Balasha is correlated with croup, and is caused by an imbalance of Vata and Kapha. Swelling of the throat with shortness of breath (dyspnea) is the primary symptom. It is treated with **Pitaka Yoga** or **Kalaka Yoga**, but is difficult to cure.

Vidari (Bubo)

Vidari is correlated with bubo, and is caused by an aggravation of Pitta. Infection of the lymph nodes on either side of the throat is the primary symptom. Although it is considered incurable it can be treated with the same remedies used for inguinal bubo (page 244).

Mansatana (Laryngocele)

Mansatana relates to a laryngocele, and is a complicated (Sannipataja) disease. Protrusion of the mucous membrane in the form of swelling of the neck is the primary symptom. It can cause blockage of the windpipe and subsequent death. It is not curable.

Shataghni (Malignant laryngeal tumor)

Shataghni relates to a malignant laryngeal tumor, and is caused by an aggravation of all three Doshas. An abnormal growth around the larynx is the primary symptom. Although it is not curable, it can be maintained with **Pitaka Yoga** or **Kalaka Yoga**.

Diseases of the Nose (Nasa Roga)

The nose corresponds with the element of Earth in Ayurveda, and is connected to the mouth and the function of taste, and thus the element of Water. Based on this combination of the Elements, disorders of the nose typically relate to Kapha Dosha and the mucus system. Disorders of Vata relate to the nose as an organ of breathing, whereas Pitta disorders typically relate to allergies and infection.

Nasasrava (Nasal catarrh)

Nasasrava is caused by Kapha Dosha. Profuse discharge (catarrh) from the nose is the primary symptom. It is treated with general measures to reduce Kapha including a medicated nasal snuff and inhalation of smoke prepared from herbs with a drying, aromatic property. A medicated nasal snuff can be prepared, either as a powder or in an oil, from remedies including **Hingu gum** (asafoetida / *Ferula narthex*), **Trikatu** *(Piper longum, Piper nigrum, Zingiber officinalis)*, **Punarnava** *(Boerhavia difusa)*, **Laksha** (lac / *Coccus lacca*), **Katphalam bark** (box myrtle / *Myrica nagi*), **Vacha** (acorus / *Acorus calamus*), **Kutaja bark** *(Holarrhena antidysenterica)* or **Vidanga** *(Embelia ribes)*. Smoke inhalation (by nose) can be done with drying herbs including **Devadaru wood** (Himalayan cedar / *Cedrus deodara*), **Danti** *(Baliospermum montanum)*, or **Shala resin** (sal tree /*Shorea robusta*)

Nasapratinaha (Blockage of the nostrils)

Nasapratinaha relates to a blockage of the nostrils, caused by an imbalance of both Vata and Kapha. Difficulty in breathing through the nose is the primary symptom. It is treated with the general measures to reduce Vata and Kapha (page 81). Specific measures include a medicated nasal snuff with **Bala Taila**, and the use of smoke inhalation (by nose) with powdered **Devadaru wood** (Himalayan cedar / *Cedrus deodara*), **Danti** *(Baliospermum montanum)*, or **Shala resin** (sal tree /*Shorea robusta)*.

Kshavathuroga (Sneezing)

Kshavathuroga relates to constant sneezing, and as a chronic disease is caused by the irritation of a sensitive nasal marma (vital point). It is treated with a medicated nasal snuff along with the wafting of steam into the nostrils and over the head. The steam should be made from boiling a decoction of the plants used for Vata diseases (page 56). **Katphalam bark** (box myrtle / *Myrica nagi*) is commonly used as a medicated nasal snuff.

Pratishyaya (Common cold)

Pratishyaya relates to the common cold, and is caused by nasal congestion that causes inflammation. It is classified into five categories as Vataja, Pittaja, Kaphaja, Sannipataja and Raktaja. It is imperative to remove nasal congestion in all types of common cold. This is accomplished by drinking cold water before bed, and the application of a medicinal nasal snuff, inhalation of steam, inhaling fumes from carminative remedies (page 175), and inhalation of smoke. A simple remedy for the common cold is powder of equal parts **Yavani seed** (wild omum / *Trachyspermum ammi*) and **Vasaka leaf** (Malabar nut / *Adhatoda vasica*) taken with **Adrakam root** tea (ginger / *Zingiber officinalis*).

Vataja Pratishyaya

Pratishyaya with the character of Vata manifests with symptoms of constant sneezing, hoarseness and watery discharge. It is treated with the general measures to reduce Vata (page 56) along with the inhalation of the fumes from carminative remedies (page 175), plenty of warm water to drink before bed, and **Mrityunjayarasa Vati**.

Pittaja Pratishyaya

Pratishyaya with the character of Pitta manifests with symptoms of fever, inflammation, and a yellowish discharge. It is treated with the general measures to reduce Pitta (page 67) along with laxative remedies (page 174), plenty of warm water to drink before bed, and specific remedies such as **Mrityunjayarasa Vati**.

Kaphaja Pratishyaya

Pratishyaya with the character of Kapha manifests with symptoms of cough, irritation in respiratory system and throat, and a thick mucus discharge. It is treated with the general measures to reduce Kapha (page 77) along with the remedies against cough (page 181).

Sannipataja pratishyaya

Pratishyaya with the character of Sannipata causes recurrent attack of numerous common cold symptoms, with runny nasal discharge and/or blockage, redness of the nose, sore throat and other related symptoms. It is treated with a combination of general measures to balance each Dosha, as well as specific remedies including **Rasanjana Taila** taken as a medicated nasal snuff, and **Katutiktasarpi**, which is any hot, bitter herb preparation made with Ghee.

Raktaja pratishyaya (influenza)

Pratishyaya with the character of Raktaja is caused by blood defects, and is correlated with influenza. Chest infection is the main identifying factor. It is treated on the same basis as pneumonia (page 186), along with laxative remedies (page 174).

Dustapratishyaya (Sinusitis)

Dustapratishyaya or sinusitis is typically caused by negligence in treating the common cold. It can be very difficult to cure. In general it is treated with the remedies used for headache or cranial arteritis. **Shirashuladivajrarasa** is a specific medicine against sinusitis, headache or cranial arteritis, given in doses of 2 pills twice daily. **Shadbindu Taila** can also be used as a medicated nasal snuff, inhaled into the nose twice a day.

Diptam (Nasal inflammation)

Diptam relates to nasal inflammation, and is caused by Pitta. Sensation of heat and burning sensation in the nose is the primary symptom. It is treated with the general Pitta treatments (page 67) along with cold water to clean and cool the sinus, and the application of a cold compress.

Nasapaka (Nasal ulceration)

Nasapaka relates an inflammatory condition of the nose that typically arises from Diptam. It manifests as a thick, yellow mucoid accumulation with inflammation and ulceration, and is caused by Pitta Dosha. It is treated with the general Pitta treatments (page 67) along with venesection (see page 92) and a plaster mentioned in the *Sushruta Samhita* made of **Kshiravrikshatwach** (barks of latex-exuding trees) with **Ghrita** (Ghee). These trees are primarily members of the *Ficus* genus, and all are very astringent. They include:

1. **Udumbara bark** *(Ficus glomerata).*
2. **Vata bark** (banyan tree / *Ficus bengalensis).*
3. **Ashwattha bark** (bodhi tree / *Ficus religiosa).*
4. **Hemakshiri bark** (swarnakshiri / *Argemone mexicana).*
5. **Vamshalochana** (bamboo manna / *Bambusa breviflora).*
6. **Kshiri bark** (rajadani / *Mimusops hexandra).*

Putinasyam (Nasopharyngeal inflammation)

Putinasyam relates to nasopharyngeal inflammation that manifests with complicated symptoms (Sannipataja). A putrid odor emanating from the nasal cavity is the most obvious symptom. It is treated with laxative remedies (page 174), emetic remedies (page 175) and a medicated nasal snuff. Hot water is advised for drinking, along with regular cleaning of the sinus with a neti pot or inhalation of steam. **Shadbindu Taila** can be used as a medicated nasal snuff.

Apinasa (Rhinosporidiasis)

Rhinosporidiasis has symptoms of Vata and Kapha imbalance. Polyps and swelling of the nasal mucous membrane develop from infestation of fleas *(Rhinosporidium seeberi)*. It is treated with remedies capable of killing fleas (taken internally or as a medicated nasal snuff), laxative remedies (page 174), and emetic remedies (page 175). Specific remedies for apinasa include **Nimbadi compound** and **Mrityunjayarasa Vati**.

Puyaraktam (Traumatic nasal infection)

Puyaraktam refers to a nasal infection that occurs as a result of physical trauma to the nose. A bloody purulent discharge from the nose is the primary symptom. It is treated with the remedies used for fistula (page 247).

Nasaparishosa (Atrophic rhinitis)

Nasaparishosa can be correlated with atrophic rhinitis (atrophy of nasal membrane), and is a Vataja disorder. Difficulty with inhalation and exhalation as well as dryness of the nose are the primary symptoms. It is treated with general measures to reduce Vata (page 56) along with a medicated nasal snuff such as **Shadbindu Taila** or **Katphalam bark** (box myrtle / *Myrica nagi)*.

Nasaraktapittam (Epistaxis / Nasal bleeding / Nosebleed)

Nasaraktapittam relates to epistaxis or nosebleeds, and is caused by same etiology of hematorrhea and is treated with the same basic remedies (page 258). In addition it is recommended to wash the nose with ice-cold water or milk. A plaster of roasted **Amalaki fruit** (Indian gooseberry / amla / *Phyllanthus emblica)* can also be applied on the forehead. Useful medicated nasal snuffs include **Palandu bulb juice** (onion / *Allium cepa)* and water mixed with a little **Sphutikarika** (purified alum).

Nasarsha (Nasal polyp)

Nasarsha or nasal polyp is caused by excrescence of the mucous membrane. It is treated with the same remedies used for hemorrhoid (page 168), including surgery.

Nasarbuda (Nasal cancer)

Nasarbuda is correlated with nasal cancer. It is caused by same factors that promote arbuda (large neoplasm), and is treated with the same remedies (page 250).

Nasashotha (Nasal edema)

Nasashotha or nasal edema is caused by same etiology as general edema, and is treated with the same remedies (page 257).

Diseases of the Ear (Karna Roga)

Although all the sensory organs are sensitive to influence, the ears in particular are considered a delicate organ in Ayurveda, and correspond with the subtle nature of the Ether Element. In this way, the ears are most related Vata Dosha, and as a result many diseases of the ear diseases are Vata in origin. To protect the delicate structures in the ear the body also tries to ensure that it is well-lubricated and protected, and hence disorders of Kapha are also commonly found. Pitta disturbance of the ear typically relate only to infection.

Karnashweda / Karnanada (Tinnitus)

Karnashweda / Karnanada is correlated with tinnitus, and is caused by aggravated nerve function (Vata) with reduced blood circulation and resultant dryness of the eardrums. The main symptoms usually seen are dryness, ear noises just such as ringing bell or bee sound, a blockage that opens and closes constantly, dizziness, headache, and sensation of heaviness in the ear region. It is commonly found in patients with Ojakshaya (page 262).

The condition is treated with the external application of warm eardrops of **Narayana Taila** (medicated asparagus oil) or a medicated oil called **Apamargakshara Taila** prepared with the alkaline ash of **Apamarga** *(Achyranthes aspera)* is boiled with water and **Tila oil** *(Sesamum indicum)*. Internally, **Yogaraja Guggulu** has been found to be helpful.

Karnashula (Otitis media / Earache)

Karnashula relates to the aggravated condition of the related nerves (Vata) causing earache. Another causative factor is inflammation or injury. Eardrops made from either warmed **Narayana Taila** (medicated asparagus oil) or warmed **Goumutra** (cow urine) is the best medicine. Slightly warmed **Lasunadi swarasa** (fresh garlic juice) or **Ardraka swarasa** (fresh ginger juice) is also helpful.

Badhira (Deafness / Hearing loss)

Ayurveda classifies badhira or deafness as either Vataja (nerve defects), Kaphaja (swelling) or Aghataja (traumatic injury). A sense of heaviness and/or blockage causing an inability to hear or very low hearing capacity is the primary symptom. Treatment based upon the cause (using general treatments) may give a positive result for Vataja or Kaphaja types in the early stage, but traumatic deafness is not curable. Specific medicines include **Bilwa Taila** eardrops and **Apamargakshara Taila** eardrops.

Karnashrava (Otorrhea)

Karnashrava is correlated with otorrhea, and is caused by aggravated function of the related nervous system. Other causative factors include head injury, dirty water inside the ear due to swimming, or, in the case of a baby, the milk of the mother getting into the ear. Ear discharge is the primary symptom. If left untreated it can cause deafness. It is treated with the general Vata treatments (page 56) along with specific remedies. A specific remedy is eardrops made from **Narayana Taila** combined with **Sphutikarika** (purified alum) or **Samudraphenam powder** (sea foam / *Sepia species*), for their drying effect in the ear. Other useful herbs prepared as a medicated Taila by cooking with sesame oil include **Apamarga plant ash** *(Achyranthes aspera)*, **Daruharidra bark extract** (barberry / *Berberis nepalensis)* and **Bhringaraja** *(Eclipta alba)* with sesame oil

Karnakandu (Ear itching)

Karnakandu relates to itching of the ear, and is a disease resulting from the local aggravation of the mucus system and a blockage of the local arteries (Kaphaja). It can be relieved with the external use of **Sphutikarika** (purified alum powder), and internally by taking **Nimba leaf** (neem / *Azadirachta indica)* or the standard formula **Nimbadi compound**.

Karnarbuda (Ear neoplasm)

Karnarbuda relates to a neoplasm of the ear and is a tridoshaja disease. It is treated with the same general methods used for cancer (page 248).

Karnarsha (Ear wart)

Karnarsha relates to ear warts, which are caused by an aggravated condition of both Kapha (arterial blockage) and Rakta (blood defects). Blood cleaning medicines such as **Alarasayana** are helpful. Externally located warts can be burned off with alkali ash treatment (page 171).

Karnaguthaka (Earwax, impacted)

Karnaguthaka relates to impacted earwax, and is a Kaphaja disorder. Blockage of hearing and a sensation of heaviness are the primary symptoms. It has to be cleaned manually by using instruments after softening first with oils.

Karnapaka (Ear infection / Ear ulceration)

Karnapaka relates to an infection of the ear, caused by the aggravated function of the related veins (Pittaja). Dirty water entering the ear canal or the accumulation of mother's milk in breast-fed infants can both cause this disease. General measures to reduce Pitta are used (page 67) along with anti-inflammatory remedies (page 154). Externally, eardrops made from **Narayana Taila** with added **Sphutikarika** (purified alum) can be used, while the standard formula **Nimbadi** can be used internally to clean the blood.

Karnapratinaha (Migraine with earwax infection)

Karnapratinaha is a Vataja disease that results from an earwax infection, causing inflammation of the local nerves resulting in headache, blockage in the ears and tinnitus. A remedy used for sinusitis called **Shirashuladivajrarasa** is used in doses of 2 pills twice daily, along with a calming medicine for the nerves such **Chandanadi Churna**, 1-2 grams twice daily. Eardrops made from **Narayana Taila** with **Sphutikarika** (purified alum) are used externally to help remove the earwax.

Krimikarna (Aural sporidiosis)

Krimikarna relates to itching and blockage of the ear with a purulent discharge. Correlated with an infectious agent ('krimi'), this is a complicated (Tridoshaja) disease. Blood cleaning medicines such as **Nimbadi** are used internally, in doses of 2 pills twice daily, along with **Bilwa Taila** eardrops externally.

Putikarna (Otitis media, purulent)

Putikarna relates inflammation and infection of the middle ear, causing blockage and exudation. It is caused by Pitta Dosha, and manifests with symptoms including burning sensation, pain, and a thick purulent discharge. Treatment consists of the same methods used for Karnapaka (ear infection).

Karnashotha (Ear swelling / Ear edema)

Karnashotha is a disease resulting from the aggravation of Kapha, causing a swelling of the ear. Internally, the anti-edema formulation **Ajamodadi Churna** is used, in doses of 1-2 grams twice daily. Externally, **Narayana Taila** can be applied.

Paripota (Earlobe swelling)

Paripota is a disease is similar to ear edema (karnashotha), and is treated in the same manner.

Karnavidradhi (Ear abscess)

Karnavidradhi relates to an abscess of the ear, and is a complex (Sannipataja) condition. It is treated with surgery.

Chapter 26: Diseases of the Eyes (Netra Roga)

According to Ayurveda the eye is created and maintained by the element of Fire. As such, the eye is adversely affected by excess heat, and just as the tears of the eye, as well as the aqueous and vitreous humors function to nourish and cool the eye, Ayurveda recommends supportive measures to balance Fire. This includes hygienic measures such as washing the face three to four times a day, taking regular baths, a healthy diet, living and working in areas with adequate ventilation or outside in the fresh air, and the ancient practice of peering at the cooling rays of the moon.

General Eye Medicines

Among the most important general eye remedies is **Triphala Churna,** prepared as an eyewash by soaking equal parts freshly dried **Amalaki fruit** *(Phyllanthus emblica)*, **Bibhitaki fruit** *(Terminalia belerica)* and **Haritaki fruit** *(Terminalia chebula)* in room temperature water overnight. In the morning the water is carefully filtered and used as an eyewash. If only the powder is used to make the infusion, filtering must be done with fine clean linen to filter out any particulate. This eyewash is good for general eye health, and can be also used for conjunctivitis.

Another common eye remedy is **Rasanjana** eye drops, made by dissolving the condensed paste extract of either **Daruharidra** (barberry / *Berberis nepalensis)* or **Darvi root** *(Berberis asiatica)* in water, used to wash the eyes every fifth day or once a week. These eye drops reduce inflammation (Pitta) and 'mucus' (Kapha), clean the eyes and help keep the duct system open.

To maintain the natural power of vision and prevent cataract formation, a collyrium (external application) made of the purified microfine powder called **Sauvira Bhasma** (purified antimony sulfide) can be painted across the entire bottom eyelid each night, making a line about 1/2 inch in width directly under the lash.

Degenerative eye diseases such as macular degeneration can be treated with eye restoratives based upon **Triphala** *(Phyllanthus emblica / Terminalia belerica / Terminalia chebula)* and other general Rasayanas. For chronic eye inflammation such as iritis and uveitis, **Triphala** can be used along with the general anti-Pitta medicines (page 67), mild laxative remedies (page 174), and anti-inflammatory medicines (page 155).

Abhishyanda (Conjunctivitis)

Abhishyanda is correlated with conjunctivitis, caused by inflammation of the conjunctiva. It is classified into four categories, with the characters of Vata, Pitta, Kapha and Raktaja.

General remedies include either **Triphala** eyewash or **Rasanjana** eye drops. **Bilwanjana** eye salve is another general remedy used for conjunctivitis as well as glaucoma. It relieves pain and subdues swelling. It is made from filtered juice of **Bilwa leaf** *(Aegle marmelos)* mixed with **Saindhavam** (mineral salt) and **Ghrita** (clarified butter / Ghee). This is ground with Ghee colored **Kauda Bhasma** (cowries), cooked and mixed with **Goukshira** (cow milk). In severe cases, laxative remedies (page 174) and venesection (page 92) can be prescribed as well.

Vataja Conjunctivitis

Conjunctivitis with the character of Vata causes painful eyes, headache, dryness and cold tears. It is treated with the general Vata treatments (page 56) along with specific remedies and laxative remedies (page 174). As an eye drop, **Netrabindu** is a specific medicine against Vataja conjunctivitis, prepared by mixing one part of **Sphutikarika** (purified alum) to 100 parts water that has been distilled with a tiny amount of **Karapura leaf** (camphor / *Cinnamomum camphora).*

Pittaja conjunctivitis

Conjunctivitis with the character of Pitta causes infection, hot sensation and hot tears. It is treated with the general Pitta treatments (page 67) along with laxative remedies (page 174), and **Rasanjana** eye drops, or **Samudraphenam** (sea foam / *Sepia* species) mixed with **Shtrikshira** (breast milk).

Kaphaja conjunctivitis

Conjunctivitis with the character of Kapha causes itching, edema and a sticky discharge. It is treated with the general Kapha treatments (page 77) along with laxative remedies (page 174), and **Netrabindu** eye drops (page 302) prepared with **Rasanjana** (condensed paste of *Berberis nepalensis* or *Berberis asiatica).*

Raktaja conjunctivitis

Conjunctivitis with the character of Raktaja causes red eyes, hot sensation and infection. It is treated with the general Pitta treatments (page 67) along with purgative remedies (page 174). **Netrabindu** eye drops (page 302) are used, after adding **Rasanjana** or **Mallayoga** {**Shankhavisha Bhasma** (purified white arsenic) with **Swarnapatri leaf** (senna / *Cassia auriculata)* and **Amalaki fruit** *(Phyllanthus emblica).*

Adhimantha (Glaucoma)

Adhimantha is correlated with glaucoma, and is caused by a severe painful pressure inside the eyes. It is classified into four categories, with the character of

Vata, Pitta, Kapha and Raktaja. All forms of glaucoma can lead to blindness if not treated properly. Without such treatment, the ancient texts state that the patient with Vataja glaucoma can be blind after six days, after five days in Raktaja glaucoma, and after seven days Kaphaja glaucoma. With Pittaja glaucoma blindness can occur at any time.

Long-term measures to preserve vision utilize a combination of general treatments and specific treatments based on the indicated Doshas. Useful herbs in all cases include **Punarnava plant/root** *(Boerhavia difusa)*, **Shatavari root** (asparagus / *Asparagus racemosus)*, **Triphala** *(Phyllanthus emblica / Terminalia belerica / Terminalia chebula)*, **Triphaladi Ghritam** and **Shirashuladivajrarasa Vati**. Externally, **Bilwanjana** eye salve can also be used, as well as **Netrabindu** eye drops (page 302).

Vataja glaucoma

Glaucoma with the character of Vata causes severe migraine-like headaches, dryness, cold tears and severe pain in the eyes. Without proper treatment, a patient at this stage can be blind after one week, and thus treatment should begin immediately after diagnosis. The first step is to prescribe **aged Ghrita** (Ghee which is at least 10 years old) to drink. Then, after applying a warm compress, the excess blood is drained from the eye by venesection (page 92). Following this, the eyes are treated with a preparation made from goat's milk mixed with water and cooked with **Hriverum plant** *(Pavonia odorata)*, **Tagara bark** *(Erytania coronarea)*, **Manjishtha plant** (Indian madder / *Rubia cordifolia)* and **Udumbara bark** *(Ficus glomerata)*. General measures to reduce Vata (page 56) are used along with laxative remedies (page 174) and enema. A medicated oil made from **Shalaparni plant** *(Desmodium gangeticum)*, milk, and a sweet plant such as **Madhukam root** (licorice / *Glycyrrhiza glabra)* is prescribed to use in the form of medicated nasal snuff.

Pittaja Glaucoma

Glaucoma with the character of Pitta manifests with a severe migraine-like headache, hot sensation, infection, hot tears and burning painful eyes. Blindness can quickly follow. Venesection operation (see page 92), cleaning the bowels with laxative remedies (page 174), eyewash with a cooling decoction, application of anti-inflammatory plasters around the eyes, and the use of medicated nasal snuffs and collyriums are all very important to apply as soon as possible. Other general anti-Pitta methods can be used (page 67). After the crisis is over, a condensed paste made from the decoction of **Trivrit root** (Indian rhubarb /*Operculina turpethum)* or **Madhukam root** (licorice / *Glycyrrhiza glabra)*, and mixed with sugar and honey is effective to use in the form of an Anjana, painted over the eyelids.

Kaphaja glaucoma

Glaucoma with the character of Kapha causes a severe migraine-like headache, itching, edema, and a sticky discharge. It is treated with general measures to reduce

Kapha (page 77) along with venesection (see page 92), laxative remedies (page 174) and specific remedies for external and internal uses, including a medicated hot compress and eye drops. Three days of fasting can be helpful, and an anti-Kapha diet, using drying foods that reduce mucus, is very important.

For the hot compress, a paste is used made from **Shyonaka root/bark** (Indian trumpet flower / *Oroxylon indicum*), **Aparajita root** (butterfly pea / *Clitoria ternatea*), **Tulsi plant** (holy basil / *Ocimum sanctum*), **Bilwa fruit** (bael / *Aegle marmelos*), **Rakta Chandanam wood** (red sandalwood / *Pterocarpus santalinus*), **Pilu nut** (wild walnut), **Arka** (milkweed / *Calotropis gigantean*), **Kapittha fruit** (wood apple / *Feronia limonia)* and **Vijaya leaf** (hemp / *Cannabis sativa)*.

The eye drops are made from **Haritaki fruit** *(Terminalia chebula)*, **Haridra root** (turmeric / *Curcuma longa)*, **Madhukam root** (licorice / *Glycyrrhiza glabra)* and **Sauvira Bhasma** (purified antimony sulfide).

Raktaja glaucoma

Glaucoma with the character of Raktaja is caused by severe migraine like headache, painful eyes, hot sensation and infection. It is treated with the general Pitta treatments (page 67) along with venesection (see page 92), laxative remedies (very important - page 174) and specific remedies for external and internal use. Also important is to cleanse the nasal passageways. In this case, a Ghee preparation made of laxative remedies with sugar is used as a medicated nasal snuff that causes discharge by sneezing. To relieve the severe pain do the following a light fomentation is used, followed by leeches applied around the eyes to suck out the blood. This is then followed by administering large doses of **Ghrita** (Ghee) internally, along with the treatments mentioned under Pittaja glaucoma.

Hatadhimantha (Acute Glaucoma / Phthisis bulbi)

Hatadhimantha is correlated with acute glaucoma has the character of Vata. The severe outward expansion of the eyeball by pressure is the primary symptom. It is not curable and causes blindness.

Netrapaka (Degenerative Ophthalmitis)

Netrapaka is correlated with degenerative ophthalmitis (eye infection), and is classified by into two categories: with edema (Sashopha Netrapaka) and without edema (Ashopha Netrapaka). Both cause complicated (Sannipataja) symptoms. Eye infection combined with inflammation is the primary symptom. It is very difficult to cure, and is treated with the remedies used for conjunctivitis (page 302) along with specific remedies including the **Jatyadi Anjanam** eye salve mentioned in the *Sushruta Samhita*, or an eye salve made from **Jati flower** (Jasmine / *Jasminum officinalis*).

Vataparyaya (Ophthalmodynia / Tic douleroux)

Vataparyaya is correlated with ophthalmodynia, and is a Vataja disorder which causes neuralgic pain of the eye. It is treated with the general Vata treatments (page 56) along with the remedies used for conjunctivitis with the character of Vata. A special Ghee preparation can be used made with the decoction of **Rasna shrub** *(Vanda roxburghii)*, **Kapittha fruit** (wood apple / *Feronia limonia)*, **Bilwa fruit** (bael / *Aegle marmelos)*, **Shyonaka** (Indian trumpet flower / *Oroxylon indicum)*, **Patala root/bark** *(Stereospermum personatum)*, **Agnimantha bark/root** *(Premna integrifolia)*, **Kashmari bark/root** *(Gmelina arborea)*, **Karkatashringi fruit gall** *(Pistacia intergerrima* insect gall) and milk. This medicine is taken internally with food.

Shuskakshipaka (Dry Blepharitis / Xerophthalmia)

Shuskakshipaka can be correlated with dry blepharitis and xerophthalmia (dry eyes), and is caused by Vata imbalance along with blood defects. Primary symptoms include difficulty opening the eyes, along with pain and burning sensations. It is treated with the general Vata treatments (page 56). A specific remedy is a Ghee preparation applied in the form of collyrium, made of **Saindhavam** (mineral salt from Sindhu), **Daruharidra bark extract** (barberry / *Berberis nepalensis)*, **Shunthi root** (dry ginger / *Zingiber officinalis)* and juice of **Matulunga fruit** (citron / *Citrus medica)* with milk and water.

Anyatovata (Ophthalmoneuritis / Optic neuritis)

Anyatovata is correlated with optic neuritis, and is caused by an aggravation of the optic nerves. Neuralgic pain of the eye is the primary symptom. It is treated with the general Vata treatments (page 56), and the Ghee preparation mentioned for shuskakshipaka (dry blepharitis).

Amladhyushita (Ophthalmia)

Amladhyushita is correlated with general ophthalmia (eye inflammation), caused by an aggravation of Pitta. Severe infection/inflammation of the eye is the primary symptom. It is treated with the general measures to reduce Pitta (page 67) along with the remedies for conjunctivitis with the character of Pitta (page 302). Venesection practice is prohibited in this case. A Ghee preparation made of **Lodhram bark** *(Symplocos paniculata)* and **Triphala** (three fruits compound) can be applied topically.

Shirotpata (Ophthalmorrhagia)

Shirotpata is correlated with bleeding in the eye, and is caused by blood defects. Redness of the eye (dilated blood vessels) is the primary symptom. It is treated with the remedies used for conjunctivitis with the character of Raktaja (page

302). A collyrium can be made of **Gairika** (red clay / ochre) ground with **Madhu** (honey).

Sirapraharsa (Chronic varicula / Neglected hyphema)

Sirapraharsa can be correlated with chronic varicula (Sirajala, see below), and is caused by neglected varicula along with blood defects. It is treated with the remedies for conjunctivitis with the character of Raktaja (page 302) along with venesection (see page 92). A condensed extract of **Daruharidra bark** *(Berberis nepalensis)* mixed with honey can be used as a collyrium. Chronic varicula can be a cause of blindness.

Shuklam (Corneal ulcer)

Shuklam is correlated with a corneal ulcer, which is a white spot that appears on the transparent cornea. It is divided into two types, traumatic corneal ulcer (Savranashuklam) and non-traumatic corneal ulcer (Avranashuklam). It is treated first by rubbing on **Saindhavam** (mineral salt), followed by the application of the seed pulp of **Bibhitaki fruit** *(Terminalia belerica)* mixed with honey to anoint the ulcer. It is very difficult to cure, if it is deep, with discharge, right in front of the pupil, or if there are double spots.

Akshipakatyaya (Corneal pannus)

Akshipakatyaya is related to corneal pannus, and is caused by complicated factors (Sannipataja). The primary symptom is a white membranous tissue that covers the eye. It is considered incurable.

Ajakajatam (Interstitial keratitis)

Ajakajatam refers to a reddish granular growth on the inner surface of the cornea is caused by ulcer. It is treated with surgery.

Pittavidagdhadrishti (Photophobia)

Pittavidagdhadrishti relates to photophobia, and is caused by defects of the sclera. The excessive or complete closing of the pupil by bright light is the primary symptom. It is treated with the general Pitta treatments (page 67) along with specific remedies. If caused by trauma, it is not curable. Some specific remedies include:

1. **Triphaladi Ghritam**, taken internally in doses of 3-6 grams, taken with milk.
2. **Gairikadi Anjanam**, eye salve, applied topically over eyelid.
3. **Gomansadi Anjanam**, eye salve, applied topically over eyelid.
4. **Swayamgupta Anjanam**, eye salve, applied topically over eyelid.

5. The stamens of **Nilotpalam flower** (Blue lotus / *Iris nepalensis*) and **Raktotpala** (red lotus / *Nymphoea rubra)*, ground to a very fine powder and applied to the eye.

Kaphavidagdhadrishti (Night blindness)

Kaphavidagdhadrishti relates to night blindness, and is caused by defects of the sclera. Normally the pupil should accommodate to low light conditions, but in Kaphavidagdhadrishti it cannot. It is treated with the general measures to reduce Kapha (page 77) along with specific remedies, including the addition of **Aja yakrit** (goat's liver) in the diet, and **Trivrit Ghritam,** prepared by cooking laxative **Trivrit root** (Indian rhubarb /*Operculina turpethum)* in **Ghrita** (clarified butter / Ghee), taken in doses of 3-6 grams. Night blindness caused by trauma is not curable.

For external use **Gairikadi Anjanam** can be used, made from **Gairika** (red clay / ocre), **Saindhavam** (mineral salt), **Pippali fruit** (long pepper / *Piper longum)*, and **Goudanta ash** (cow tooth ash). **Gomansadi Anjanam** is another useful external remedy, made from **Gomansa** (cow meat), **Maricham seed** (black pepper / *Piper nigrum)*, **Shirisha seed** *(Albizzia lebbeck)*, and **Manashila Bhasma** (purified realgar). The *Chakradatta* recommends **Chandrodayavarti** eye salve.

Dhumadarshi (Unclear vision / Amblyopia)

Dhumadarshi relates to unclear vision, without refractive error, and is caused by heat from high fever or sun exposure. In this condition, the lens can be seen afflicted with a smoke like coloring. It is treated with the general Pitta treatments (page 67), along with the remedies for hematorrhea (page 258) taken with **Ghrita** (clarified butter / Ghee).

Hraswajadya (Photophobia)

Hraswajadya relates to photophobia, and is caused by defects in the lens. Difficulties in seeing during the daytime and objects appearing smaller in size are the primary symptoms. It is considered incurable.

Nakulandhya (Defective vision with colorful illumination)

Nakulandhya relates to defective vision characterized by constant colorful illuminations, and is caused by defects in the lens. It is considered incurable.

Gambhirika (Contraction of the lens / Hypermature or calcific lens)

Gambhirika relates to the contraction or atrophy of the lens, caused by an aggravation of the optic nerve (Vata). Severe pain and defective vision are the main symptoms. It is considered incurable.

Linganasha (Cataract)

Linganasha is correlated with cataract, causing the opacification of the lens. It is classified into six categories: Vata, Pitta (Mlayi and Nilam), Kapha, Raktaja and Tridoshaja. Cataracts of all types are very difficult to cure. In the beginning stage cataracts can be treated with remedies for conjunctivitis (page 302 – according to differentiation) along with **Chandrodayavarti** eye salve. Advanced cataracts are not curable, nor are those caused by continual exposure to the bright light of the sun.

Vataja cataract

Cataract with the character of Vata causes a pink opacification of the lens. It is treated with venesection (see page 92), laxative remedies to clean the bowels (page 174), **Purana Ghrita** (old Ghee), and **Triphala Churna** (standard powder compound) taken mixed with sesame oil.

Pittaja cataract

Cataract with the character of Pitta is divided into two categories called Mlayi and Nilam. Mlayi causes yellowish opacification of the lens whereas Nilam causes a bluish opacification. Both are treated with venesection (page 92), laxative remedies to clean the bowels (page 174), **Purana grhita** (old Ghee) and **Triphala Churna** (standard compound) taken with **Ghrita** (Ghee / clarified butter).

Kaphaja cataract

Cataract with the character of Kapha develops with white patches or white opacification of the lens. It is treated with venesection (see page 92), laxative remedies to clean the bowels (page 174), **Purana grhita** (old Ghee) and **Triphala Churna** (standard compound) taken mixed with **Madhu** (honey). It is treated also with surgery.

Raktaja cataract

Cataract with the character of Raktaja causes reddish opacification of the lens. It is treated with the remedies used for cataract with the character of Pitta.

Tridoshaja cataract

Cataract with the character of Tridoshaja causes a variegated opacification of the lens. It can be controlled but not cured with the general treatments for cataract.

Timira (Errors of refraction / Eyecoat illnesses)

Timira relates to errors of refraction of the eye caused by defects in the structures of the eyeball. Ayurveda states that the internal part of the eyeball (vitreous body) is covered by four coats or layers called patalas:

1. The outermost coat, called prathama patala, is made of the white sclera.

2. The second layer, called dwitiya patala, consists of the vascular uveal tract, including the choroid up to the ciliary body.
3. The third coat, called tritiya patala, is the retina and optic nerve tissues.
4. The innermost fourth coat, chaturtha patala, consists of the lens.

Based upon this differentiation, eyeball defects are classified into four categories: Prathama patalagata Dosha, Dwitiya patalagata Dosha, Tritiya patalagatadosha and Chaturtha patalagata Dosha. During the treatment of Timira symptomatic treatments (based on Vata, Pitta Kapha, etc.) should be prescribed along with one or more of the specific remedies mentioned below.

Prathama patalagatadosha (Scleral defects / Scleritis / Scleromalacia)

Defects of the outer sclera can cause errors of refraction. Such defects include thinning or hardening of the sclera (changing its shape), as well as scleritis caused by inflammation in the adjacent fatty tissue lining the orbit. Symptoms include problems such as the patient can see when the eyes turn upwards, but cannot see when the eyes turn downward, as well as diplopia (double vision).

Dwitiya patalagatadosha (Retinitis / Uveitis / Iritis / Pars planitis / Choroiditis / Hypermetropia)

Any pathogenic defect of the choroid at the rear of the uveal tract up to the muscle of the lens chamber can be the cause of hypermetropia (the sense that far objects are more clear than near objects), with the additional symptoms of disturbed vision with floaters, thread lines, nets, etc.

Tritiya patalagatadosha (Myopia / Macular degeneration)

Defect of the retina causes poor vision. In this condition, the patient cannot see clearly (myopia) and can later develop gradual loss of vision (macular degeneration). The placing of these two diseases in the same category is due to the fact that Vata natured patients tend to develop myopia early in life, and macular degeneration later in life.

Chaturtha patalagatadosha (Lens defects / Myopia / Hypermetropia)

Any pathogenic defect of the lens can be the cause of myopia or hypermetropia. If serious, such defects can cause blindness.

Specific Remedies for Timira

All types of eyecoat illness or refractory problems are treated with specific remedies:

1. **Triphaladi Ghrita**, taken internally in doses of 3-6 grams.

2. **Triphala** eyewash.
3. **Sukhavativarti** eye salve, applied topically.
4. **Chandrodayavarti** eye salve, applied topically.
5. **Haritakivarti** eye salve, applied topically.
6. **Shatavari payasa** *(Sushruta Samhita)*.
7. **Amalaki payasa** *(Sushruta Samhita)*.

Payasa means 'pudding medicine', and the last two medicines mentioned above are puddings made with either **Shatavari root** (asparagus / *Asparagus racemosus)* or **Amalaki fruit** (Indian gooseberry / *Phyllanthus emblica)*.

Lens Defects (Sthiladosha)

Sthiladosha or defects of the lens are four in number, and are treated with the same remedies used for Timira. Adhasthiladosha (near-blindness) is caused by a defective bottom of the lens. Uparisthiladosha (distance-blindness) is caused by a defective upper surface of the lens. Paraswasthiladosha (side-blindness) is caused by defective side of the lens. Tiryasthiladosha (double vision / diplopia) is caused by defective vertical line of the lens.

Arma (Pterygium)

Arma or pterygium is divided into five types, all of which are treated with surgery. Prastariarma ('spreading pterygium') is a complex (Sannipataja) condition of red and blue colored thin patches on the bulbar conjunctiva. Although not painful, it tends to spread. Shuklarma (white pterygium) is a Kaphaja disorder manifesting as soft white patches thickened developing on the conjunctiva that grow very slowly. Raktarma (red pterygium) is caused by pathogenic defect of the blood, manifesting as a red patch in the thickened conjunctiva. Adhimansarma (fleshy pterygium) is a complex (Sannipataja) condition manifesting as colored, thick, soft, and fleshy patches developing on the conjunctiva. These purplish or liver colored patches have the nature of spreading. Snaywarma (dry pterygium) is a complex (Sannipataja) condition manifesting as dry thickened patches, pale in color, developing on the bulbar conjunctiva. Pterygiums in the beginning stages can also be treated with the remedies used for corneal ulcer (page 306).

Shuktika (Episcleral blue spots / Nevus of Ota / Axenfeld's Loops)

Shuktika relates to an episcleral blue or brown spot caused by an inflammatory (Pittaja) condition. They are treated with the remedies used for yellow conjunctivitis (Pittabhisyanda, page 302). Venesection (venesection) is prohibited.

Arjunam (Episcleral red spot)

Arjunam refers to an episcleral red spot caused by pathogenic blood defects (Raktaja). It is treated with the remedies used for conjunctivitis characterized by blood defects (Raktabhishyanda, see page 302).

Pistakam (Episcleral white spot)

Pistakam relates to an episcleral white spot (transparent or colored like rice) caused by both Vata and Kapha. Dimness of the episclera with edema is the main symptom. It is treated with specific remedies including **Mahousadhayoga Anjana**.

Sirajala (Varicula / Telangiectasia)

Sirajala or varicula is caused by pathogenic defect of blood. Redness of the eyes with net-like enlarged veins of the conjunctiva is the main symptom. It is treated with the remedies used for conjunctivitis characterized by blood defects (page 302). Surgery is used in advanced cases.

Sirajapidaka (Angioma of the conjunctiva)

Sirajapidaka refers to an angioma of the conjunctiva, and is a complex (Sannipataja) disease. A vascular tumor surrounded by vessels located on the conjunctiva is the primary symptom. It is treated with surgery.

Balasakakhya (Concretion / Bitot's spot)

Balasakakhya refers to a shiny blister or pimple (concretion) that appears on the conjunctiva. It is a Kaphaja disorder, and is treated with the measures used for Kaphaja conjunctivitis along with specific remedies.

One specific medicine used externally is an alkali. Wheat with blue mold is soaked in **Goukshira** (cow milk), then ground roughly with **Arjaka leaf extract** (white mint plant / *Mentha spp.*), **Aparajita seed/root** (butterfly pea / *Clitoria ternatea*), **Kapittha fruit** (wood apple / *Feronia limonia*), **Bilwa fruit** (bael / *Aegle marmelos*), **Kirundi plant** (*Vitex negundo*, white), and **Jati flower** (Jasmine / *Jasminum officinalis*). This combination is burnt, and the alkali ash produced is dissolved in water and cooked (to condense) with **Tutthakam Bhasma** (purified copper sulfate), **Saindhavam** (mineral salt from Sindhu) and **Goupitta** (cow bile).

Puyalasa (Dacryocystitis)

Puyalasa or dacryocystitis relates to an infection of the nasolacrimal sac, and is a complex (Sannipataja) disease. At the beginning stage a painful swelling develops with infection, which then breaks and discharges pus. To treat puyalasa, venesection is performed (page 92), after which a warm poultice is applied. Treatment then follows that mentioned under ophthalmitis, using the remedies for conjunctivitis (page 302) along with an eye salve called **Jatyadi Anjanam** (*Sushruta Samhita*) made from **Jati flower** (Jasmine / *Jasminum officinalis*). Finally, a collyrium can be applied made from **Kashisa** (ferrous sulfate), **Saindhavam** (mineral salt from Sindhu) and **Shunthi root** (dry ginger / *Zingiber officinalis*), mixed with honey.

Upanaha

Upanaha refers to a hard, painless, pink glandular growth located between the joint of the iris and the lens is called upanaha. It is not infectious, but causes itching and is a Kaphaja disease. It is removed with surgery.

Netrasrava (Eye diseases with epiphora)

Netrasrava refers to an overflow of tears (epiphora) related to different eye diseases. It is classified into four categories: Puyasrava, Shleshmashrava, Raktasrava and Jalashrava. Netrasrava in general is treated by washing the eyes with an infusion of **Triphala** (three fruits compound) and pasting a bit of **Triphala plaster** (mix **Triphala** with water) on the corner of the eyes, near the nose.

Puyasrava (Dacryocystitis)

Puyasrava is a complex (Sannipataja) disease related to puyalasa, manifesting first as a painful swelling with infection, which then breaks with a discharge and pus-filled tears. It is considered very difficult to cure, and is best treated with venesection (see page 92) along with specific remedies, including **Triphala** (three fruits compound) used internally, and **Kajjali Anjana**, and eye salve made from purified mercury powder ground with sulfur.

Shleshmasrava (Dacryoblennorrhea)

Shleshmasrava is related to dacryoblennorrhea, and is a Kaphaja condition that causes edema of the lacrimal duct system, promoting a painless, white, thick, viscid discharge of mucus from the lacrimal sac. One treatment is to wash the eyes with decoction made of **Triphala** *(Phyllanthus emblica / Terminalia belerica / Terminalia chebula)* with **Pippali fruit** (long pepper / *Piper longum).* It can also be treated with **Rasanjana** eye drops or **Netrabindu** eye drops (page 302). It is considered very difficult to cure.

Raktasrava (Dacryohematorrhea)

Raktasrava relates to dacryohematorrhea, and is caused by pathogenic defects of the blood. Shedding of hot tears with blood is the primary symptom. It is treated with specific remedies used for hematorrhea (see page 258) or the methods used for Raktaja conjunctivitis, including the general Pitta treatments (page 67) along with purgative remedies (page 174), and **Netrabindu** eye drops (page 302). Internal intake of a decoction of **Triphala** (three fruits compound) with honey is also recommended, as well as use of **Bilwanjana** eye salve. It is considered very difficult to cure.

Jalasrava (Dacryorrhea)

Jalasrava or dacryorrhea is a Pittaja inflammation, and manifests as an excessive flow of hot yellowish tears caused by inflammation of the lacrimal sac. It is treated with **Netrabindu** eye drops (page 302) along with an internal intake of decoction of

Triphala (three fruits compound) with **Madhu** (honey). It is considered very difficult to cure

Parvani (Dacryolith)

Parvani or dacryolith is caused by pathogenic blood defects. A tumor like painful swelling of the lacrimal duct is the main symptom. It is treated with surgery.

Alaji (Dacryoma located toward the iris / Scleral nodule / Scleritis)

Alaji is a complicated (Sannipataja) local inflammation, generally large in size, located between the joints of the conjunctiva and iris. It is caused by pathogenic blood defects, and the affected area develops a grape-shaped boil. It is very painful and also has the problem of epiphora. It is considered incurable.

Krimigranthi (Parasitic blepharitis)

Krimigranthi refers to parasitic blepharitis, and is a complex (Sannipataja) disease. A glandular suppurative growth develops between the joint of the external and internal parts of the eyelids, with itching and parasites such as Trichinosis *(Trichinella spiralis)*. It is treated with surgery.

Utsangapidaka (Chalazion, small)

Utsangapidaka is correlated with chalazion, and is a complex (Sannipataja) disease. A small tumor like boil develops inside or outside of the eyelid, usually in the meibomian glands. It is treated with surgery.

Kumbhika (Melanoma on eyelid)

Kumbhika is correlated to melanoma and is a complex (Sannipataja) disease. A dark pigmented growth in the corner of the eyelid forms, appearing as the seed of a pomegranate prior to when it breaks and discharges, after which the swelling goes down. This repeated swelling, breaking and discharging is the primary symptom. It is treated with surgery.

Pothaki (Trachoma / Viral follicular conjunctivitis)

Pothaki is correlated with trachoma and is a Kaphaja disease. Granular pimples appearing like red mustard seeds are located in the conjunctiva of the eyelids, manifesting with pain, itching, discharge and a sense of heaviness. A specific external medicine used is made from the powders of **Saindhavam** (mineral salt), **fruit** (long pepper / *Piper longum*), **Kustha root** *(Saussurea lappa)*, **Prishniparni plant** *(Uraria lagopoides)* and **Shalaparni plant** *(Desmodium gangeticum)*, boiled in a decoction of **Triphala**. It is also treated with surgery.

Vartamasharkara (Squamous blepharitis / Staphylococcal blepharitis)

Vartamasharkara relates to squamous blepharitis, and is a complex (Sannipataja) disease. A local inflammation located in the margin of the eyelids surrounded with small crusty pimples is the primary symptom. It is treated with surgery.

Arshovartma (Blepharoncus)

Arshovartma relates to blepharoncus, and is a complex (Sannipataja) disease. A small, hard, painless tumor located inside or outside of the eyelid is the primary symptom. It is treated with surgery.

Shuskarsha (Dry Blepharoncus)

Shuskarsha relates to a dry blepharoncus, and is a complex (Sannipataja) disease. A large, dry tumor located inside the eyelid is the primary symptom. It is treated with surgery.

Anjananamika (Sty / Hordeolum)

Anjananamika refers to a sty or hordeolum, and is a disease caused by blood defects. A copper colored small sized soft boil located in a sebaceous gland of the eyelid is the primary symptom. It is treated with surgery, followed by application of a plaster made from **Rasanjana** mixed with **Madhu** (honey).

Bahalavartma (Xanthelasma / Blepharopachynsis)

Bahalavartma relates to xanthelasma, and is a complex (Sannipataja) disease. Thickening of the eyelid with pimples is the primary symptom. It is treated by steaming, rubbing the eyelid with **Manohwa Yoga** to remove keratin and debris, washing with hot water and then applying a plaster of **grhita** (clarified butter / Ghee). Scarification surgery is also used.

Vartmabandhaka (Blepharitis, complex / Eyelid swelling)

Vartmabandhaka relates to a complex blepharitis, and is a chronic, complicated (Sannipataja) swelling of the eyelids, manifesting with itching, mild pain and other complications. The eyelids cannot close completely due to swelling. It is treated by steaming, rubbing the eyelid with **Manohwa compound,** laxative remedies (page 174), washing with warm water and then applying a plaster of **Ghrita** (Ghee) with **Rasanjana**. Scarification surgery is also used.

Klishtavartma (Allergic blepharitis)

Klishtavartma refers to an allergic blepharitis caused by blood defects. The main symptom is a sudden reddening of the eyelid. It is not painful, and the eyelids become soft and floppy over time. It is treated with the remedies used for blepharitis along with the remedies for allergies (page 151 or page 294).

Vartmakardama (Ulcerous blepharitis / Blepharoconjunctivitis, exudative)

Vartmakardama refers to an ulcerous blepharitis caused by Pitta and blood defects. The primary symptom is inflammation of the eyelid margins with a serous discharge. It is treated with the remedies used for blepharitis (above) along with a plaster of **Rasanjana**. Scarification surgery is also used.

Shyavavartma

Shyavavartma is a complex (Sannipataja) disease of black or blackish eyelids with severe inflammation. Swelling inside and outside of the eyelids, pain, burning sensation, itching and discharge are the primary symptoms. It is treated with remedies of blepharitis (above) along with laxative remedies (page 174). Scarification surgery is also used.

Praklinnavartma / Klinnavartma / Pilla (Allergic edema)

Praklinnavartma, klinnavartma and pilla all relate to an allergic edema of the eyelids, caused by a vitiation of Kapha. A painless watery edema outside of the eyelids with simultaneous inflammation of the conjunctiva is the primary symptom. It is treated with the astringent **Kashisa Yoga** (ferrous sulfate - *Sushruta Samhita*) for external application, along with remedies for allergy and hay fever (see page 151). An eye salve called **Samudraphenanjanam** is also used.

Aklinnavartma (Ankyloblepharon / Symblepharon)

Aklinnavartma relates to both ankyloblepharon and symblepharon, and is a complicated (Sannipataja) disease. It manifests as a recurring fusion or joining of the upper and lower ciliary edges of the eyelids. It is treated with **Samudraphenanjanam** eye salve.

Vatahatavartma (Blepharoplegia)

Vatahatavartma relates to blepharoplegia, and is caused by a vitiation to the related nerves (Vataja). It causes paralysis of the eyelids and can be treated with the remedies used for paralysis (page 230). It is very difficult to cure.

Netrarbuda (Cancer of the eyelid)

Netrarbuda relates to cancer of the eyelid, and is a complicated (Sannipataja) disease. A red irregular growth located in the conjunctiva of the eyelid is the primary symptom. It is treated with the remedies used for external neoplasm, including surgery (page 250).

Nimesam (Blepharospasm / Myokymia)

Nimesam relates to blepharospasm, and is caused by irritation of the related nerve (Vata). Repeated brief twitching or blinking of the eyelid is the primary symptom. It is can be treated with the general Vata treatments (page 56) but is very difficult to cure. The *Chakradatta* states that this disease is curable with the treatment of snorting pure diluted **Purana grhita** (old Ghee), or by washing the eyelid with a paste of old Ghee.

Shonitarsha (Angioma of the eyelid / Melanoma of the eyelid)

Shonitarsha relates either an angioma or melanoma of the eyelid, and is caused by blood defects. It manifests as a malignant red-pigmented bud-like soft lump located in the middle part of the eyelid. As it grows again and again, even after removal by operation, it is considered incurable.

Lagana (Chalazion, large)

Lagana refers to a large chalazion, and is a Kaphaja disease. A hard tumor-like painless growth located at the eyelid margin is the primary symptom. It is first cleaned with surgery, after which it should be burnt with either a corrosive alkali (page 171) or a heated surgical instrument.

Vishavartma (Ulcerative edema of the eyelid)

Vishavartma relates to the ulcerative edema of the eyelid, and is a complex (Sannipataja) disease. Visha means the stem of lotus, and the Sanskrit writers noted that this eyelid swelling resembles the lotus stem with its cavities. Edema with discharge from the ulcerated lesions is the primary symptom. It is treated with surgery along with the remedies used for sty (anjananamika, page 314).

Kunchanam (Blepharoptosis / Ptosis)

Kunchanam relates to Blepharoptosis, and is a complex (Sannipataja) disease. Drooping of the upper eyelid is the main symptom. It is difficult to cure, but can be treated with the remedies used for paralysis (page 230).

Pakshmakopa (Trichiasis)

Pakshmakopa relates to trichiasis, and is a Vataja disease. Growth of the eyelashes into the conjunctiva or cornea with pain and inflammation is the primary symptom. It can be treated with surgery, with the abnormal hairs carefully extracted with forceps, after which each root has to be burnt out very carefully with a heated golden rod. It is very difficult to cure.

Pakshmashata (Eyelid alopecia)

Pakshmashata relates to a loss of eyelid hair caused by Pitta. An ulcerative blepharitis causing itching and a mild heat sensation in the eyelid are the early symptoms, followed by a falling out of the eyelashes. It is treated with the remedies used for blepharitis (page 314).

INDEX

www.ingramcontent.com/pod-product-compliance
Lightning Source LLC
Chambersburg PA
CBHW021850020426
42334CB00013B/261